Child Health Guide

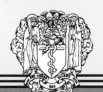

ROYAL SOCIETY
of MEDICINE

Child Health Guide

DR RICHARD WEST
MD, FRCP
PROFESSOR, UNIVERSITY OF BRISTOL

HAMLYN

CONTENTS

PREFACE

Good health is much more than freedom from illness: it is complete physical, mental and social wellbeing. For children to be fully healthy they need to be physically healthy, to be loved, and to be emotionally secure. They have to be taught to socialize and be able to form sound and rewarding relationships. They require, too, sufficient stimulation and encouragement to enable them to fulfil their potential for personal development.

Considered in this way, it is apparent that parents have the major role to play in making and keeping their children healthy. This book has been written primarily for parents in the hope that the information and guidance it provides will asssist them in their role of promoting the health of their children. It also aims to help parents teach their children the importance of following a healthy lifestyle, and of continuing to look after themselves and their bodies throughout life. Essential information on all aspects of health maintenance is included, as are descriptions of most of the common and important diseases of childhood and their treatment. Routine aspects of child care are not covered, unless they have health implications.

The book is not intended (and should not be used) as a substitute for seeking advice and help from health care professionals. Rather, it is intended to provide parents with a better understanding of the requirements that children have if they are to be healthy, and of the role that health professionals can play in assisting with this.

In writing this book I have been very conscious of the help I have received from others. As a children's doctor I have learnt much from my professional colleagues in all branches of health care. Chris Bungay and Mary John are two such, both of whom have contributed to the text. Even more have I learnt by being privileged to observe and to share in the family life of many of my patients. My own family have taught me most of all.

Richard West, Merton, 1990

CHILDHOOD DEVELOPMENT

Providing Healthcare for the Growing Child, from Babyhood to Adolescence

Understanding the needs of children is one of the essentials of good parenting. With this aim in mind, Part One looks at the ways in which children develop between pregnancy and puberty and explains how they can be kept healthy both physically and emotionally. The knowledge of how to achieve a healthy lifestyle and thereby avoid many of the health problems of adult life is an invaluable legacy for parents to impart to their children, as this section demonstrates. Not all medical problems are preventable, however, and guidance on the care of children who are chronically sick or disabled can also be found here.

CHAPTER

1

PLANNING FOR PARENTHOOD

When a couple decide they would like to start a family some preparation is needed. Planning for parenthood should start before conception and continue throughout pregnancy. Part of this process is acquiring some medical knowledge of what happens during pregnancy and how the baby develops. This not only adds to both parents' enjoyment and interest, but also means that they will have a better understanding of the factors which are important for mother and child.

Pregnancy is not an illness, and the aim should be for the mother to stay healthy throughout, and if possible to have a normal delivery. Supervision of the pregnancy by the doctor or midwife is to determine whether everything is progressing well, in which case no medical intervention is necessary. However, if there is any indication that things are not ideal, early corrective measures can be taken to try to maintain mother and baby in the best of health.

The baby's health during the pregnancy is indeed closely linked with that of the mother, and some maternal conditions can seriously affect the baby's well-being. However, it is outside the scope of this book to deal with the effects of pregnancy and childbirth on the mother, and only those aspects which are of particular importance to the child are covered.

PRE-CONCEPTION COUNSELLING

People are increasingly aware that planning to have a baby is not just a matter of deciding when to become pregnant, and many doctors now provide a pre-pregnancy counselling service. This is directed partly at educating potential parents about pregnancy and labour, and partly at finding out whether there are any medical problems that would be better sorted out before the pregnancy is started. For example, the mother may not have been vaccinated against rubella (German measles), which can seriously damage a developing child; immunization when she knows she is *not* pregnant will prevent her developing rubella when she is.

Obviously it is in the interests of both mother and baby that the mother should start the pregnancy healthy, and if any medical conditions are detected in the pre-conception medical they can be treated or discussed. Preparation for pregnancy involves both parents and a couple should ensure that their lifestyle is healthy, and should learn together about the needs of the expectant mother; about how the progress of the pregnancy is monitored by doctor or midwife and the purpose of the various checks and investigations that will be carried out; and about the basics of labour and delivery.

As part of the routine, enquiries will be made about any diseases or disabilities in other members of the family, with the aim of finding out whether there are any special genetic implications that the couple should be aware of; if necessary people can be referred to a genetic counselling clinic (see page 111).

If a couple are not already aware of the dangers of smoking and drinking, the doctor at the pre-conception clinic will talk about them. Heavy smoking can have an adverse effect on the fertility of both men and women, and could cause problems in conceiving in some couples. Both tobacco and alcohol can be harmful in pregnancy (see page 12). Ideally, women who smoke should give up the habit before becoming pregnant.

There is some evidence, not yet conclusive, that vitamin and mineral supplements taken before pregnancy may lessen the likelihood of having a baby with spina bifida. Until more is known about this it is not possible to make firm recommendations, except to say that if vitamins and minerals are taken they should be kept to the recommended dose; excess amounts may be harmful.

CONCEPTION AND GROWTH

At the time of conception the sperm and ovum (egg) unite to form the fertilized ovum, a single cell which has the potential to develop into a baby. This cell starts to divide to form other cells. Initially these are apparently identical, but later they begin to show differences: this is the first indication that they are going on to form either different

body structures or the placenta (afterbirth).

Within a week of conception the small cluster of cells becomes attached to and then implanted in the wall of the uterus (womb), and the placenta gradually develops. This is the organ which conveys oxygen and nutrients from the mother to the developing embryo, and removes any waste products from the embryo. Once implantation occurs, cell differentiation takes place rapidly, and over the first twelve weeks all the major organs and parts of the body are formed. During this period the developing baby is known as the 'embryo', and the formation of the various organs is called 'embryogenesis'. After twelve weeks the term 'fetus' is used; growth continues, but now development takes place within the individual organs.

Doctors always refer to the stages of pregnancy in weeks, calculating from the date of the last menstrual period. Although conception usually occurs about two weeks after the start of the last period the date is often uncertain, so cannot be used as a reference point. Some women cannot remember the date of their last period, or may have had irregular cycles. Calculations of fetal maturity are then made by examining the size of the uterus or by using ultrasound to estimate the size of the fetus (see page 13). The duration of a normal pregnancy is around 39–41 weeks.

At conception spermatozoa (**1**) penetrate to the upper part of the Fallopian tube, where fertilization occurs (**2**). The fertilized ovum (**3**) undergoes cell division as it progresses down the tube to the uterus (**4**), and eventually attaches itself to the uterine wall (**5**).

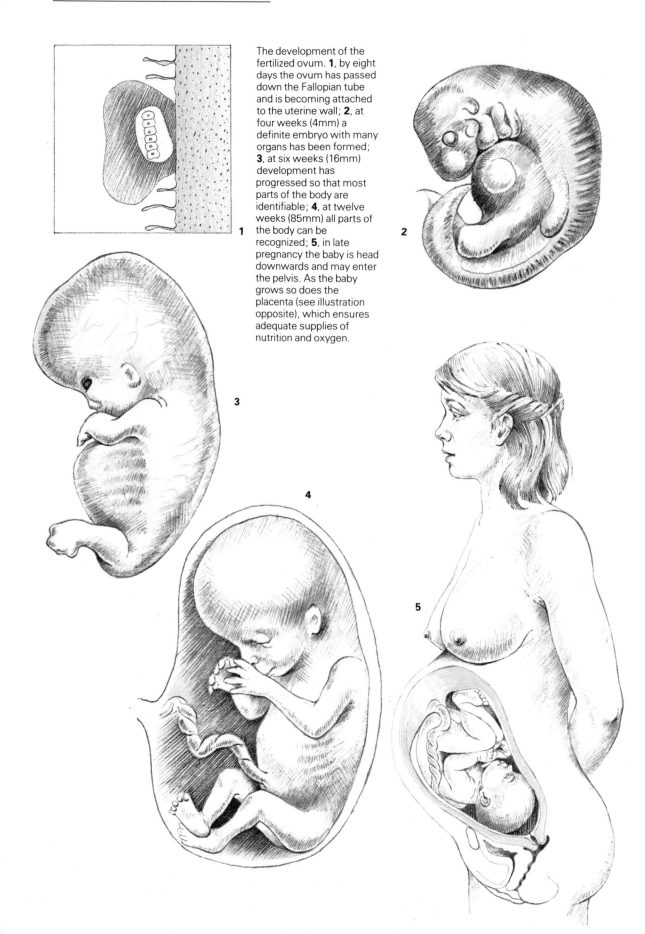

The development of the fertilized ovum. **1**, by eight days the ovum has passed down the Fallopian tube and is becoming attached to the uterine wall; **2**, at four weeks (4mm) a definite embryo with many organs has been formed; **3**, at six weeks (16mm) development has progressed so that most parts of the body are identifiable; **4**, at twelve weeks (85mm) all parts of the body can be recognized; **5**, in late pregnancy the baby is head downwards and may enter the pelvis. As the baby grows so does the placenta (see illustration opposite), which ensures adequate supplies of nutrition and oxygen.

The placenta

The fetus gets all its nutrients and oxygen from the mother's circulation via the placenta; the placenta also transfers carbon dioxide and other waste products from the fetal circulation into the maternal circulation so that they can be excreted by the mother. The growth of the baby in the uterus is thus dependent on the proper functioning of the placenta. (The increase in size and weight of the fetus can be seen from the illustrations, left.) Usually the placenta functions well

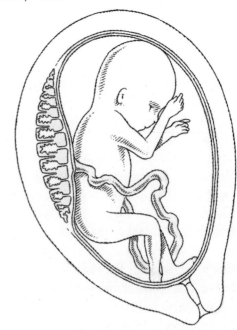

Maternal and fetal blood vessels are adjacent in the placenta (see section), permitting the exchange of oxygen, nutrients and waste products.

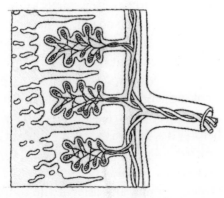

throughout pregnancy, but its efficiency may be impaired as a result of high blood pressure, toxaemia of pregnancy (characterized by high blood pressure, protein in the urine, and excess weight gain), smoking, partial separation of the placenta from the wall of the uterus, or postmaturity (longer than normal pregnancy; ie beyond forty-one weeks).

In situations where there is concern about placental function one of the tests performed is repeated ultrasound to measure the rate at which the fetus is growing. If the rate is slower than normal it may indicate that the baby is not receiving sufficient nutrients across the placenta. A fetus that has become growth-retarded because of undernutrition is at risk of dying in the womb if the condition is prolonged, and is particularly susceptible to a reduction in the amount of oxygen in the circulation. If poor placental function persists or worsens it may be neces-

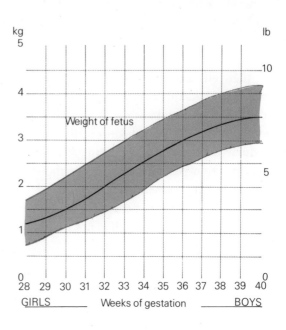

As can be seen from this chart, the fetus gains weight rapidly during the last third of pregnancy.

sary to induce labour early. With improvements in the care of premature babies, being born early is a less severe hazard than receiving inadequate nutrition in the womb.

DURING PREGNANCY

Eating and drinking

Most mothers have some nausea and sickness in early pregnancy. This usually settles by the end of the first three months. Once the period of morning sickness is over, the mother's appetite is likely to increase. Weight is put on steadily during pregnancy, with a total gain of about 22–28 pounds (10–13 kg). Some of this is due to the weight of the baby, the surrounding fluid and the growth of the uterus, but some represents an increase in the mother's fat stores. Provided this is not excessive, it is both normal and healthy: these stores are important for the maintenance of breast feeding, as nursing mothers have to produce food for the baby for several weeks or months after birth.

There are no special foods that have to be eaten during pregnancy, but it is important that the diet is varied, as this helps to guarantee that all necessary nutrients will be consumed in adequate quantities. During the second half of pregnancy it is as well for a mother to increase her intake of milk or dairy products, as these are important sources of calcium. Non-pasteurized cheese, though, such as brie or camembert, should not be eaten during pregnancy because of the danger of Listeria (see page 283). It is not necessary to drink large amounts of milk; bread can provide an alternative source of dietary calcium for mothers who do not like milk. The fetus needs calcium from the mother for bone growth, and taking plenty of milk, dairy produce or bread ensures that her body does not become calcium-depleted.

Drinking alcohol may cause problems for the baby. Even modest drinking (1–2 glasses daily) on a regular basis seems to increase the likelihood of a miscarriage, so that alcohol is best avoided altogether in early pregnancy. Heavy drinking at any stage may affect the development and well-being of the baby. It has particular repercussions for the developing brain, and can cause brain damage.

Smoking and medication

Mothers who smoke during pregnancy are more likely to have low birth weight babies than mothers who do not, as one of the effects of tobacco smoke in the bloodstream is to reduce the amount of blood flow through the placenta. Mothers should try to give up smoking when they become pregnant. Even if a woman has tried unsuccessfully to stop before, it is in both the baby's interest and her own to try again. At the very least smoking in pregnancy should be severely curtailed. Giving up may be easier if the couple do it together.

Medicines and drugs taken by the mother during pregnancy may also affect the baby. Although a few drugs are known to have definite adverse effects, there is inadequate evidence for most to be able to say that they are completely safe. It is therefore important in pregnancy to restrict medicine-taking to essentials. Iron and vitamin preparations which are prescribed to pregnant women do not have any harmful effect on the baby and should be taken as directed. Other medications should only be taken if expressly indicated, and if a doctor is giving you a prescription remind him or her that you are pregnant. It is not only medicines that can harm the baby: recreational and addictive drugs have a direct effect on the baby and can be harmful. They should not be used during pregnancy.

In the same way that some medications

could be harmful to the baby if taken by the mother, some chemicals could also be toxic. Work in an industrial or laboratory setting which involves handling solvents and other chemicals or exposure to industrial fumes is best avoided. Working with X-rays and other ionizing radiation may also put the fetus at risk. There is no evidence that using a VDU is harmful. If you think your workplace may be a hazard in early pregnancy you should discuss this with the personnel officer or a union representative. It may be that you can be moved to an alternative job if there is a significant risk.

ULTRASOUND

Nearly every woman now has at least one ultrasound examination during pregnancy. This is a way of showing what is happening inside the womb, providing parents with the first glimpse of their baby.

Ultrasound consists of sound waves which are beyond the range of human hearing, but otherwise have similar properties to other sound waves. The images are formed electronically from the echoes that are sent back as the ultrasound waves pass through the different layers of tissue underneath the probe. Unlike X-rays, ultrasound does not have any measurable harmful effect on either mother or baby: its safety was rigorously tested before it was introduced into routine use. It is therefore a very useful tool for the obstetrician: not only does it produce high-quality pictures of inside the womb, but the investigation can be repeated as often as necessary without risk.

There are several reasons for using ultrasound in pregnancy. It can be employed from about six weeks after the last period for the very early diagnosis of pregnancy, if there is a particular need. It can detect twins early in pregnancy: the fetal head can be identified by ultrasound by about ten weeks, so that if two heads are found the diagnosis of twins is established.

One of the most common reasons for using ultrasound in pregnancy is to determine the maturity of the baby, and to check on his growth. The test is usually carried out at around sixteen weeks, and is now mostly routine. The width of the baby's head is measured at its widest part, because at this stage of pregnancy this correlates well with the age of the baby in weeks. This allows a check to be made on the mother's dates, if they are known. It also provides a reference for use later if there is concern about the baby's growth.

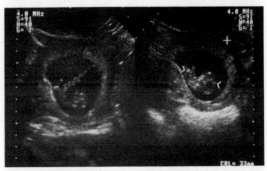

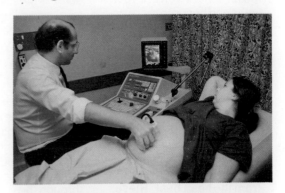

Top: The use of ultrasound has revolutionized antenatal care. During an ultrasound examination ultrasound waves pass through the mother's abdomen as the probe moves over it and the echoes received back are decoded as images of the baby's features.

Above: This close-up of an ultrasound result shows two views of a ten-week old fetus inside the uterus. The fetus can be seen best in the picture on the right. The umbilical cord is clearly visible in the picture on the left. The arrow heads are used to measure the fetal head, which is a useful indicator of age.

Actions and Sensations in the Fetus

As the fetus develops in the womb the ability to perform different actions gradually develops.

Limb movement

The mother does not become aware of fetal movement until around 17-20 weeks of pregnancy. The use of ultrasound has enabled the fetus to be studied throughout pregnancy. Kicking movements are apparent from twelve weeks. As pregnancy progresses, movements involve all four limbs and become more co-ordinated.

Breathing movements

In the second half of pregnancy the use of ultrasound can be used to detect movements of the chest wall. Respiratory movements occur between 40 and 70 times a minute, and can be differentiated from the heart beat. These rapid breathing movements can sometimes be seen through the mother's abdomen.

Sucking and swallowing

The fetus can both suck and swallow. Sucking of finger or thumb has been detected both by ultrasound and by amnionoscopy. As well as showing that the fetus has the ability to suck these monitorings also suggest that the feeling of touch is well developed. Amniotic fluid surrounds the fetus and some is swallowed. The swallowed fluid passes first into the stomach and then to the intestine where it is absorbed.

Sensation

Occasionally it is necessary to give a fetus a blood transfusion in the later stage of pregnancy. This involves passing a needle through the mother's abdominal wall, through the wall of the uterus, and into the abdominal wall of the fetus, using ultrasound control. Blood can then be injected into the abdominal cavity of the baby where it is absorbed into the circulation. The fetus moves as the needle goes through the abdominal wall, suggesting that the fetus feels the prick of the needle.

Hearing

Although the fetus is surrounded by fluid the uterus is not a silent place. There seems little doubt that sounds of the mother's heart beats, arterial pulsation and of bowel contractions are heard by the fetus in late pregnancy. Recorded sounds from inside the mother's abdomen have been used to provide a soothing tape to help newborns get off to sleep.

TESTING FOR FETAL ABNORMALITY

At around sixteen weeks, ultrasound can be used to check on the baby's development, and is able to detect some serious congenital abnormalities. Conditions such as spina bifida or hydrocephalus (see pages 301 and 277) may be recognized, as can some heart and kidney defects, and some other problems. Early detection enables a couple to be counselled. In cases of severe fetal abnormality parents can make a decision as to whether they wish to continue with the pregnancy or have an abortion (sometimes called a termination). With correctable problems, such as some forms of severe congenital heart disease, arrangements can be made for investigation and surgery immediately after birth. In a few instances, such as obstruction in the flow of urine from the bladder, which can damage the kidneys, it is possible to operate on the baby during pregnancy.

There are other tests that can be done to detect fetal abnormality. Amniocentesis is a technique which involves inserting a needle into the womb and removing a small amount of fluid, which contains fetal cells. These cells can be studied for chromosomal disorders and some biochemical defects. Down's syndrome (see pages 104 and 259) is a chromosomal abnormality which occurs more commonly when mothers are over the age of 35, and in many antenatal centres older mothers are offered amniocentesis for detection of this disorder. In cases of severe fetal abnormality an abortion might have to be considered.

A considerable disadvantage of amniocentesis is that it has to be done relatively late in the pregnancy, which may have reached eighteen weeks before the test results are available. A newer technique, called chorionic villus sampling, involves removing a very small piece of the placenta at around ten weeks for chromosomal or biochemical testing, and this enables abnormalities to be detected at an earlier stage. Fetal blood can be obtained from the placenta if there is a high risk of thalassaemia (see page 303) or other inherited blood diseases.

Some centres do blood tests on the mother for spina bifida, Down's syndrome and some other fetal abnormalities as a matter of routine; the mother should always be informed of their purpose. The tests themselves are not diagnostic, and an abnormal result has to be followed by amniocentesis, chorionic villus sampling or ultrasound examination. In mothers of the rhesus negative blood group a blood test to see if there are antibodies to the rhesus factor is done routinely during pregnancy. Rhesus disease (see page 294) is now very uncommon, but it is important to know if there is any likelihood of it affecting the baby, so that the best treatment can be planned for him.

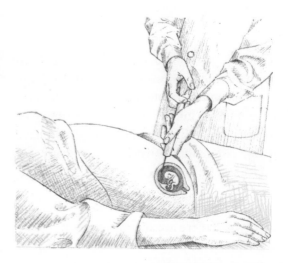

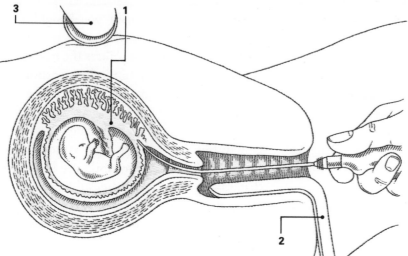

Above: In amniocentesis a needle attached to a syringe is inserted through the abdominal wall and through the wall of the uterus under ultrasound control. When the needle is in the amniotic cavity around the fetus, a small amount of fluid is withdrawn.

Left: Chorionic villus sampling involves removing a small piece of placenta (**1**) by means of a speculum (**2**) aided by ultrasound. The ultrasound probe (**3**) allows the obstetrician an interior view of the mother's womb.

HOME OR HOSPITAL?
PLANNING THE BIRTH

Only about 1 per cent of deliveries are now planned to take place in the home, the rest taking place mainly in district general hospitals or in family practitioner units. Hospital deliveries are now advocated on the grounds that women should be encouraged to have their babies in well-equipped and well-staffed units where facilities exist to cope with any emergencies which could endanger the life or health of either mother or child. Unfortunately, big units are sometimes perceived as impersonal and unfriendly: large numbers of women attend antenatal clinics and go into hospital, and there are so many staff that there is little opportunity for people to get to know each other as individuals. There is also some concern among both mothers and professionals that in a large hospital setting women are more likely to have medical intervention to start labour or to speed the delivery, when they could have had a safe natural birth, as it is easier for midwives to involve doctors in the labour and delivery. (In general, midwives take care of normal deliveries; doctors may be involved if there are any problems.)

While home delivery has the advantage of being a family affair in well-known surroundings, fewer facilities are available should serious problems arise. The move towards hospital deliveries in recent years has been associated with a progressive fall in the perinatal mortality rate, and the virtual abolition of maternal mortality. Some mothers would like to have their babies at home. If the family doctor and midwife feel that the likelihood of serious problems arising is small, they can support this.

In many areas a midwifery service is no longer available for home deliveries, as facilities have been concentrated in the district general hospitals where almost all births take place. For most mothers, therefore, there is no possibility of a home delivery, although it may be possible to arrange for antenatal care to be shared between the community midwife, family practitioner and hospital.

There have been, however, welcome changes in the service provided by hospitals. The same midwife may now be present at antenatal visits throughout the pregnancy and may also be involved when the new baby arrives; a birth plan may be arranged with each mother, so she can record her preferences about labour and delivery; and more varied routines for labour and delivery may now be possible. A more personalized form of hospital care will be welcomed by all mothers, and could provide the ideal combination of a safe labour and delivery in an emotionally supportive and warm atmosphere.

Your family doctor will know what facilities are available in your area for antenatal care and delivery, and you should make a point of discussing the options with him or her early in pregnancy.

INFANT FEEDING:
BREAST OR BOTTLE?

When you are pregnant you should give some thought as to how you would like to feed your baby. Breast milk is the best available food, containing in ideal proportions all the requisite nutrients for growth in the first few months of life. Modern artificial infant formulae are designed to imitate breast milk closely but are still not quite as good. The protein and fat in breast milk are in a form that makes them very digestible; the milk also contains various proteins secreted by the mother which increase the baby's resistance to infection.

In antenatal classes mothers learn about pregnancy, labour, birth and baby care. Appropriate exercises and relaxation techniques are also taught.

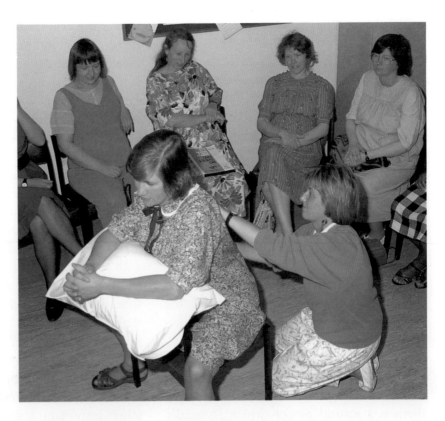

Although there are nutritional advantages to breast milk, manufactured baby milks are perfectly satisfactory, and babies will thrive if artificially fed. There is, however, more to infant feeding than just nutrition. What is unique about breast feeding is the closeness it brings between mother and baby. Being pregnant and feeling the baby growing and moving inside your body is the beginning of a unique relationship; breast feeding is an equally close, but very different partnership in which mother and baby are both actively building a loving intimacy with each other. If there are difficulties in getting breast feeding started, this relationship may not seem a very relaxed one at first, but most mothers find persisting is worth while, and problems can usually be overcome.

If a baby is to be bottle fed, then mothers should try to foster an equally close and loving bond, and not lightly let friends and other family members do the feeding instead,

particularly during the first few weeks.

If you do decide to breast feed, or think you would like to try to see how you get on, you are more likely to be successful if you are well prepared, and have talked through what it entails with the midwife or a breast feeding counsellor. Furthermore, if your nipples are flat or inverted, massaging them and wearing breast shells inside your bra during pregnancy to draw them out gradually, will make feeding easier. This is something on which the midwife will be able to advise.

Any decision made about feeding during pregnancy can be changed when the baby is born. If you only decide after the delivery that you would like to breast feed, you still stand a good chance of being successful. Alternatively, if you wanted to breast feed but find that, even after help from the midwife or counsellor, you cannot manage for some reason, you can always change to artificial feeding.

THE BABY DURING LABOUR

The onset of labour is signalled by the establishment of regular contractions of the uterine muscle, which gradually increase in frequency and strength. During the first stage of labour these contractions lead to the gradual opening of the cervix, the neck of the womb. When the cervix is fully open and the lower end of the uterus and the vagina form a continuous birth canal, the contractions become stronger, and are propulsive in character. The baby gradually moves down, the head passing through the mother's pelvis. The head is born as it passes out of the pelvis, and the rest of the body follows rapidly.

The birth attendants have to keep a close watch on the condition of mother and baby, as well as assessing the progress of the labour. Birth is a natural process which is usually accomplished smoothly without the need for medical intervention. However, complications can occur which put at risk the life of the baby or the mother, and careful observations are needed to ensure that both baby and mother remain well.

With every contraction of the uterus the amount of blood flowing through the placenta is reduced, as the muscular contraction of the uterine wall temporarily obstructs the flow of maternal blood. During early labour, when the contractions are not particularly forceful, this has few repercussions for the baby, but as labour progresses the effect is more pronounced. The amount of blood getting to the fetus during a contraction is reduced, and this may cause a temporary slowing of the fetal heart rate.

Sometimes during labour, particularly where there has been previous placental insufficiency, the baby may not receive enough oxygen. The first manifestation of this is the fetal heart rate becoming more rapid, but if the oxygen shortage becomes more severe it has other effects on the heart, including a marked slowing of the rate with each contraction. As shortage of oxygen could lead to asphyxia of the baby, the delivery may be speeded up, by forceps delivery if the second stage has begun, or by Caesarean section if earlier in labour.

The main way of assessing the condition of the baby during labour is by monitoring the fetal heartbeat, and how the heart responds to uterine contractions. Listening to the heart with a stethoscope is simple, and enables a check to be made on the rate from time to time. It is difficult or impossible to use a stethoscope during a contraction, however, and it is precisely then that the baby is most likely to show the signs of oxygen shortage. Furthermore, the baby's heart is only being listened to intermittently. There are two other important ways of monitoring the baby's heart. In early labour a device acting like a microphone may be strapped to the abdominal wall and attached to a recorder, so that a continuous trace of the heart action is obtained. The second and better method is to use an electrode to pick up the electrical activity of the heart, which can then be recorded as a continuous trace. This can only be done once the opening of the uterus (the cervix) has begun to dilate. A small electrode is attached by a clip to the baby's scalp. As well as recording the fetal heart rate the electrode also measures the strength, timing and duration of contractions, so that any alterations in heart rate pattern can be interpreted in relation to the progress of labour.

Monitoring the baby's heart rate enables the attendants to keep a close check on his condition. If all is straightforward, only observation is needed. If the condition of the baby seems to be deteriorating, an informed decision to speed up delivery can be made.

CHAPTER 2

THE NEWBORN BABY

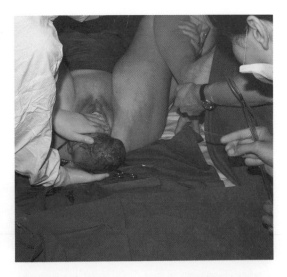

During the last stage of labour the contractions gradually propel the baby down the birth canal. The head is born as it passes out of the pelvis. Once the head has been delivered gentle pulling ensures that the rest of the baby's body follows quickly afterwards.

The birth of a baby is a deeply emotional experience, both for the mother and father and for others present at the delivery; for the baby it is the moment of achieving an independent existence. The birth should be conducted in such a way that parents can experience the naturalness and the wonder of it and also so that, should anything not be straightforward, adequate help is on hand.

To survive separately from her mother, a baby must rapidly adapt from life in the womb, where the oxygen supply came through the placenta, to breathing in air. Changes in circulation occur as the lungs are used for the first time, and the baby will lose heat very quickly if not kept warm.

Emerging from the warm, dark and relatively quiet life suspended in amniotic fluid in the womb, into the bright, colder and noisier world outside acts as the stimulus for the necessary adaptive changes. Very often a baby will make facial grimaces as soon as her head is born, and most babies take their first breath and start to cry as soon as they are delivered. Shortly afterwards the eyes open.

Liquor runs out of the mouth and nose, and the baby is initially held head downwards to help drain it. Mouth and nose are gently cleared of fluid with a small suction tube. At the time of delivery the baby appears blue, because the amount of oxygen in the blood is reduced as she passes through the birth canal. As breathing is established the face and body become pink; arms and legs often remain blue for several minutes. The umbilical cord is clamped and cut, and the baby is wrapped for warmth and can be passed to the mother.

ASSESSING THE BABY'S CONDITION AT BIRTH

If the baby takes her first breath within seconds of being born there is no doubt that adaptation to life outside the womb is proceeding satisfactorily, and that she is in good condition. Not all babies cry immediately, but this is not necessarily a cause for concern. Very often having the airways cleared of liquor and mucus with a suction tube will be enough to stimulate breathing.

When the baby has been delivered a small suction tube is used to suck out the airways and remove fluid from the nose and mouth.

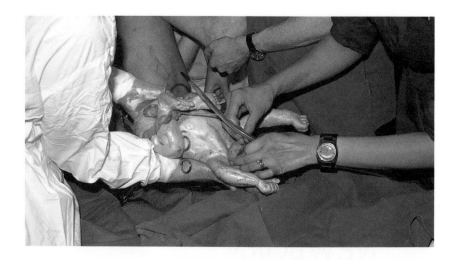

The midwife or doctor will assess the condition of the baby, and if this is satisfactory the first breath can be waited for calmly. If, on the other hand, it looks as if her condition has become depressed by lack of oxygen during birth or by sedative drugs given to the mother further steps will be necessary (see 'Resuscitation', below).

The assessment, often done at one minute and five minutes after delivery, is based on five factors: the baby's heart rate, respiratory effort, muscle tone, response to stimulus (a nasal catheter or tube) and colour. This quick form of appraisal is known as the Apgar score (see table, right), named after the paediatrician who devised and validated it. Each of the five factors is given a score from 0 to 2, and the individual figures are added together to produce the Apgar score. Babies with scores between 6 and 10 in the first minute after delivery are in satisfactory condition, and are likely to start breathing on their own; babies with lower scores are likely to need resuscitation.

RESUSCITATION

If the baby has a low Apgar score at birth it is better to help establish respiration than to wait hopefully. Far and away the commonest reason for a low Apgar score is that the baby is short of oxygen; this depresses the signals from the brain which are needed to start the respiratory muscles working. The newborn can tolerate being short of oxygen for longer periods than older babies. However, while the baby is not breathing the shortage of oxygen in the body becomes progressively more serious. Severe oxygen deficiency may prevent the respiratory effort happening at all. The rapid availability of effective resuscitation has been one of the great advances in perinatal care over the last thirty years, and is one of the main reasons why stillbirth is now much less common than formerly.

How the Apgar score is calculated

Factor	0	1	2
Heart rate	Absent	Below 100	Above 100
Respiratory effort	Absent	Slow, irregular	Good, crying
Muscle tone	Limp	Some limb flexion	Active
Response to nasal catheter	Nil	Grimace	Cry
Colour	Blue or pale	Body pink, limbs blue	Pink

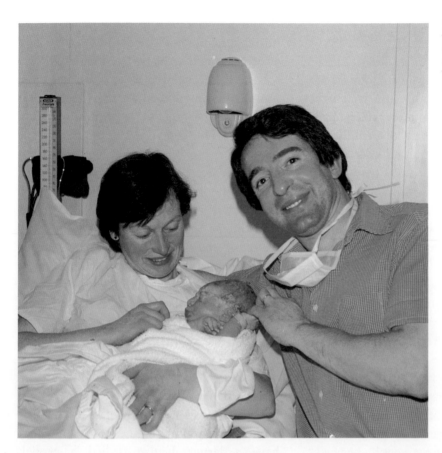

It is an emotional moment when a couple hold their baby for the first time, and share the experience of welcoming the new member of the family.

During resuscitation it is important to keep the baby warm as her condition will be made worse if her temperature falls below normal. First of all the nose and mouth are sucked out to remove mucus, if this has not already been done. Only if the baby is taking some gasps will oxygen be given via a face mask; oxygen would be ineffective if she is not, because it would not reach her lungs. small plastic tube may be inserted through the mouth into the windpipe (a procedure known as intubation) so that oxygen can be delivered straight into the lungs. The oxygen is given intermittently so that the lungs repeatedly expand and then partially deflate, as in normal breathing. This immediately increases the amount of oxygen in the blood,

If the baby makes no effort to breathe, a and usually the baby starts to breathe spontaneously and her general condition improves. If facilities for intubation are not available, mouth-to-mouth resuscitation can be performed; this forces air into the baby's lungs, and thus increases the oxygenation of the blood.

The usual reason for a baby not breathing spontaneously after birth is that the level of oxygen in the blood has become so low during labour that respiratory effort is depressed. However, painkilling drugs given to the mother during labour can also produce the same result; if this is thought to be a factor the baby will be given an injection to counteract it.

If the shortage of oxygen in the baby's circulation is severe, the heart may be affected, and for babies with a very low Apgar score at birth resuscitation efforts will include stimulating the heart with external heart massage and possibly with drugs.

THE NEWBORN EXAMINATION

This will take place at a convenient time soon after birth, when breathing is well established and mother and father have had a chance to hold their newborn child. The purpose of this first examination is to weigh and measure the baby, check her temperature, determine whether the labour and birth have affected her condition, and detect any obvious abnormalities. It also includes a check for common congenital anomalies: the midwife or doctor will examine the mouth and palate, the head and ears, the back, limbs and fingers, the genitalia and anus, and listen to the heart. A further examination should be done a few days later.

If there is any cause for concern, or if the infant is of low birth weight (below 2.5 kg/ 5½ lb), a decision may be taken to send her to the neonatal nursery for treatment or observation; otherwise the baby should stay with her mother and have a cot by her bed.

During labour the baby is squeezed through the mother's birth canal, and certain effects of this may be noted. There will be a soft swelling over the part of the scalp that was pushed first down the birth canal, which is known as the 'caput succedaneum', or 'caput' for short. This disappears in the first couple of days. All babies, except some born by Caesarean section, will have some degree of moulding of the head, which is often asymmetric. This moulding is caused by adjustments in the alignment of the bony plates of the baby's skull during labour which enable the head to squeeze through the maternal pelvis. Sometimes this is very marked, particularly in big babies or if labour has been prolonged. Over the first two or three days after birth the head gradually resumes its proper shape.

Bruising is common after birth, and with forceps delivery there may be some marks left on the face by the blades. These fade within a couple of days. Some babies may have a larger bruise, called a cephal-

In the newborn examination the doctor notes the general level of alertness of the baby. Persistent drowsiness could indicate a difficult delivery or the presence of infection. The doctor checks the hands, feet, genitalia and the following: the head circumference is measured and the fontanelle (soft spot) felt – see illustration, below; the ears are checked to make sure they are properly formed as minor congenital anomalies are common; the mouth is examined, particularly the tongue and palate; various reflexes are tested to gauge how the nervous system is functioning – for example, an object placed in the baby's mouth should induce reflex sucking (see page 54 for illustrations of other newborn reflexes); listening to the heart sometimes detects other sounds, known as murmurs (see page 145), which may indicate congenital abnormality; the hips are examined carefully. Dislocation of the joint is easy to treat if it is diagnosed early (see page 259).

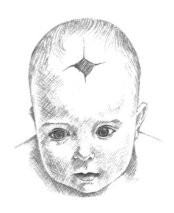

haematoma, over one side of the head; it is deep in the scalp and appears like a squidgy swelling with no discoloration of the overlying skin. A cephalhaematoma is due to bleeding because of injury during delivery, and will disappear in one or two weeks.

Babies that have been relatively short of oxygen during labour or delivery usually improve rapidly once they are born and have started breathing. Some remain drowsy or rather inactive and will require gentle handling for a few days, possibly in a special care nursery. Babies of low birth weight are also likely to require a stay in a special care nursery, as they have more difficulty than other babies in keeping body temperature stable, in feeding and sometimes in breathing.

When the medical examination is repeated after a few days, the doctor will carry out another full check. He or she will also look for jaundice (see page 28), anaemia (page 149) and skin infections, and examine the state of the umbilicus (page 26) and also the hips, looking for potential dislocation (page 28).

The other routine medical check, done around the fifth day, is a blood test known as the Guthrie test. This is performed by pricking the heel and absorbing the blood on a piece of special blotting paper. This blood is tested for various uncommon but serious metabolic diseases, including phenylketonuria (see page 291) and thyroid deficiency (see 'hypothyroidism' on page 278).

DEVELOPING A RELATIONSHIP

Holding your baby and performing activities like feeding, washing or nappy changing provide the foundations of the relationship between you. You should talk to the baby, touch and stroke her and establish frequent eye contact. This gradually builds up a closeness between the two of you and increases the baby's awareness of you, of other people and of the surrounding environment.

If the baby feels secure and loved and is provided with plenty of opportunity for social interaction, the effect on her personality and all aspects of development will be markedly beneficial. As babies grow, their relationship with their parents becomes deeper, and mutual love develops. This affection makes communication easier and more rewarding; a good relationship can grow better and better, and the child can develop in an optimal emotional environment.

In the 1970s a series of experiments was performed which looked at the development of the mother-baby relationship. Mothers who had their newborn infants with them all the time in the first few days were compared with mothers who fed their infants but were separated from them between some feeds. The results of these experiments were interpreted as showing that these first few days of life were a critical period during which the quality of the future relationship was determined. There was enthusiastic and widespread interest in this research. The term 'bonding' was applied to the mother-child attachment that developed during the 'critical first few days' and exaggerated claims were made for its importance.

Subsequent research has refuted these earlier findings. The relationship between mother and child will be good if it is relaxed and rewarding: the quality of the contact is more important than the quantity. The more anxieties or disappointments a parent has (for example, with a newborn child that is premature or ill), the more the relationship will be under stress. However, once the anxieties are overcome, the relationship can flourish and be just as good as if there had been no setback.

DAY-TO-DAY CARE

Feeding

The choice between breast and bottle feeding is discussed on page 16. However you have decided to feed your baby, if you are doing it for the first time you will need some help. It is important that the midwife or feeding counsellor can spend time helping you, and you should ask if you need advice.

The breasts do not produce ordinary milk in the first two or three days, but provide instead small quantities of a yellowish fluid called colostrum. Colostrum is rich in protein and various substances that help the baby to resist infection. The baby will not be able to suck for long at a time in the first few days. You should try to find a position for feeding that is comfortable for you, and equally so for the baby, and where you can watch her feeding. Some women are more at ease semi-recumbent or lying down, while others prefer to be sitting up in a comfy chair.

With bottle feeding you also need to work out a routine, including making up feeds and testing the temperature of the milk, and to establish the most comfortable and closest way of holding the baby. Only small amounts of feed are taken at first, but this builds up rapidly. General guidance only can be given on how much a baby should take each day, as

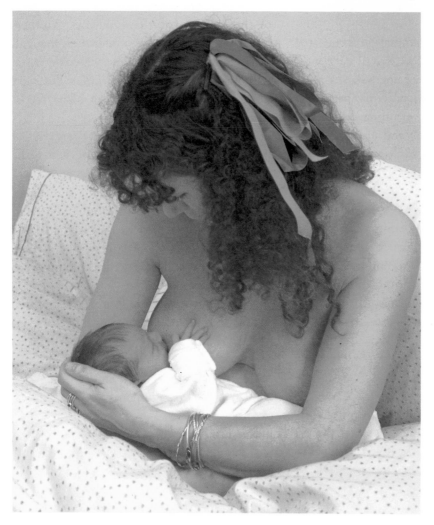

Left and right: Feeding brings mother and baby together and helps them develop a close relationship. Breast feeding is unique in this respect and the mother who bottle feeds should try to foster an equally close and loving bond. Whichever method is chosen, it is important that the baby is held comfortably and in a position where eye contact with the mother is easy.

If the baby is gaining weight satisfactorily and is content after feeds, enough milk is being taken in.

The bowels

Babies usually open their bowels shortly after birth, and certainly should do so in the first twenty-four hours. The stools passed for the first 2–3 days of life are sticky and dark green and are known as meconium. Thereafter the stools change in colour and consistency to soft and yellow. Once feeding is established, babies normally pass 2–6 stools a day, usually shortly after a feed is taken.

Occasionally babies are born with a bowel obstruction, and this is first recognized when the infant does not have a bowel action following birth. Recording the fact that a new baby has passed meconium is an important indication of normality.

Weighing and weight gain

The baby will be weighed at birth, and every day for the first week. This is one measure of progress and how the baby is doing. Over the first few days you should expect a small loss of weight of a few ounces each day, but by about the fourth or fifth day this trend is reversed, and birth weight is normally regained by about the eighth day. If the initial daily loss seems excessive or weight gain appears slow, the midwife or doctor will discuss possible causes with you. Slow weight gain may indicate inadequate milk intake but this may be due to the baby having a depressed appetite as much as you having an inadequate milk supply or poor feeding technique, and the reason should be found and corrected. Weight gain and growth are further considered on pages 48-9.

Preventing infection

Newborn babies are very susceptible to infection, and do not develop good resistance

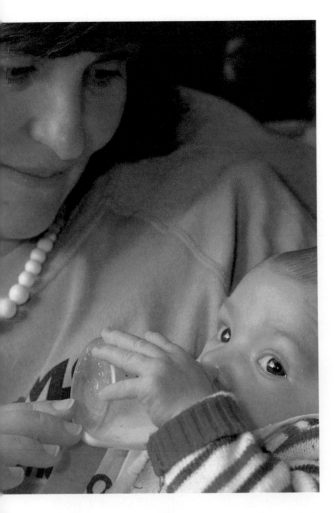

every child is different and some need slightly more milk than others. By the end of the first week the baby should be taking approximately 130–160 ml per kg body weight (4½-5½ fl oz per pound body weight) per day. This will be split up between feeds, which at first are likely to be about every three hours, including during the night.

In general it is better to feed babies on demand than to try to do it by the clock. If a baby wakes and cries for a feed nothing is to be gained by waiting, and the baby's crying can be upsetting. Similarly, if babies are asleep there is little point in waking them to give a feed for which they are not yet ready. Within a few weeks most babies have a routine that is fairly regular.

until they are around 6 months old. Even after this, children are more likely than adults to pick up infections. Hands should be washed before young babies are handled, and babies should not be passed around indiscriminately for everyone to hold, although obviously they will be cuddled by close family members. Many of the germs that cause infections in infants are common bacteria, which children and adults often carry without knowing on the skin as well as in the nose, mouth or bowel; hence the importance of hand washing. If somebody obviously has an infection, such as a cold, sore throat or septic spots, he or she should not be handling the baby.

Particular care is required over feeding, as infection of the alimentary tract, gastro-enteritis, is both prevalent and potentially dangerous (see page 266). There is little risk for breast fed babies: breast milk is fresh and will not contain harmful bacteria. Breast feeding leaves no opportunity for the baby to pick up infection from an inadequately cleaned and sterilized bottle or teat, and breast milk contains antibodies that give the baby increased resistance to infection. Bottle fed babies are at particular risk and so great care should be taken to protect them; feeds must be made up carefully in hygienic sur-

roundings, cleaning and sterilizing bottles and teats must be done correctly, feeds should not be made up more than twenty-four hours in advance, and once it has been warmed, any unused feed should be discarded.

It used to be common to bath babies soon after birth to remove the fatty material known as vernix, and any blood; the current practice is to leave the vernix to be absorbed into the skin, as it helps to provide protection against infection. The baby is initially cleaned by 'topping and tailing', wiping first the face and then the nappy area with cotton wool moistened with warm water. One bath before the baby leaves hospital is now the norm, so that the mother can learn how to do it, and have help available if she needs it. At home it is not necessary for the baby to be bathed every day, although if you both enjoy bathtime you may want to. Bathing on alternate days makes sure the baby stays clean, and helps to prevent infection.

The umbilicus

After the baby is born the midwife reclamps the umbilical cord, and cuts it off short. The stump dries out and falls off about a week after birth. It is important that it is kept both dry and clean, as the cord can provide a way in for infection. An antiseptic dusting powder

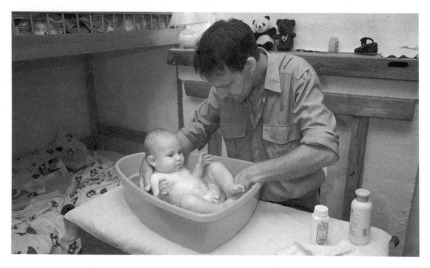

Most babies enjoy bathtime and the opportunity it provides for play and socialization.

may be used to help dry out the cord and keep it free of infection. When the stump falls off it leaves a clean umbilicus which soon becomes completely skin-covered and usually retracts below the surface of the abdominal wall.

COMMON MEDICAL PROBLEMS

Birth marks

Some babies have marks on their skin when they are born, and these are known as birth marks, or naevi; there are several types.

Very common, particularly in fair-skinned infants, is a triangular red patch on the forehead, accompanied by a red patch at the back of the neck. The medical name for this is naevus flammeus (flame-shaped birth mark), but the patches are commonly called stork-beak marks, from the fanciful idea that the stork that brought the baby held the head in its beak, marking the forehead and the nape of the neck. They persist for a few months and gradually become less marked.

Also very common in Chinese, Asian or Afro-Caribbean babies is a blue-black pigmentation over the lower back, which sometimes extends all over the back. This is often called Mongolian blue spots as it is very common in Chinese babies, but in fact it appears frequently in all pigmented races. To the uninitiated these blue spots may look like bruises. They gradually become less marked with time, and disappear by the time the baby is 2 years old.

Pigmented brown birth marks are common. Usually they are relatively small, but may be multiple; sometimes they are rather larger, and may also be hairy. They persist throughout life.

Flat red birth marks known as port-wine stains may occur, although they are rare.

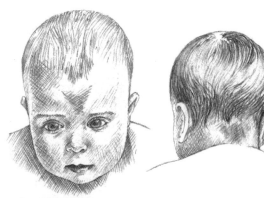

Stork-beak marks are a very common type of birth mark and can occur on the forehead and nape of the neck as red patches.

They are most common on the face, but can be found anywhere, and may be extensive. They are due to dilatation of some of the tiny blood vessels in the skin.

Strawberry naevi (cavernous haemangiomas) are usually considered to be birth marks, although they may not be apparent at birth and are often first noted when the baby is a few weeks old. They consist of a patch of blood vessels in the skin which are dilated, and appear as a raised red spot. They often enlarge over the first few months of life, and may be unsightly. However, they gradually shrink in size and eventually disappear completely without needing treatment. They always fade by the age of 5 years, and very often much sooner.

Treatment may be possible for unsightly birth marks, and a skin specialist can be consulted when the baby is bigger.

Breast enlargement and vaginal bleeding

Some degree of breast enlargement in newborn babies is common, and sometimes very pronounced. It can occur in both girls and boys, and is due to the stimulation of breast tissue before birth by the high levels of female sex hormones, called oestrogens, which were present in the mother's circulation and have crossed the placenta. In some cases a few drops of milk are produced by the baby's breast. No treatment is required. It is important that the breasts are not repeatedly handled or squeezed as this could predispose them to infection. Left alone, they gradually reduce in size over the first two or three weeks.

Occasionally, girl babies lose a small amount of blood from the vagina in the few days after birth; during pregnancy, oestrogen from the mother stimulates the baby's uterus, and as the oestrogen level falls after birth, there is slight bleeding from the uterus. It is of no medical significance.

Clicking hips

As part of the newborn examination, the hips are checked to see if they are normal. Some babies are born with dislocated or unstable hip joints. If this is recognized early and appropriately treated there is no lasting effect (see page 259); when it is not discovered until the child has started to walk, treatment is more difficult and success less certain.

In examining the hips of newborn babies the doctor tries to put the joints through a full range of movements to see if there is any limitation or instability. Sometimes the doctor can feel the hip slipping in and out of

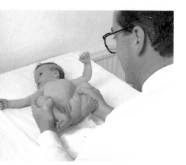

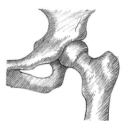

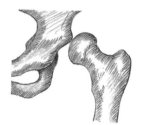

One of the purposes of the newborn examination is to detect dislocated or unstable hip joints. This is done by putting the joints through a full range of movements to see if there is any limitation or instability.

The artworks show a normal joint (**left**) and one that is dislocated (**right**).

its socket, which makes a palpable clunk. In the course of the test some hips make a click, rather like the noise that is sometimes heard when the knees are bent. If this is the case, the doctor may well want to keep an eye on the baby until he or she is sure the hip is normal.

Jaundice

Jaundice is a yellowish discoloration of the skin and the whites of the eyes due to a build-up in the blood of a yellow pigment called bilirubin, which is formed as red blood cells break down. About half of all newborns develop some degree of jaundice on the third or fourth day without there being any underlying disease. This normal or physiological jaundice occurs because the normal baby is born with more blood than she needs for life outside the womb, and the excess is broken down in the first few days. The iron from the blood pigment haemoglobin is stored in the body, but the rest of the haemoglobin is converted to bilirubin, which is excreted by the liver into the intestine.

Whereas mild physiological jaundice is of no medical significance, severe jaundice is important and its cause should be established, as it can adversely affect the baby.

Babies who are born prematurely may develop moderate or severe jaundice, as their livers are not fully mature and may not be able to excrete the bilirubin which is building up in the blood; this is described on page 36. Other causes of moderate or severe jaundice in the newborn period include infections, and forms of anaemia (see page 149) in which red blood cells are first damaged and then broken down. Rhesus disease (see page 294) used to be a common cause of severe jaundice and anaemia but is now rarely seen.

If a baby is more than slightly jaundiced the doctor may arrange for blood tests to check the level of bilirubin in the blood to make sure it is not high enough to need treatment with phototherapy (see page 37).

Skin rashes

The skin of a newborn baby is very thin and delicate, and mild rashes are common. Small white spots over the nose and cheeks are known as milia, and are quite normal. A fine red rash consisting of a few small red spots may be caused by the baby getting a bit hot, or by her skin rubbing against bedding. Such rashes are often called sweat rashes, and are not important.

Skin infections do occur quite frequently, however, and have to be taken seriously. A rash due to skin infection may consist of minute septic spots, or a blotchy red rash, or of spreading areas of redness. If your baby develops spots and you are not sure of their significance, ask the opinion of the midwife or doctor.

Some degree of nappy rash may occur in newborns, but is more common in older babies. This is a reddening of the skin, or discrete red spots, caused by prolonged contact of urine with the skin. The use of a

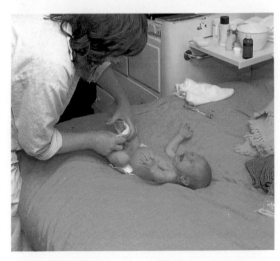

Young babies have very delicate skin, which is prone to mild rashes. Nappy rash occurs in both newborn and older babies and can be prevented by using a barrier cream.

cream such as zinc and castor oil in the nappy area acts as a preventative. (For more on nappy rashes, see page 63.)

Sticky eyes

Babies' eyes are very susceptible to infection; pus may form, making the edge of the eyelids sticky. If the infection is more severe, the eye will be reluctant to open; if the eye is forced open, pus will be seen inside the lids. The eyes may become infected either during delivery, from germs present in the mother's vagina, or after delivery. The doctor will want to take a swab from the eyes to find the cause of the infection and may want a vaginal swab from the mother as well. Treatment will be started with eye drops, and if the infection is severe, irrigating the eye regularly with drops may be necessary. Usually sticky eyes will clear up after a couple of days of treatment.

Sticky umbilicus

The umbilical stump may become infected, in which case it will appear moist and purulent (pussy) material may be obvious. A swab will be taken to find out which bacteria is causing the infection. If it is marked, the infection may be treated with an antibiotic given by mouth or injection to prevent it spreading to other parts of the body.

Thrush

Thrush is a fungal infection which in babies can affect the mouth and interfere with sucking. Mild thrush looks like milk curd on the tongue or inside the cheeks, but the patches are attached to the mucous membrane and cannot be wiped off. If the infection is more severe, the whole tongue and inside of the mouth may look white, and at this stage the baby may be reluctant to feed. Thrush is very easy to treat with nystatin or amphotericin drops.

CHAPTER

3

SPECIAL CARE FOR NEWBORN INFANTS

At birth or in the newborn period, some babies need more than routine care. This may be because they are of low birth weight, or because they have additional medical problems.

Around 5–10 per cent of babies are born weighing less than 2.5 kg (5½ lb), and are referred to as 'low birth weight' (LBW) babies. The term 'very low birth weight' (sometimes abbreviated to VLBW) is applied to children weighing less than 1.5 kg (3 lb 5 oz).

Until relatively recently all low birth weight babies were classified as premature, but it is now realized that, while many low birth weight infants *are* born early and are immature, for others gestation has continued for the appropriate time of around forty weeks. Low birth weight babies are now identified either as pre-term (that is, born early), or as born weighing less than expected for the length of the pregnancy. Some babies are both pre-term and light for gestational age ('small for dates').

Babies of low birth weight have special needs in the newborn period because of their small size; if they are also pre-term, they need special help because of the immaturity of many of their body systems and organs. Low birth weight babies are also more prone to medical problems than those born at term and who have grown well throughout the pregnancy.

While the majority of babies requiring special care are of low birth weight, some babies of normal birth weight also have problems, including asphyxia or injuries sustained in labour or delivery, serious congenital abnormalities, infections or jaundice (see page 28).

Some babies needing special care will be able to stay with their mothers while being kept under extra observation and given treatment by the doctors and nursing staff. Others will need to be cared for in a neonatal nursery, where there are staff specially trained in caring for the sick and frail newborn, and where special equipment is available.

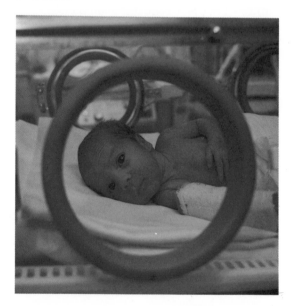

Incubators are among the most common forms of equipment used for babies in need of special care. Low birth weight or pre- term babies are unable to control their body temperature and so the incubator maintains this within the normal range.

THE NEONATAL NURSERY

All maternity units have a neonatal nursery where babies requiring special care can be looked after, observed and given treatment by experienced staff. For many low birth weight babies, particularly those born after the thirty-third week of pregnancy and of expected weight for gestational age, the necessary procedures are routine, and the baby progresses steadily without incident. A few babies need very careful management and may require specialized care, including prolonged treatment on a ventilator (see page 41) to assist their breathing. This level of care, often referred to as intensive neonatal care, is not available in all neonatal units, and some babies will need to be transferred to a regional intensive care unit. Very low birth weight babies almost always need intensive care.

Transfer to a regional intensive care unit may be arranged after the baby is born or even during labour. If the baby is to be moved after the birth, the regional unit medical team will come with a transport incubator and all the necessary back-up equipment to convey him to the intensive care unit. This ensures that the baby's condition is not worsened by the journey. Sometimes, when a mother goes into labour very prematurely, it may be obvious that the baby is going to be tiny and immature, and will require immediate intensive care. In such cases, if at all possible, the mother is transferred during labour to the centre where the intensive care neonatal unit is situated, to ensure that her baby is born in the place where he will have the best chance of survival.

As well as trained and experienced staff, the neonatal nursery will have special equipment to monitor the baby's condition and to assist in treatment. Babies that are of low birth weight, and particularly those that are immature or sick, need to be monitored closely, so that if anything starts to go wrong the nurses or doctor can take corrective action immediately. Much of this monitoring is done automatically, utilizing machines to record heart rate, breathing, blood pressure, temperature and the amount of oxygen in the blood.

Frequent blood tests are needed to check on the working of many of the baby's internal organs, and in some babies X-rays or swabs may need to be taken frequently. Parents should be informed of the purpose of the various monitors and recorders, and be familiar with the way in which they work.

In addition to monitoring equipment, the neonatal unit will have other aids to help in the care of the baby. Most babies will be nursed in incubators, or under heat cradles, which have an overhead heater to keep the baby warm. At some stage of their stay in the nursery many babies will require a very fine tube to be inserted into a vein, either for taking blood samples or to deliver fluid, drugs or nutrients. Because this intravenous tube (often referred to as the intravenous line) is so narrow, a pump is necessary to maintain a flow. Some babies will need ventilators to help with their breathing, and others with jaundice may need treatment with fluorescent light from a phototherapy unit (see page 37).

The surroundings and equipment in the neonatal nursery may be upsetting for many parents. In addition parents are bound to be anxious about having a baby who needs special or intensive neonatal care. The more you can understand what is going on, and what the different machines and procedures are for, the less intimidating the experience should be. The staff should do their best to help you understand, but you should always

A general view of a neonatal nursery, showing incubators and some of the monitoring equipment.

Here, babies requiring special care are looked after, observed and treated by skilled staff.

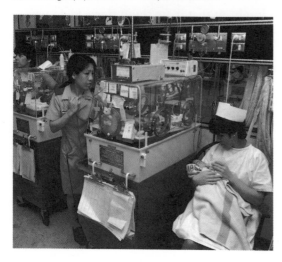

ask about anything that is worrying you. As you become used to the nursery you will be able to help the nurses in the care of your baby.

Having a baby who requires care in a neonatal nursery is often a disappointment to parents. They will have looked forward to the birth eagerly, and made plans in the expectation that their baby would arrive at the appropriate time and be healthy. Instead, the baby may arrive before all the preparations are complete and then have to be separated from his mother. The infant may look thin and scrawny and not how the parents had pictured their new baby. Furthermore there may be serious concerns about the baby's health, and parents are bound to worry, perhaps feeling that they should keep their distance emotionally in case the baby does not survive.

Parents should *not* feel guilty if their initial reaction is one of disappointment rather than joy. Most parents of low birth weight babies and other babies needing to be in a special care nursery initially experience negative feelings. Once the shock has been absorbed, parents can get to know their child

and join in with providing the special care that he requires. Gradually a full relationship can develop.

If low birth weight and other sick babies are cared for in neonatal units that provide special care, and if adequate intensive care is available for those babies that need it, the chances of a baby surviving are very good. For very low birth weight babies, weighing between 1 and 1.5 kg (2 lb 3oz and 3 lb 5 oz) at birth, survival is achieved in around 85 or 90 per cent of cases, and figures are even better for bigger babies. For babies weighing less than 1 kg (2 lb 3 oz) the survival figures are not so good, but even babies born at around twenty-six weeks of gestation and weighing only about 700 g (1½ lb) stand a chance of survival.

One of the questions that concerns everyone who is involved in providing intensive care for very small and very sick infants is whether, if the child survives, he will be normal or handicapped. The incidence of handicap is higher than normal in surviving very low birth weight babies, but long-term follow-up shows that the majority have no handicap, and only about 6 per cent of the survivors are unable to attend a normal school. Since intensive neonatal care was introduced, there has not been an increase in the numbers of handicapped children, because providing good neonatal care prevents the development of disabilities in many children who would otherwise have had a handicap.

LOW BIRTH WEIGHT BABIES

The pre-term baby
Pre-term babies are those born before the thirty-seventh week of pregnancy. Babies may be born early, either because the mother

goes into labour spontaneously or because the doctor induces labour when the health risks to mother and/or baby in allowing the pregnancy to continue are greater than in caring for a low birth weight baby.

Going into premature labour spontaneously can be caused by weakness of the neck of the womb (known as incompetence of the cervix), or by an infection of the mother associated with fever. It is usual in twin pregnancies for delivery to be a few weeks early, and also if there is too much fluid around the baby, a condition known as polyhydramnios. Occasionally accidents and emotional stress may lead to the onset of labour, but in many cases the cause of the early onset of labour is not known.

Medical indications for inducing labour early include high blood pressure or toxaemia of the mother which can impair the health of mother and baby, maternal diabetes, poor growth of the fetus (as shown by ultrasound), and bleeding from early separation of the placenta, all of which can threaten the survival of the baby.

In general the shorter the period of gestation the more likely the baby is to suffer from problems of immaturity. All pre-term babies are likely to have problems with maintaining body temperature, and initially will not be strong enough to take feeds from the breast or a bottle. Most will develop jaundice during the first week, and some will have breathing difficulties. Pre-term babies are particularly prone to hernias and to undescended testicles (see page 307). Babies that are born earlier than thirty weeks of gestation are likely to have major problems because most of the body's systems have not developed to the stage where they are fully functional and can enable the baby to maintain an independent existence outside the womb. All the problems mentioned above are discussed later in this chapter.

The baby who is small for gestational age

A baby who weighs less than usual for the length of gestation has not grown properly during intra-uterine life (life in the womb). This may be because the baby has not received adequate nutrition through the placenta during the pregnancy (see page 11), or because he is genetically very small, or because there is a disease or abnormality which is affecting him.

Poor placental function which leads to inadequate nutrition of the fetus (referred to as placental insufficiency) can have many causes. It occurs in mothers who have high blood pressure or who smoke, and in those with toxaemia of pregnancy, or premature separation of part of the placenta (see Chapter 1). Sometimes there is no obvious cause. As some of the causes of placental insufficiency are also causes of premature labour, some babies are born both small for gestational age and pre-term.

The first effect of placental insufficiency is on the growth of the fetus. Less than optimal amounts of nutrients reach the baby, resulting in a degree of starvation. If placental function continues to deteriorate, the fetus stops growing, and the oxygen supply to the baby also becomes impaired. If this happens the baby may die if not delivered early. After birth babies who have suffered from placental insufficiency often exhibit 'catch-up growth': putting on weight faster than normal to make up for the period during which growth was impeded.

Using ultrasound to monitor the growth of the baby during pregnancy enables poor intra-uterine growth to be detected. With placental insufficiency the growth rate of the baby slows, whereas the baby who is genetically small will have grown slowly but steadily throughout the pregnancy.

Some fetuses grow poorly because of

abnormality or disease. Some chromosomal defects (see Chapter 8), intra-uterine infection due to rubella (German measles) or other viruses, and other diseases can all lead to poor fetal growth. Such babies do not show catch-up growth after delivery.

Babies who are small for gestational age do not usually have problems with breathing or jaundice in the newborn period unless they are also pre-term, but they are particularly liable to develop a low blood sugar (hypoglycaemia) after birth, and are also prone to infections (see pages 25 and 42).

CARING FOR LOW BIRTH WEIGHT BABIES

Pre-term infants make few spontaneous movements, and spend a lot of the time asleep. They do, however, have to be fed, turned and have nappy changes just like other babies, and will probably be dressed even if inside an incubator. Because of their special needs they will require close observation and therefore they are likely to need to be connected to machines which monitor body functions like pulse and breathing. They also require blood tests and other procedures that term babies do not.

Most pre-term babies favour a 'frog' posture when they are lying flat in an incubator, lying on their tummy with their legs flexed; they can also be nursed on their side, but are likely to require a rolled-up cover as a wedge to help keep them in position. Pre-term babies should be handled gently when they need to be moved, and it is important that they do not get cold. If the doctors or nursing staff have to keep the baby out of the incubator for any length of time for a special procedure, warmth is provided by an overhead heat cradle.

At first parents may be inhibited from touching the baby or having much to do with

him because of the unfamiliar surroundings of the special care baby unit, and because he is small and in an incubator. The staff should encourage parents to open the portholes on the incubator and reach in to touch and hold their child; later mothers and fathers can share the care of their baby with the nurses when they visit the unit, and if appropriate have periods of holding and cuddling him.

The immediate needs of low weight babies are maintaining body temperature, feeding, controlling jaundice, and treating any breathing or digestive problems. In the longer term it is important to prevent or treat any infections, and to ensure that growth is adequate.

Body temperature and incubators

Babies who are born earlier than about thirty-seven weeks, and those weighing less than about 2.5 kg (5½ lb) need to be observed closely in the newborn period to see if special care is required. Most low birth weight babies are unable to control their body temperature, and unless they are kept warm their temperature will drop. A fall in body temperature to below 36°C (97°F) is harmful for a baby. For some of the bigger low birth weight babies keeping them well covered in a warm nursery may be adequate, but most need to be in an incubator.

An incubator is designed to maintain the baby's body temperature within the normal range, and at the same time enables the baby to be closely observed. Some incubators provide a thermostatically controlled, constant-temperature environment that can be set at the appropriate level, small babies needing higher temperatures than large ones. Some sophisticated incubators have a temperature control that is regulated by the baby's own temperature (measured by a probe inserted into the baby's rectum) so that

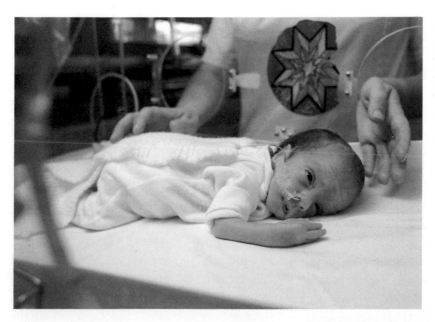

Pre-term babies have to be fed, turned, changed and dressed just like other babies and with even greater care. Babies who are too young to be able to suck adequately are fed by means of a naso-gastric tube which passes through the nose or mouth into the stomach.

body temperature is maintained within a very narrow range. These incubators have been a great advance in the care of very small babies.

As well as controlling the baby's temperature, an incubator has to ensure that the air the baby breathes is humidified, and if necessary enriched with oxygen (see page 41).

Feeding

Low birth weight babies need nutrients soon after birth, as they do not have reserves to enable them to withstand more than a few hours without food. Babies who are small for gestational age are likely to have dangerously low levels of sugar in the blood (hypoglycaemia) if they are not fed adequately. Part of the routine care of small babies is measuring blood sugar regularly to ensure that the level remains satisfactory.

The more immature and poorly a baby is, and the lower his weight, the more difficult feeding is likely to be. Such babies, however, are in urgent need of adequate nutrition, not only to give them strength to withstand their current problems but to enable them to grow and develop.

Small newborns are unlikely to tolerate milk feeds straight away, and for the first day or two glucose solutions are given to combat dehydration and hypoglycaemia (see page 43). Babies who are only a few weeks premature may be able to tolerate ordinary formula feeds, or feeds specially made for pre-term infants. If a mother wants to breast feed she can express her milk until the baby is old enough to be able to feed from the breast. Expressed breast milk in sufficient amounts can provide adequate nutrition for the pre-term baby in many instances. Special formulae are available which have been designed to meet the particular needs of the low birth weight infant.

The method of feeding low birth weight babies and what is given both need to be determined individually for each baby and reviewed regularly. Babies of around thirty-six weeks of gestation or older, if otherwise well, may be able to feed from breast or bottle. They readily become fatigued, and this is to be avoided. Breast feeding requires more sucking ability from the baby than does bottle feeding, and so some babies who are not ready to take the breast may be able to manage a bottle, or may manage to suck alternate feeds, provided they are tube-fed for the interim one.

Babies younger than around thirty-six weeks will not be able to suck adequately, and will need to be fed using a tube which is passed through the mouth or nose into the stomach (naso-gastric tube). Feeds may be given via the tube every two or three hours, or in more immature babies may be run in slowly but continuously, the nursing staff making sure that the baby is not given more feed than can be absorbed.

Very low birth weight babies and others who are sick may not be able to absorb nutrients from the intestine in adequate amounts for life and growth. It may be necessary to give them intravenous nutrition either to supplement or replace tube feeding.

For intravenous nutrition specially prepared basic nutrients are infused through a vein into the baby's circulation.

Low birth weight babies do not have adequate stores of iron and vitamins A, B, C and D when they are born, and they need to be given supplements for the first few months of life.

Jaundice of prematurity

Jaundice during the newborn period is described in Chapter 2 (see pages 28-9). Pre-term babies are very likely to become jaundiced in the first few days of life as the immaturity of the enzyme systems in the liver means the baby cannot get rid of the bilirubin pigment which builds up in the blood. It is the high amounts of bilirubin in

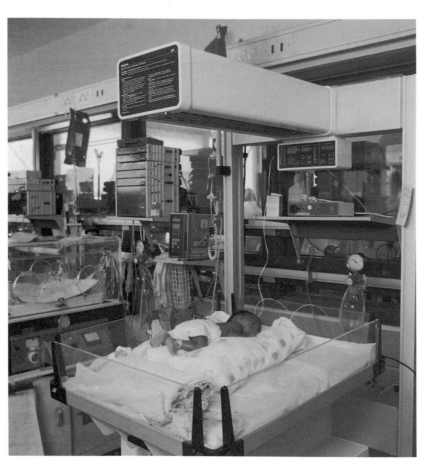

The overhead heat cradle enables a pre-term baby to be nursed out of an incubator. This makes it easier to carry out medical or nursing procedures.

the blood that give rise to the yellow skin coloration known as jaundice. The level of jaundice must not be allowed to become too high, as it could cause brain damage. An important aspect of the care of pre-term newborns is monitoring the level of the bilirubin by frequent blood tests, and treatment is aimed at keeping the level within safe limits.

If the jaundice looks as though it is becoming marked, phototherapy will be used. Phototherapy consists of laying the child in a fluorescent light source which is rich in ultraviolet rays. The eyes need to be covered, but otherwise the baby is naked. If a jaundiced child is exposed to ultraviolet light, the light breaks down the bilirubin in the blood circulating through the skin, and lessens the jaundice. One of the effects of the treatment is to make the child lose more water through the skin, so babies having phototherapy are given extra drinks of water.

In some babies phototherapy alone is not enough to prevent the level of jaundice rising dangerously high. If this is the case then treatment with an exchange transfusion may be needed. A small amount of the baby's blood is removed, and replaced with blood from a donor; this is repeated many times until most of the baby's blood has been removed and replaced with donor blood. As the donor blood does not contain the bilirubin which causes the jaundice, the baby's jaundice improves as the procedure progresses.

Within about a week of birth the baby's liver is likely to be functioning fully, and jaundice is not likely to continue to be a problem beyond this stage.

Growth

Babies who are born pre-term and are of appropriate weight for gestational age ideally should continue to grow at the same rate as they would have done if they had remained in the womb until term. To do this requires that they are healthy, and that they receive adequate amounts of all the right nutrients.

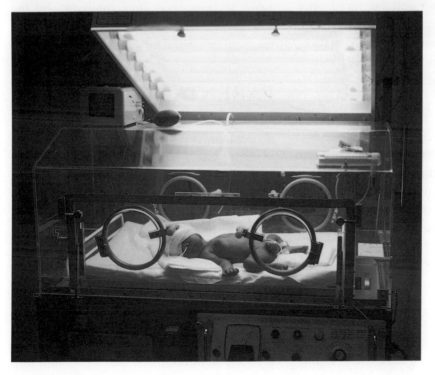

Pre-term babies often become jaundiced in the newborn period. Phototherapy using fluorescent light is the treatment given to lessen the jaundice.

This can be achieved for babies born after about thirty-three weeks who remain well. Given either breast milk or pre-term formula in adequate amounts, together with vitamins A, B, C and D and iron supplements, they grow well, and growth can be expected to continue normally throughout childhood.

It is much harder to attain normal growth in pre-term babies of very low birth weight (below 1.5 kg/3 lb 5 oz). Their alimentary tract is not fully mature, and may be unable to absorb adequate amounts of food; even when these babies are fed intravenously, growth is sub-optimal and is further interfered with if they become ill. As a consequence, weight gain may be very slow in the first few weeks, but gradually improves as the child becomes bigger and more mature.

Growth in newborn babies who were small for gestational age is influenced by the cause of the poor intra-uterine growth. Where placental insufficiency has led to a restriction of nutrients reaching the fetus, catch-up growth may well be rapid after birth. Where the baby was inherently small, or underweight because of illness or malformation, the poor growth pattern is likely to continue in early childhood.

Going home

Many neonatal nurseries will recommend that babies are discharged when they are medically fit, are feeding well, can maintain their body temperature, and are gaining weight satisfactorily, whatever their weight. Others will require the baby to have attained a weight of around 2.2 kg (5 lb).

In addition to the baby meeting these requirements, parents need to feel confident that they have mastered all the necessary skills to look after their child. When babies are in special care parents have little opportunity to handle and look after them. Some-

times, however, arrangements can be made for the mother to stay in the hospital for one or two days before the baby's discharge; in these circumstances she can ask advice if necessary.

Physical care of the baby who comes home from a neonatal nursery is essentially the same as for any other baby, as discharge is not arranged until the baby is thriving on what is, for all practical purposes, normal baby care.

For the parents, however, excitement is likely to be mixed with anxiety. Provided all goes well, confidence soon builds up, but it is important for parents to be given support and advice if there are problems or worries. Many neonatal units have liaison staff who will visit families at home in the few days after discharge, and this system works well. Alternatively, a telephone call to the neonatal unit may be all that is needed. The family doctor or health visitor will provide other resources. Most babies who have been cared for in a neonatal nursery will usually be seen again at least once after discharge by the medical staff to ensure that progress continues to be satisfactory.

PARENTAL STRESS

Parents of a child who requires treatment in a neonatal unit are aware when the baby's life is in danger, and will obviously be upset and anxious. With very immature or very sick babies the period in which the child's condition is critical, and it is uncertain whether he will survive, may be very prolonged and go on for days or weeks.

Parents may be further troubled by the feeling that they are losing contact with their baby. Because the infant is being looked after by the neonatal unit staff and is in an incubator connected to monitors, it is difficult to develop the sort of relationship that would come from caring for a healthy baby. In addition parents may have feelings of failure as their baby is not healthy, and of disappointment that having the baby was not as joyous an event as had been anticipated.

The stress on parents can be considerable, and may go on for a long time. Prolonged worry can affect their own health and their relationships with each other and with other people; such stress should be acknowledged, and ways of coping with it found. Friends and relatives have an important role in providing support and comfort.

The staff of the neonatal unit will understand the anxieties of the parents; in fact, nurses caring for these sick infants experience many of the same feelings. The staff try to help parents to cope, by arranging opportunities for mothers and fathers to express their worries, by explaining what is going on, by arranging meetings with other parents who have had the same experiences, and by giving counselling and support. It is important that parents feel they are an integral part of the caring team. Staff can teach mothers and fathers how to handle, care for and feed their baby, and to understand the purpose and workings of all the monitors and other equipment used in providing special care. Many parents will have an initial reluctance to handle the baby in this way, but with encouragement they will be able to play an important part in providing loving care for him.

THE DYING BABY

Some babies are born too early, or become too ill to respond to medical treatment. In other babies with severe congenital abnormalities, or in babies who become severely brain damaged due to oxygen lack or brain haemorrhage, all those involved in the care of the baby may consider that it is not justified to continue intensive medical support.

When a baby is dying, parents will be severely affected. Some prefer to be present when the baby dies; others would rather be away from the neonatal unit, or in a quiet room by themselves. If they are with the baby they may like to cuddle him or hold a hand, and they should feel free to hold the child for as long as they want to after the death.

There will follow a time of great emotional upheaval, with mixed feelings of sadness and loss, and possibly also anger or guilt. The support of friends and relatives is invaluable. Gradually the emotions become calmer, although the loss and some sadness will remain. Some inexperienced and unthinking friends and acquaintances may consider the loss of a small baby who has not had the chance to become a full member of the family easier to get over than other bereavements. The infant has, however, held a very special and central role in the thoughts and feelings of the parents for several months, and they are likely to be deeply moved by both the brief life and the death of their baby.

Losing a child is discussed further in Chapter 12.

MEDICAL PROBLEMS OF PRE-TERM AND OTHER NEWBORN BABIES

In all newborns serious or life-threatening conditions may occur. Genetic disease, congenital abnormalities, infections or placental insufficiency *in utero*, and asphyxia or birth injury are all potential causes of serious ailments. Furthermore, the newborn has little resistance to infections and even with optimal care serious infections sometimes occur.

The baby born prematurely is at even

greater health risk; the shorter the pregnancy, the more likely the baby is to have medical problems. Very immature babies, born two or three months early, are likely to have many major problems. Even with the very best available neonatal care some babies will die.

Breathing

One of the most profound changes that occurs with the birth of a baby is the taking of the first breath. Breathing is the fundamental new activity that initiates the baby's independence from his mother, and the baby cannot live unless it is established. However, in pre-term babies the control and mechanism of breathing may not be adequately developed.

During fetal development some respiratory movements occur as early as around eighteen weeks of gestation, and from then on there are more frequent movements in which the chest expands and contracts and small amounts of amniotic fluid, which surrounds the baby in the womb, move in and out of the lungs. Development of the lungs themselves to the stage at which they can function outside the womb is not accomplished until about 24–26 weeks, development continuing over the next ten weeks.

Some degree of breathing difficulty is common in pre-term babies born before thirty-six weeks, as until that stage the lungs may not be sufficiently developed to sustain the profound change that comes with birth: obtaining oxygen from the air via the lungs, rather than from the mother's circulation via the placenta. The earlier a baby is born, the more likely there is to be breathing difficulty, but not all babies born early develop symptoms.

Before birth the lungs contain no air, and have only a small blood supply. With the first breath they expand as they fill with air, and the circulation changes: the baby's blood is now directed through the lungs to be oxygenated, before it returns to the heart to be sent around the body. After the first few breaths regular respirations become established; the rate and depth of breathing are controlled by reflex by the respiratory centre in the brain to regulate the amount of oxygen and carbon dioxide in the blood. In very immature babies the respiratory centre is not sufficiently developed to maintain regular respirations, and such babies may have episodes in which breathing stops. These occurrences are known as apnoeic attacks (see page 42).

The main functions of the lungs are to transfer oxygen from the inspired air into the bloodstream, and to remove carbon dioxide from the blood and eliminate it from the body in the expired air. With each inspiration the lungs expand and air is taken in; with expiration some of this contained air is breathed out, and the lungs contract. However, even at the end of expiration a lot of air remains within the lungs, and oxygen and carbon dioxide exchange between the blood and air goes on continuously.

The lungs stay partially inflated at the end of each expiration because the fluid that lines the air passages contains a special substance, called surfactant, which lowers the surface tension. Without surfactant the lining fluid would make the lungs collapse, so that most or all of the air would go out of the lungs at the end of each expiration.

Respiratory distress syndrome (RDS)

It is a deficiency of surfactant in the lungs of pre-term babies that causes the commonest respiratory problem – the respiratory distress syndrome, or RDS. An alternative name for the same condition is hyaline membrane disease.

In RDS the lungs deflate completely after each breath because of the surfactant deficiency, and every inspiration requires a lot more effort than usual. In addition the amount of oxygen passing into the blood is reduced as some of the blood flows through uninflated lung which contains no air.

In the fetus surfactant is present in small quantities in the lung fluid from about twenty-eight weeks of gestation, but not in normal amounts until around thirty-five weeks. The earlier the baby is born, the more likely the amounts of surfactant to be inadequate, and the more likely the baby to develop some degree of RDS. Production of surfactant is increased once the child is breathing air, and in the mildest cases of RDS symptoms will only last for a couple of days; after this, adequate surfactant is available in the lung fluid.

The clinical features of RDS are very variable. In most children symptoms are mild, and may only consist of slightly laboured breathing which persists for a few hours or a few days; in others RDS is life-threatening, and intensive treatment is needed. In a pre-term baby the first indication that RDS is going to develop is that at some stage in the first twelve hours of life the baby's breathing becomes difficult, the rate increasing and the baby having to put more work into each breath. The baby may also become rather dusky or blue in colour as the amount of oxygen in the blood falls. The earlier symptoms of RDS start, the more likely it is to be severe.

If the baby does begin to develop symptoms, the nursery staff will monitor breathing and may do a blood test to establish the amount of oxygen in the blood. Extra oxygen may be introduced into the incubator. It is very important with low birth weight babies, whenever oxygen is being given, to assess regularly how much oxygen is getting through to the blood. The aim is to raise the amount of oxygen to normal values, but if the levels become higher than normal this too can be dangerous. Prolongèd high oxygen concentrations may lead to damage of the retina of the eye (see Retrolental fibroplasia, page 294).

Adding oxygen to the air in the incubator only slightly raises the oxygen concentration of the air breathed in, but for many babies with mild RDS, this is the only treatment needed. Further surfactant is produced in the lungs in the days after birth, and in these babies respiratory distress symptoms only last for a few days.

If the RDS is more severe, the baby may need to breathe air that is more enriched with oxygen than can be achieved just by running oxygen into the incubator; in this case a 'head box' may be used to deliver oxygen to the baby. This consists of a perspex hood that covers the baby's head, but only fits loosely around the neck. Running oxygen into the head box means that the oxygen concentration in the air around the baby's head can be much higher than in the rest of the incubator. The symptoms of RDS may be improved if the baby has to breathe out against a slight resistance; this may be achieved by using a head box which fits closely around the neck, or by giving oxygen by tube into the nose; the baby breathes out of the mouth, but as the lips remain together they create a slight resistance.

If the RDS is even more severe and the baby is having to put a great deal of effort into breathing, it may be necessary for him to be connected to a ventilator which takes over the work of breathing. A small plastic tube (known as an endotracheal or ET tube) is passed through the mouth or nose into the baby's windpipe (trachea). Once the baby has been intubated in this way the ET tube is connected to a ventilator. Modern ventilators can be adjusted so that each baby can be given the correct amount of air, at the rate of pressure and oxygen concentration appropriate for his individual needs. The amount of oxygen reaching the baby's blood is measured regularly and the ventilator adjusted accordingly.

Most babies who require ventilator treatment only need it for a short time; with very premature babies it may be necessary to continue ventilation for several weeks.

The main principles in managing RDS are to maintain the amount of oxygen in the baby's bloodstream, and to provide other support while waiting for the RDS to improve; the baby should eventually start to make surfactant in adequate amounts to enable the lungs to function normally. Specific treatment, with artificial surfactant being put into the lungs, has been developed and is useful for some babies.

Pneumothorax Babies with RDS have to make a great effort to expand and contract the lungs, and the pressures involved sometimes cause a small rupture of an air sac on the outer side of the lung; this means that air escapes from the lung into the space around it, the pleura. This is known as a pneumothorax. Resuscitation and ventilation (see pages 21 and 41) also sometimes cause a pneumothorax. When a pneumothorax is present it inhibits the full expansion of the lung and increases the difficulties the baby has in breathing. The pneumothorax can be treated by inserting a tube into the pleural cavity so that the escaped air drains out, and the lung can then re-expand.

Apnoeic attacks Some very immature babies are not able to maintain regular respirations, and may have episodes in which they stop breathing. These apnoeic attacks are most common in the first week of life. In some small babies regular respirations may be initially satisfactory, but apnoeic attacks start if they become unwell in any way, such as developing an infection.

Because apnoeic attacks are relatively common in very premature babies, all such babies have their breathing monitored by a recorder, which will sound an alarm if breathing stops. Most apnoeic attacks can be arrested and regular breathing re-established by stimulating the baby in some way. Very often just touching the baby will cause breathing to start again, or it may be necessary to give extra oxygen and press on the chest, or to stimulate the tongue or the back of the mouth.

If a baby has repeated apnoeic attacks, or if the attacks themselves are prolonged and difficult to stop, it could be dangerous, as with each attack the level of oxygen in the baby's blood falls and this affects all the vital organs. The baby may be given a drug to stimulate breathing, which may stop the attacks. If attacks persist it may be necessary to put the baby on a ventilator so that breathing is maintained regularly. Ventilator therapy can be continued until the baby has outgrown the tendency to apnoeic attacks, which is unlikely to last longer than a few days, or a week or two.

Infections

All babies are liable to infection. They have delicate skin and mucous membranes which means that bacteria can readily gain access to the body, and the body's defence mechanisms against infection are not well developed in the first months of life. Babies who are born prematurely and those who are otherwise ill are particularly prone to infections.

Because they have little resistance newborns should not be exposed to unnecessary risk of infection. Only a small number of people should handle the baby, and anybody harbouring an infection should keep away.

Babies need to be kept clean, and strict hygiene is necessary for preparing feeds.

When a newborn baby does develop an infection, it can easily become serious and is likely to spread around the body. Urinary tract infections (see page 171), gastroenteritis, pneumonia, septicaemia and meningitis (see A-Z section, which starts on page 228) occur commonly in this age group. Furthermore, because the body has not developed all the systems for combating infection, there may be few signs to indicate that the baby is infected. It is rare for newborns to develop a temperature if they are infected, and there may not be any signs of local inflammation. Instead, infection may be suspected if the baby is off feeds or vomiting, is perhaps rather grey in colour, or developing episodes of drowsiness or apnoea (when breathing stops). His temperature may be low rather than normal or high.

If doctors suspect infection in a newborn baby they will take blood and urine samples, and swabs for the microbiologist to look for bacteria, and they may do a chest X-ray and lumbar puncture (see pages 145 and 157); all these are to detect evidence of infection. Because of the hazards of untreated infection in young babies, treatment with antibiotics may be started before definite evidence of infection has been found.

The developing brain

The brain has many different functions, including controlling heart rate, respiration, body temperature and appetite, receiving and interpreting touch, visual and sound stimuli, controlling body posture and movement, and thinking. Development of all these functions and many more takes place gradually, and some are not complete until adult life is reached. Growth in size and the development of structure, however, occur mainly before birth and in the first year.

The brain can grow and develop normally in the low birth weight baby, but there are some hazards that can occur in early life that have the potential to cause brain damage; part of the management of the baby in the neonatal nursery is designed to reduce the risks of problems developing.

Although there are several different factors that are common in pre-term and small-for-dates babies and that put them at risk of brain damage, the vast majority of such babies are of normal intelligence and have normal brain functioning.

Hypoglycaemia, or a low level of glucose sugar in the blood, is very common in the newborn period of low birth weight babies, particularly in those who have suffered from placental insufficiency and are small for gestational age, as described on page 33. One of the dangers of hypoglycaemia is that it can cause brain damage, so it is important that the blood sugar level is monitored regularly, and the baby receives adequate nutrition to prevent the level becoming too low.

The low levels of oxygen in the blood that can occur in babies who are asphyxiated at birth or who develop respiratory distress syndrome can give rise to brain damage if they are prolonged. Short periods of hypoxia (low oxygen in the blood) are usually tolerated without problem. Measuring the amount of oxygen in the blood regularly and using ventilator therapy to maintain it within normal limits are important in maintaining brain function.

Infection, particularly meningitis (see page 285), is another threat to normal brain development. As has been emphasized above, low birth weight newborns have little resistance to infection, and any infection is potentially serious.

A further possible hazard to the developing brain is bleeding inside the fluid-filled part of the brain; this is called intraventricular haemorrhage. The cause of intra-ventricular haemorrhage is unknown, but it is more common in babies who are pre-term and have been hypoxic. It occurs without warning, and is signalled by a sudden worsening of the baby's condition. The haemorrhage can be diagnosed and its severity assessed using ultrasound. Full recovery is likely from small intraventricular haemorrhage, but if the haemorrhage is large or repeated, brain damage is likely, and many such babies do not survive.

All very small babies are carefully followed up after discharge from the neo-natal unit to check on their growth and development. Part of the reason for this is to detect early any signs of impairment of brain function, however minor. Impaired function may affect body posture or movement, hearing, vision, intellect or any other area of brain activity. Early treatment of any functional impairment is necessary as it minimizes the resultant disability.

The alimentary system

The alimentary system in very small and immature babies may not be developed enough to digest and absorb adequate amounts of feed. Initially small amounts of feed are given by tube (see page 36) into the baby's stomach, and a careful watch is kept to make sure that the stomach or the intestines do not become distended by fluid which is not absorbed. If no fluid is absorbed or the amounts absorbed are inadequate, the baby needs to be fed intravenously using specially prepared basic nutrients.

Sometimes babies who are initially able to absorb feed or fluid from the intestine suffer a subsequent deterioration in gut function. The abdomen may become distended, and fluid will collect in the stomach; this can be drawn off by the naso-gastric tube.

Alimentary function may become depres-sed because the baby's general condition worsens, due to such problems as developing RDS or infection. It may also occur because the inner lining of the intestine becomes damaged, a condition known as necrotizing enterocolitis.

The cause of necrotizing enterocolitis is uncertain, but it is common in very small babies. The intestine stops working, be-comes distended and the inner lining starts to peel off. Sometimes the whole wall of the intestine is involved and the intestine perforates. In many cases of necrotizing enterocolitis, transferring the baby to intra-venous feeding and aspirating the intestine through the feeding tube to prevent the build-up of fluid will allow the condition to settle down and the gut to recover, but in more serious cases surgery to repair the intestine may be needed.

Patent ductus arteriosus

Before birth the lungs are non-functional and have only a small blood supply. Most of the blood is diverted through a large vessel called the ductus arteriosus into the general circulation. After birth the lungs expand and start to absorb oxygen. The ductus arteriosus normally constricts so that blood does not pass through it and then gradually changes from a blood vessel into a fibrous band.

In some pre-term babies, particularly those with respiratory distress syndrome, the ductus does not close naturally, or re-opens in the first few days of life. If it remains open it is known as patent. An open ductus increases the work of the heart, and this may further worsen the baby's condition. It is sometimes possible to induce the ductus to close using a drug injection, but if the duct remains open, surgery is required. The chest is opened, and the ductus is identified and then tied off. Although this is major surgery it is usually well tolerated, even by tiny babies.

4

INFANCY AND CHILDHOOD

BECOMING A PARENT

The first few days of being a parent, particularly if this is the first baby, are filled with new experiences. It is also a very busy time: the mother is still recovering from the delivery, the baby needs feeding and looking after, there are midwives and ward staff to talk to, and probably lots of visitors to be seen. In the

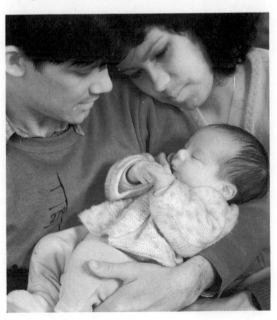

midst of this activity parents have to start to learn how to look after their new baby. Inexperienced or worried parents should always seek support and help from others. Caring for a baby is a skill which has to be learnt, and advice from someone trusted can be invaluable, whether it is supplied by a friend or neighbour, a member of the family or a health care professional.

In the post-partum period (the first few days after birth) doctor, midwife, nurses and breast feeding counsellors are available for practical advice and, because they also have a lot of experience of the feelings and anxieties of new parents, they will be able to help if anything is worrying you. Beyond the newborn period the family doctor, health visitor, child health clinic or well baby clinic can all provide support. Some couples are reluctant to consult them, as they feel that they should work everything out for themselves, or that seeking help is a sign of weakness, but an essential part of being a good parent is knowing when to ask for advice.

What becoming a parent actually means cannot be fully foreseen and, as all babies are different, the experience is unique each time. Parents have to come to terms with the realization that they are responsible for this totally dependent new person who needs continuous care. It is usually some months before they adjust and feel relaxed and confident in their new role.

The relationship between father and mother is also different after the baby arrives, and a new and mutually satisfactory arrangement has to be worked out. This is a time of great emotion, with high peaks and many troughs. Both parents are likely to feel stressed and may also feel guilty that at times their feelings towards the baby are not as positive as they had expected.

One is brought up with the concept that parents naturally love their child, starting from the instant the baby is born. Love is not an instant emotion, however, but something that grows gradually as two people get to know each other. Each person invokes changes in the other, and the bond between them grows and strengthens with time. It is therefore not surprising that there will be occasions when parents do not feel affection for their baby. This is not something to feel guilty about, nor an indication of being a poor mother or father.

During this period of readjustment it is important that parents try to support each other and communicate their feelings, remembering to share the positive as well as the negative.

Being a good parent

Being a satisfactory parent requires a caring manner, commitment, some knowledge of children's various needs, and a range of parenting skills. There are lots of right ways to be a good parent and everyone does it differently.

For some women motherhood is totally engrossing and highly rewarding; caring for and bringing up children gives them complete fulfilment, and they have no wish to work outside the home. Their career is being a mother and they are usually excellent at it. Similarly, some fathers are absolutely committed to caring for their family.

Few people are so wholly absorbed by their children, however. A couple need some time alone away from the family, the mother wants to work outside the home, or one or both parents wish to follow a sport or hobby. Provided they do not provoke conflict within the family, and the children's essential needs for love, caring, communication, stimulation and support continue to be met, such activities outside the home are to be encouraged.

A mother who goes out to work should not feel guilty, provided she has made fully adequate arrangements for her children to be looked after. For a child, having fulfilled and contented parents is more important than having them within earshot twenty-four hours a day. At times of illness or family crisis children will require more attention from their parents, and appropriate plans must be made for this.

Being a parent is not competitive. While some people are clearly in the 'Supermum' or 'Superdad' class, what is more important is that both parents make sure they come into the 'good enough' class, good enough every day, and rising to 'excellent' when needed.

WHERE TO GO FOR ASSISTANCE

There is a network of services available to help with your child's health needs. Foremost is your family doctor, who is there for consulting about any illnesses your child develops, or worries you may have about such things as weight gain, growth or development. The family doctor can also advise on any specialized medical services.

You will also have a health visitor who may be based in the surgery or health centre with your family doctor, or in the child health clinic. Wherever she is based, she will make visits to your home to see how you are getting on. Health visitors do most of their work with babies and small children, but will remain in contact, and can be called on if needed, until children are 5 years old.

Child health clinics are run by the community health services of the local health authority. They are staffed by health visitors, specially trained community medical officers or community paediatricians, and support staff. The clinic provides a readily accessible resource centre for babies and children. Its functions include:

Choosing a family doctor

When children are small they are going to have to visit the doctor frequently, both for routine developmental checks, for immunizations, for treatment of illness and if you are worried about their progress. While all family doctors look after children, some have a special interest and training in child care. Such doctors are likely to organize well baby clinics in their practice, rather than sending parents to see the staff at the child health clinic.

It is important that you feel confident of your doctor's skills with and attitudes to children. If you are worried about your children's health you will need to be reassured that everything necessary has been done for them. If you do not feel happy with your doctor's manner, both with children and with you as a parent, it is better to arrange to see someone else.

- Weighing and measuring babies
- Advising on any problems
- Selling baby foods
- Arranging regular developmental checks
- Arranging vision and hearing tests
- Referring for specialist opinions.

If you need help with housing, finance or other problems, or want nursery provision for your child, the social services may be able to help. There will be an office near you, and you can make an appointment to go and see someone to discuss your problem.

There are also various voluntary groups which you may find helpful. These will vary with locality, but are likely to include organizations to help with establishing and maintaining breast feeding, to provide a meeting place for young mothers, to set up play-groups, or perform other useful and beneficial functions.

FEEDING

Milk is the natural food for babies and provides all the essential nutrients until infants reach about 6 months. If the baby is breast fed, drops containing vitamins A, B, C and D are recommended in case the mother's milk is vitamin deficient. Commercial baby formulae all have vitamins added in adequate amounts.

Very few infants need introducing to solids before 3 months, and it is usually unwise to make the attempt. Babies are too young to be able to chew solids, and at this age they are reluctant to experiment with new flavours and textures. Solid foods contain calories in a very concentrated form, and babies introduced to them early may well become overweight. Furthermore, the body's immune system is not fully developed in the first few months, and eating a lot of different foods may predispose to allergies.

Most babies should start mixed feeding by the age of 5 or 6 months. Beyond 6 months milk alone does not provide enough iron and other nutrients for the baby's needs. Mixed feeding has to be introduced gradually, and parents need to be prepared for the first offerings to be spat out. To start with, most parents only provide solids once daily, often at the midday feed.

The choice of first weaning food is wide. Probably best is a small amount of puréed vegetable or fruit prepared at home without added salt or sugar. Alternatively there are cereals such as powdered rice, and a whole range of commercially available weaning foods. Wheat-containing cereals are used less frequently than formerly because they contain gluten. The majority of children tolerate gluten with no problems at all, but a few children with a rare condition called coeliac disease (see page 252) develop symptoms earlier if they are fed gluten-containing foods in infancy.

As more solids are added to the diet, milk intake will be reduced and the pattern of feed times will gradually change to three meals a day with drinks in between. The foods eaten will also be increasingly varied and puréed food will be replaced by more solid types as the baby develops teeth and learns to chew.

There is no need to stop breast or bottle feeding just because a baby has been weaned, and many mothers enjoy continuing with a breast feed at least once a day up until about 1 year. For the formula-fed baby, the change to pasteurized cow's milk can take place at any time between 6 months and a year. Children should be given whole milk, not skimmed or semi-skimmed which do not contain enough

calories; milk remains an important source of protein and calcium throughout early childhood. Cow's milk, unlike formula infant milks, is not a good source of vitamin D, and all children should be on vitamin drops in the recommended dose from the time of stopping formulae until at least the age of 2 years.

GROWTH IN INFANCY

In the first few days after birth babies lose a little weight, but thereafter gain weight and grow. In the average baby, birth weight is regained by around 8 days; the baby is double her birth weight by about 5 months, and treble her birth weight by the age of 1 year. Growth in length also proceeds rapidly. In the first year the baby's length increases by

Below left: Normal range of supine length in girls and boys between birth and the age of 2 years.

Below right: Normal range of weight in boys and girls between birth and the age of 2 years.

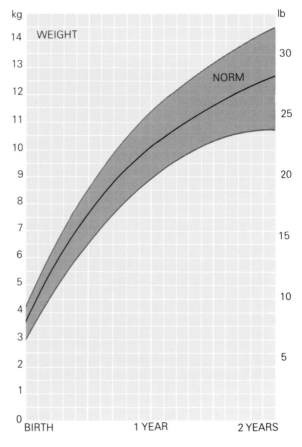

are best interpreted by plotting them on growth charts.

Growth charts are derived from the study of large numbers of normal babies, and give a range of normality against which other babies can be compared. The charts are designed so that the upper and lower figures at any age represent the limits within which about 94 per cent of normal children will fall. Three per cent of normals will be below the lower point, and 3 per cent above the upper point. While children may be below the lower point and still be normal, it is more common to find something interfering with growth, and the doctor should review such children to make sure there is nothing requiring treatment.

The charts can be used for a single measurement of weight or length, but they are more informative used with a series of measurements. This enables the rate of growth to be assessed. If the measurements show a rate of growth parallel to the lines on the chart, the rate is normal. If the rate is slower, it requires assessment and the doctor should be consulted; if it is faster, it may either suggest catch-up growth, or be an early indication that the baby is too fat.

Although birth is marked, the chart extends before birth and starts at thirty-two weeks' gestation. For babies born prematurely it is more meaningful to relate growth to gestational age than to actual day of birth. For a baby born six weeks early, six weeks should be deducted from her actual age before plotting her growth measurements on the chart. This correction is only really necessary in the first year: growth charts for children over 1 start at birth and actual age is plotted.

You can use the charts opposite to gauge how your baby is growing. The child health clinic or your doctor is likely to employ similar ones.

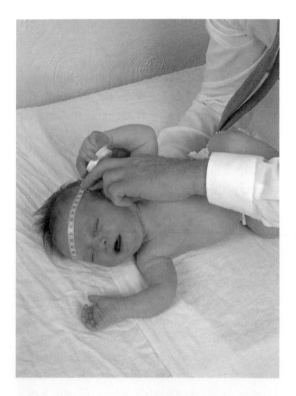

Measuring head circumference is one of the three factors needed to assess growth accurately, the other two being length and weight.

about 50 per cent and head, body and limbs all increase proportionately.

While talking about the average baby gives some idea of the rate at which growth occurs, of more practical value is knowing the range of normality for individual babies. Babies are born at different weights, at different stages of maturity, to parents of different heights. All of these factors are going to influence how a baby grows in the first year. Breast fed babies tend to gain weight at a slightly slower rate than bottle fed ones.

Growth in the first year is most commonly assessed by considering weight and rate of weight gain because weighing is easy; other measurements, such as length or head circumference, are more difficult to do accurately. To assess growth fully, however, all three should be measured. Once the baby has been weighed and measured, the results

Poor weight gain

Weighing a baby regularly in the first few months of life provides a useful check on how she is progressing. Over this period weight gain is usually rapid. Measurements must be accurate, and should preferably be taken on the same scales, as differences of only a few ounces cause confusion. Weighings should not be too frequent: although the trend in infancy should be a steady weight increase, there is often variation from week to week. Furthermore, weight will depend on how long it is since the last feed, and on the state of bladder and bowels. Some weeks there is little or no weight gain, and other weeks the gain is greater than average. Unnecessary anxiety can arise from frequent weighing if too much attention is paid to temporary hesitations.

If your baby is gaining weight poorly you should discuss this with your health visitor or doctor who will want to know about feeding and whether you and the baby are healthy. The first consideration will be whether the baby is getting enough milk. How well is the baby sucking? How frequent are the feeds? Does there seem to be enough milk in the breast? What quantity of milk is being taken? All babies regurgitate a small amount after feeds, and this is known as possetting. However, if the baby vomits significant quantities after a feed and is not gaining weight well, this will require investigation. Some babies on formula feeds are overfed, and they may vomit after meals also, but they continue to gain weight at a normal or increased rate.

In babies who are gaining weight rather slowly because they are inherently small individuals, growth in length and head circumference will be equally depressed. Alternatively, if there is inadequate calorie consumption, whether because of low milk intake or disease, growth of the head usually continues at a normal or near-normal rate. Brain growth is protected even if growth of other parts is slowed.

When a breast fed baby does not seem to be gaining weight as well as she should, the mother is likely to be anxious as to whether she has enough milk. Provided breast feeding has been well established, and the mother is healthy and eating adequately, it is unlikely that the supply is deficient in the early weeks of life. It is a pity to transfer the baby to the bottle on the assumption that poor weight gain is due to inadequate supply unless this is definitely the cause.

Apart from the above, there are other causes of failing to gain weight and thrive in infancy and the doctor will carry out an examination to see if a baby has any abnormalities. She may simply have developed an infection, which interferes with appetite. This is easily noticeable when a baby has a cold with a runny nose – sucking is difficult and little feed is taken – but other infections may not be so obvious. Urinary tract infections in babies are relatively common and do not usually produce very obvious signs; a urine specimen should be checked for infection if poor weight gain persists.

Poor weight gain may be due not only to physical factors, but also to emotional problems within the family. Even very young babies are sensitive to tensions, and in families where there are difficulties the baby may miss out on love and stimulation, which are as necessary for growth as adequate food intake.

Postnatal depression in mothers is very common, at least in minor degree. A mother who is feeling wretched and apathetic may not be able to respond and interact with her baby properly, and this may cause the baby to lose interest in feeding. Maternal insecurity, where the mother feels isolated and unsupported, may have a similar effect. Persistent tensions and disharmony between parents, or between parents and neighbours or in-laws, also destroy the secure, relaxed atmosphere the baby needs. Obviously the occasional family row is not going to have any lasting effect, but babies cannot develop fully unless brought up in a caring way by parents responsive to their physical and emotional needs.

Poor weight gain precipitated by adverse social factors, or emotional or relationship problems, needs to be tackled and solved just as much as physical illness. It is likely your doctor or health visitor can help or else will put you in touch with someone who can. Alternatively, seeing a social worker may be useful. Even seeking help and sharing the problem is likely to improve matters although the difficulties may take some time to resolve.

DEVELOPING NEW SKILLS

As well as growing in length and weight, babies are continually developing and acquiring new skills and abilities. Many of these achievements are common to all children: learning to fix vision on an object, to follow with the eyes, to turn the head, to sit and to crawl, to vocalize and to acquire language. The way many of these skills evolve, however, is not just determined by a child's innate genetic make-up, but is influenced by her interactions with those around, particularly parents. This is obvious when one considers something like learning how to talk, but it applies equally to many other areas of development.

Parental stimulation provides a child with a good start in life, but encouragement has to

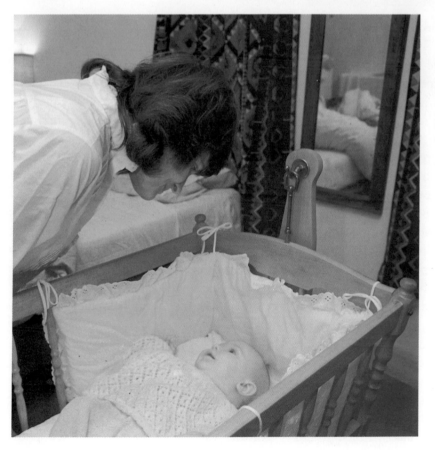

Babies begin to interact with those around them at a very early age. By two months, for example, most babies will have established eye contact and be able to follow movement. Parents can stimulate this awareness by responding to it positively.

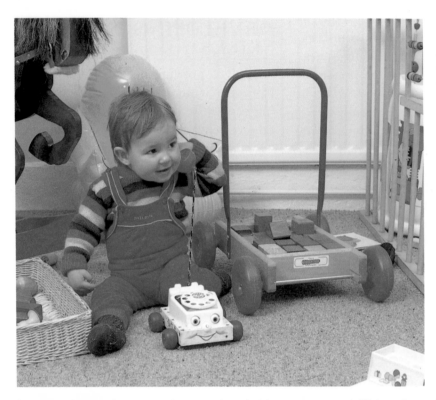

Playing with toys appropriate to their age enables children to practise the developmental skills that they are gradually acquiring.

be sensitive and appropriate to the child's developmental stage. In acquiring any new ability there are three phases: the first time something is done, repeating the action many times until it becomes familiar and more competent, and then the stage when an action can be carried out in a skilled and relaxed way. Parents take great pleasure in their child's new skills, and part of their contribution lies in the repeated rehearsals of each stage until an action is performed so smoothly that it becomes automatic.

For descriptive purposes, development in infancy is often considered in separate categories: motor abilities, vision and fine movement, social and emotional development, and hearing and speech. This division is helpful in discussing how development takes place and the stages it goes through, but it is important to realize that these various aspects all interact. Obviously the development of language is influenced by social and emotional factors as well as by hearing, and

motor abilities depend to some extent on having adequate vision.

The harmony of development is individual for everyone; every ability the child acquires fits together and makes her the person she is at any given time. It is important for parents to recognize this harmony at every stage of childhood. No one activity should be pursued to the detriment of other aspects which are vital to the development of the person as a whole.

The table opposite summarizes some of the developmental stages that a child passes through during the first two years. The ages at which each child masters a skill will vary; those in the table are approximate averages – that is, when about half of a group of children of a particular age have that ability. It follows that many normal children will not have reached a given stage by the age shown. Furthermore, because all children are different, the sequence of acquiring new abilities varies; this is more marked as the

Development Chart

MONTH	MOTOR SKILLS	SOCIAL SKILLS	HEARING AND SPEECH	VISION AND FINE MOVEMENT
1	Holds head erect for a few seconds	Is quieted when picked up	Startled by sounds	Follows light with eyes
2	Holds head up when face downwards	Smiles	Listens to bell or rattle	Follows object up, down and sideways
3	Kicks well	Follows person with eyes	Searches for sound with eyes	Glances from one object to another
4	Lifts head and chest when face down	Returns a stranger's smile	Laughs	Clasps and retains cube
5	Holds head erect with no lag	Frolics when played with	Turns head to sound	Pulls paper away from face
6	Rises on to wrists	Turns head to person talking	Babbles and coos to voice or music	Takes cube from table
7	Rolls from front to back	Drinks from a cup	Makes four different sounds	Looks for fallen object
8	Tries to crawl vigorously	Looks at herself in mirror	Shouts for attention	Passes toy from hand to hand
9	Turns around on floor	Helps to hold cup for drinking	Says 'mama' or 'dada'	Manipulates two objects at once
10	Stands when held up	Smiles in mirror	Listens to watch	Clicks two bricks
11	Pulls up to stand	Feeds with fingers	Can use two words	Makes a pincer grip
12	Walks or side-steps around play pen	Plays pat-a-cake	Can use three words with meaning	Retains three cubes
13	Stands alone	Holds cup	Looks at pictures	Favours one hand
14	Walks alone	Uses spoon	Knows own name	Holds four cubes
15	Climbs upstairs	Can point to shoes	Uses four to five clear words	Places one object upon another
16	Pushes pram, toys, and so on	Tries to turn doorknob	Uses six to seven clear words	Scribbles freely
17	Climbs on to chair	Manages cup well	Babbled talk	Pulls cloth to get toy
18	Walks backwards	Takes off shoes and socks	Enjoys pictures in book	Constructive play with toys
19	Climbs up and down the stairs	Knows one part of body	Uses nine words	Makes a tower of three bricks
20	Jumps	Bowel control	Uses twelve words	", of four bricks
21	Runs	Bladder control by day	Makes two-word sentences	Circular scribble
22	Walks upstairs	Tries to tell of experiences	Listens to stories	Makes a tower of five or more bricks
23	Seats herself at table	Knows two parts of body	Uses twenty words or more	Copies vertical strokes
24	Walks up and down the stairs	Knows four parts of body	Can name four toys	Copies horizontal stroke

child gets older and the number of skills and abilities increases.

Motor development

At the time of birth a baby is able to move all her limbs, will grasp a finger put in her palm (the grasp reflex) and can turn her head to one side if placed face downwards. She does not have enough muscle strength or control to support her head if she is lifted up, and parents have to learn to provide that support when handling her. Various reflexes are present, and these form a basis for future development.

Another important reflex present in small children is the so-called rooting reflex, which operates when the cheek is touched. The head turns so the mouth is directed towards the touch. The ability of babies to find the nipple with their mouths if they become detached initially depends on this. The rooting reflex too gradually becomes less marked, as with increased awareness and control the infant performs the act voluntarily. The newborn baby also has the ability to suck if something is put in her mouth, and to stretch out her arms and legs and give a cry if startled.

Some basic reflexes take time to develop, and such things as co-ordination and the maintenance of posture depend on reflexes which gradually evolve as the nervous system matures. Because many stages of motor development cannot be reached until the nervous system has developed the requisite control, parental stimulation of the child should be directed towards encouraging the practice of already acquired motor skills rather than trying to make the child acquire new ones.

Control of the head develops gradually. By about 6 weeks a child will probably be able to hold her head in line with her body for a short time if she is lifted up in the prone (face downwards) position. By 8 weeks she is

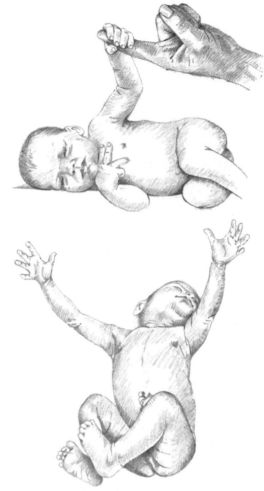

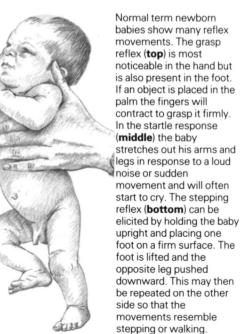

Normal term newborn babies show many reflex movements. The grasp reflex (**top**) is most noticeable in the hand but is also present in the foot. If an object is placed in the palm the fingers will contract to grasp it firmly. In the startle response (**middle**) the baby stretches out his arms and legs in response to a loud noise or sudden movement and will often start to cry. The stepping reflex (**bottom**) can be elicited by holding the baby upright and placing one foot on a firm surface. The foot is lifted and the opposite leg pushed downward. This may then be repeated on the other side so that the movements resemble stepping or walking.

likely to be able to raise her head slightly if lifted prone, and by 4 months will raise her head well. Holding the head steady when lifted in the supine (face upwards) position is possible by about 3 months, although the head will still be a bit wobbly if the child is moved suddenly.

Head control is essential before many other movements can be mastered. Lying on her tummy, the baby who can lift her head up soon learns to kick her legs, and by about 6 months will support herself on her hands. By about 7 months she can roll over from her front to her back. Soon the arms are co-ordinated and can be used in a reciprocal manner, and the body may be pulled forward in a commando crawl, with the legs trailing. Some babies push themselves backwards rather than forwards. Within a short time the ability to bring the knees up develops, and at around 9 months true crawling starts. Before long the child is pulling herself upright by holding on to cot-side or furniture, soon moves around in the upright position holding on to the furniture, and then, as co-ordination and balance improve, is able to stand unsupported for a few seconds. The average age for reaching this stage is around 13 months, and within another month the child takes her first steps.

Development is a gradual and continuing process but when some skills are acquired the change is marked: smiling, crawling, sitting, pulling up to stand, and walking, for example. In assessing child development the ages at which such changes occur are used as reference points, so they have become known as developmental milestones.

The skill of sitting up unsupported is acquired at around 8 months. For a couple of months before this the baby will enjoy sitting propped up so that she can look about. True sitting requires a fairly straight back. When newborn babies are at rest their backs are curved, as they were in the womb. Their spines straighten as they lie on their backs, but in the first few months of life they are not strong enough to support their weight in an upright position.

If baby seats or buggies are used for children under 6 months the child should not sit upright, but at an angle of about 45 degrees, and the curve of the spine should be supported. Slings for carrying small babies close to the mother's or father's chest are designed so that the spine is well supported in the sling.

Sitting unsupported opens up new opportunities to the baby. She can look around and will reach out to pick up close objects, most of which are put into her mouth. It is not long before the desire to pick up out-of-reach objects stimulates mobility; the baby will try either turning into a crawling position, shuffling along on her bottom, using her legs and hands to make progress, or lying down and rolling over and over to get nearer to her goal.

As strength and co-ordination improve the baby gradually progresses through a developmental sequence of movement which starts from prone lying, then crawling, next pulling up to stand, followed by cruising around holding on to the furniture, then standing alone, and finally walking unaided. Although this is the commonest sequence, it is not the only one.

About 10 per cent of normal babies never go through a crawling stage, but follow a different sequence of motor development. Instead of crawling, these children get about in a sitting position. Developmental paediatricians therefore call them 'bottom-shufflers'. This pattern of development is often familial, and grandparents may be able to recall that a parent followed the same sequence. Such babies can often be identified early, as they dislike lying on their tummies

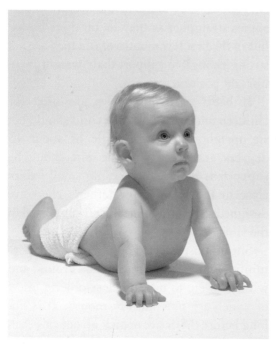

By the age of 6 months a baby should be able to push up with the wrists. He or she will try to crawl at 8 months, but true crawling does not begin until about a month later.

motor ability is being acquired, the child is also learning how to make fine movements and how to hold and manipulate objects.

Trying to separate the acquisition of these skills from the development of vision is somewhat artificial. Whereas a non-seeing child, with no other handicap, will not be much delayed in learning to sit and to stand, fine hand movements will almost certainly be delayed.

Vision and fine movement

Within the first week of life babies fix their eyes on faces that come near their own. By 1 month they will follow with their eyes a face that moves across their field of vision. At this stage not all the nerve cells of the visual system in the brain have developed, and the image perceived by the baby is not detailed. Visual acuity, the ability to perceive fine detail, does not reach adult standard until about the age of 2 years. By 3 months the baby uses her eyes to follow moving objects in all directions, and will be able to glance from one thing to another.

The hands start to be used for reaching out and grasping at around 3 months and by 4 months a child can hold a small wooden brick or other object. At this stage the two hands do not work together. By 6 months the baby can pick up a brick, by 8 months she is passing it from hand to hand, and by 9 months can cope with an object in each hand. At this stage the palm and all the fingers are used together, but initially the action of picking up is not very controlled; the child tends to sweep her hand round until it comes to an object, and then grasp it with the edge of the palm. The child watches the hand to control its movement, and gradually learns to reach out directly to what she wants. By about 1 year she has progressed to using the thumb and forefinger for picking up, and has good fine control.

As well as developing fine motor control,

and become very distressed if put face downwards. When awake they prefer to lie on their backs, in which position they take an interest in what is going on around them and often start to develop communication skills early. They are reluctant to take weight on their feet, and usually learn to sit unsupported at around 10 months. Although this is later than for most babies, it is normal for bottom-shufflers and does not represent developmental delay. Once they can sit unsupported, these children learn a way of progressing in this position, sometimes using both legs, sometimes only one, to propel themselves. Bottom-shufflers are often later than crawlers to stand alone and walk, the average age of starting to walk being around 16 or 17 months.

The development of mobility in the child, which requires control of many of the major muscles of the body, has been briefly considered. At the same time that this gross

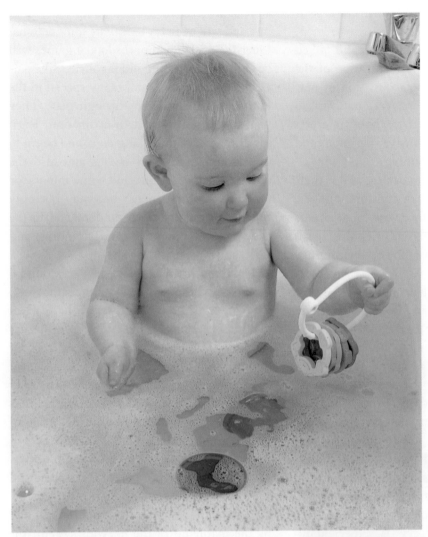

Left: Vision and fine movement are closely linked developmental factors in the early stages of childhood. A baby aged 9 months will use his palm and fingers to pick up an object and will watch his hand to control his movements.

Below: Self-awareness and the ability of the child to make sense of his environment grow rapidly from about the age of 1 year.

the child is also learning about the nature of the world. Before 6 months only objects within the visual field hold the attention. By about 7 months a child will look for a toy that falls off the edge of the table. By 1 year she will look for and find a toy that she sees being hidden, perhaps covered by a cup. The child progresses from being an observer, to understanding that objects have an existence even when not visualized, to starting to control the environment.

Social development

From birth babies are socially responsive. With the very premature baby response is

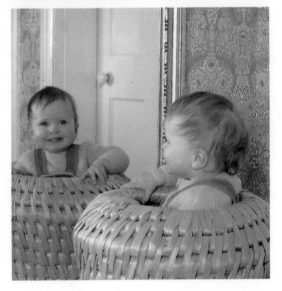

limited, but the baby born at term can cry for attention when uncomfortable or distressed, and quietens on being picked up and talked to. Although the gradual maturation of the brain plays a part in the acquisition of new social skills, these, by their very nature, can only develop properly if the baby interacts with caring and responsive parents, and others in the family grouping.

Crying is very basic to babies, as it is their way of expressing pain, discomfort, hunger, anger and distress. Before very long parents can often identify different cries that mean specific things; these are the very beginnings of language.

The sound of a baby's cry is almost impossible to ignore, and if it lasts for more than a minute it is best to respond. Leaving a baby crying is distressing to the caring adult, and although having to attend to the baby may be inconvenient, she needs to be made comfortable or picked up. The baby who repeatedly starts to cry again after being settled down causes great stress for the parent, and it may be difficult to avoid anger. However, parents must realize that the baby is in pain or unhappy, has only one way to express this, and does not want to be alone. A baby that is left to cry is experiencing rejection. If this happens once or twice it will not have any lasting effect but, if often repeated, it could interfere with social interaction.

The first smile is seen between 3 and 6 weeks in most babies. At first, smiling is an expression of pleasure, but is not directed at anyone in particular. Within a few more weeks the infant interacts and learns to return the smile of a parent or other person. By 5 months the baby takes pleasure in frolicking games that involve talking, laughing and being picked up and joggled gently. Before long she joins in the laughter.

At about 6 months of age the baby shows a lot of interest in what is going on around her, and will even try to imitate some actions. Over the next few months lots of games will be enjoyed, including old favourites like pat-a-cake and peep-bo, and many special to the family. Children learn through play. They gain motor ability and co-ordination, learn social interaction and language, and begin to understand their own bodies and also the outside world. To the adult some infants' or toddlers' games may become boringly repetitive, but they are fundamental to the child's development of understanding and skills appropriate to her age.

Drinking from a cup is learnt at around 6 months, and chewing at about the same time. By 9 months a child will try to help when drinking by holding the cup, and by 1 year she will be feeding herself with a rusk or biscuit, even if in rather a messy fashion.

Developmental changes in the first year result in the transformation of the helpless newborn baby into a child on the verge of walking and talking, with all that entails in the acquisition of new skills and understanding. Although much of the pattern and timing of development is determined by growth, by increased physical strength, and by the maturing of the nervous system, the quality of parenting that a child receives determines whether each stage reaches its full potential. Having someone who loves and cares, stimulates and takes an interest, talks and plays, forms a sound foundation for later development as a whole, but particularly for emotional, social and language progress.

Hearing and speech

The newborn reacts to loud sounds with a startle response, throwing out the arms and legs, and often starting to cry. By 2 months the baby is aware of soft noises; if crying, she will often become quiet and still at the sound of a voice and will listen to a bell or soft

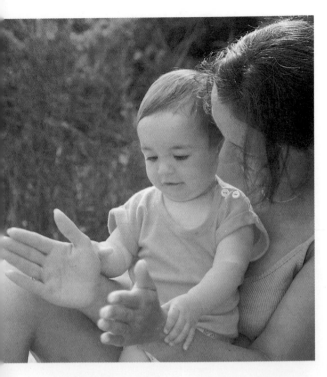

Games are very important in helping children to learn. Clapping helps to teach rhythm and coordination while both parent and child are enjoying themselves.

rattle. By 3 months she will try to find the source of a sound with her eyes. If a baby has a serious hearing problem parents will usually be aware of it by 2 months and should seek expert advice by asking the clinic or their doctor to refer them to a specialist.

Babies will turn their heads towards sounds at around 5 months or so, and babbling and cooing to music or voices follow soon after. With appropriate cues from an adult the baby learns in babbling the concept of turn-taking: each person responds to the other and takes it in turns to vocalize and then to listen. This is another of the fundamentals of language and speech. Being able to make different sounds is another basic, and by about 7 months most children have four or five noises in their repertoire.

By about 8 months most children understand 'no' and 'bye-bye', and they are likely to say their first word, usually 'mama' or 'dada', during the ninth or tenth month, although not always using it appropriately. By 1 year two or three words are likely to be used with meaning. Thereafter, understanding of the spoken word grows apace, as does vocabulary.

The development of language is much more fundamental than just knowing the names that are applied to various objects. Before a child can understand the concepts of speech — like joining words together, and using different types of words such as nouns, verbs and adjectives — she must grasp the more basic aspects of reality. Knowing oneself to be an individual and that other people also are individuals is crucial. There is a need to investigate the form and function of one's body, and to discover the immediate environment, how it is organized and how it changes. Without such basic understanding words cannot be joined together in any meaningful way.

Once again the inter-relationship of different aspects of development is involved. Language is dependent on the mastering of gross motor skills to enable exploration of the environment, on vision to comprehend surrounding objects, on social interaction, and on manipulative skills to investigate both one's own body and the world around. Each phase of learning is built on the foundation of previous stages.

Learning also depends on help from those around, and the provision of a secure and loving home is the most important requirement. The child who feels frightened or unwanted will not learn effectively, and her future personality may be damaged. The more that parents can positively interact with a child, the more that child's development will be fostered. Whether at play, on outings or during the daily routine, talking to the child, pointing out objects and happenings, and encouraging various activities all help, and the experience brings rich rewards to both parent and child.

GROWTH IN LATER CHILDHOOD

During the last few weeks of pregnancy the growth of the fetus is very rapid, more so than at any other time of life. Rapid growth continues in the first year (see the charts on page 48), the birth weight trebling and the length increasing by around 25 per cent.

Although growth is most often measured by considering the changes in weight and height, all parts of the body are involved. During the second year the rate of weight and height gain is also rapid, but somewhat slower than in the first year.

Growth from 2 years

From the second birthday until the onset of puberty, the average increase in height each year is about 5-6cm (2-2½in), the rate lessening slightly in each successive year.

The measurement of weight in children is relatively simple if reliable scales are available, but it must be realized that weight varies even during the same day, depending on what has been eaten or drunk, and whether the bladder and bowels are full or empty. It is best not to weigh children too often, or the fluctuations in weight from day to day may give an erroneous impression.

Measurement of height is more difficult,

Below left: The average height gain in boys and girls aged between 2 and 16 years.

Below right: The average weight gain in boys and girls aged between 2 and 16 years.

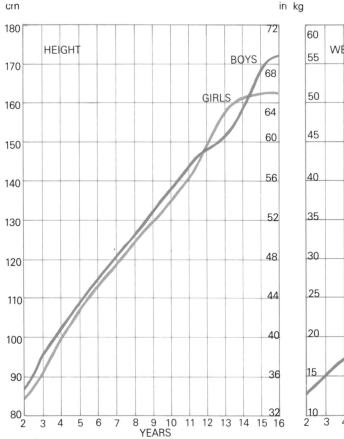

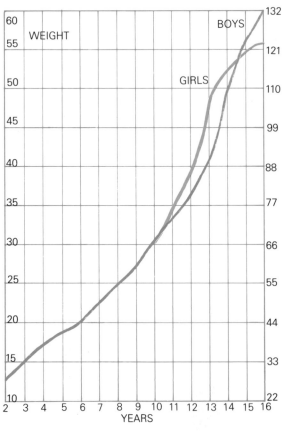

particularly in small children who find it hard to keep still. Until the age of around 2 years children are best measured lying down on a rigid surface with one person holding the head steady and another holding the feet. This gives a length measurement. Over the age of 2 height is measured with the child standing up against a rigid surface.

In any group of normal children of the same age there will be variations in height and weight. Growth charts (see preceding page) can be used to help in determining whether or not growth is normal.

The rate of growth is as important in assessing the child's progress as the actual measurements of height and weight. This rate of growth can be expressed as the number of centimetres or inches grown in a year if measurements are available. If the rate of growth is within the normal range for that age, even if the child is excessively short or tall, there is not a current problem with growth; the child's position on the growth chart is explained by earlier events. For example, a child who had a period of growth retardation *in utero* and was born small may continue to be small after birth. While many such children will show catch-up growth and will attain normal height and weight for age, some will remain smaller than their peers. Nevertheless, if the rate of growth is normal after birth, even though height and weight are below normal, there is no problem.

The relative proportions of different parts of the body change during childhood. The newborn has a relatively large head, and less well grown legs; in later childhood the trunk and legs lengthen in proportion to the head and arms. Individual parts of the body also grow at different rates. The appearance of the face changes. The middle part becomes more prominent because of the growth of the sinuses in the cheeks, and the secondary dentition is much larger than the milk teeth.

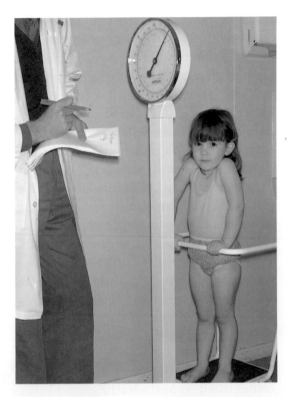

Scales for weighing children must be accurate, and the child should be undressed.

Lymphoid tissue, including the tonsils and adenoids, grows faster than other tissues in the first few years. Conversely there is very little growth in the size of the gonads or genitalia in the first half of childhood, but in later childhood and puberty their growth rate is much faster than the growth of other parts of the body.

Factors affecting growth

For children who are healthy and well nourished, size is mainly determined by genetic factors. If both parents are short the child is likely also to be short; if both are tall, the child is likely to be tall. If one parent is short and the other tall the child may well be of average height. At any given age the child's height will also be influenced by the rate of growth. Some children are early developers, and grow rather more quickly than average. A slow rate of growth may either be inherent in the individual – so-called constitutional slow development – or may be a result of illness or poor nutrition. Delayed growth can be recognized by taking an X-ray to assess the maturity of the bones of the wrist and hand. A bone age can then be calculated to indicate skeletal maturity. If the bone age is significantly behind the chronological age, there has been a delay in growth. Constitutional slow development often runs in families, and parents may remember that they themselves entered puberty later than average, or were always among the smallest in the class at school even if they are now of average height. Any child who is short for her age or is growing slowly should be assessed by the doctor. If there is a problem the cause must be found and, if possible, treated.

Some girls who are very tall may be concerned that their final adult height is likely to be significantly above average. If this is a cause for concern they can be assessed in a growth clinic in mid-childhood; if the predicted final height is excessive it may be possible to stop the action of growth hormone.

COMMON MEDICAL PROBLEMS

Colic

Colicky pains are due to waves of contraction in the muscles of the intestine or other internal organs. The pains are intermittent, building up and persisting for one or two minutes, and then fading, only to recur in a few minutes' time.

In their first few months, some babies seem to have colicky abdominal pains following feeds, particularly after the evening one. They cry and draw their legs up, and this lasts a minute or two, then they gradually calm down, only to have a repeat attack a few minutes later. The episodes of colicky pain may last at least an hour before disappearing.

Getting up the wind and giving gripe water may help, as may rubbing the tummy gently, but more commonly the only thing that gives any relief is a cuddle. Parents should realize that this evening colic is not due to any underlying disease, but is probably related to an immaturity in the regulation of intestinal activity.

If evening colic is severe your doctor may be able to advise, and may give an antispasmodic medicine; also see page 166.

Constipation

Most babies have two or three bowel actions a day. The stool is soft and the baby does not have to strain to pass it. However, some breast fed babies have much less frequent stools, either once a day or even every two days. Provided the stools are soft and the baby does not have to strain there is no need to worry. The breast milk may be so well absorbed that there is little residue to be passed.

Constipation is much more common in bottle fed babies. Stools are infrequent and hard, and the baby has to strain and seems in discomfort. Constipation may be due to underfeeding, and increasing milk intake may help. If it persists, adding a teaspoonful of brown sugar to each feed should ease matters, as may giving a daily drink of orange juice. The sugar should be discontinued as soon as the bowels return to normal.

If the baby is old enough to start weaning, giving a little puréed prunes or other fruit can also help to soften the stools. If, in spite of sugar and fruit, the constipation persists, using milk of magnesia as a laxative may be indicated. It should only be taken for a short period and if the problem continues you should consult your doctor.

The crying baby

As already discussed, babies cry when they are hungry, distressed or in pain. Mothers soon learn to distinguish the different types of crying and know how to respond. Sometimes it is enough to turn the baby over for her to settle, or she will be calm after being fed and changed.

More troublesome is the baby who cries in obvious distress, but without apparent cause. She may stop on being picked up, only to start on being put down again, or may carry on crying even when being cuddled. Parents are likely to feel worried in case there is something wrong with the baby. They may also be on edge themselves because of the incessant crying, because it is impossible either to relax or to get on with other things, and possibly because they are concerned about the noise upsetting the neighbours.

If parents do become anxious or annoyed the baby senses it and reacts by becoming more tense and less likely to relax. As a result, the crying is likely to continue. Whatever the cause, it is important to try to remain calm. If the baby does settle on being cuddled, then it is best not to try to put her down until she is completely relaxed and a bit sleepy. This makes it difficult to do any other tasks, but is preferable to incessant crying. A sling for carrying the baby can be helpful: she will feel secure, and you are better able to get on.

Continued crying may be due to the baby being uncomfortable or in pain. Colic, for example, often causes prolonged crying each evening (see page 62). Some babies have periodic bouts of prolonged crying for which a serious medical problem is seldom responsible. If the baby has been otherwise well until the crying started, it is unlikely to be due to anything serious, particularly if the crying stops shortly after she is picked up and cuddled or rocked. The doctor may need to be consulted if a previously contented baby continues to cry and can not be consoled.

You should ask your doctor or health visitor for advice if your baby has repeated episodes of prolonged crying. If it is getting on top of you and you worry that you might harm the baby, you should say this too. The doctor or health visitor will not be shocked, as it is a common worry, and talking about it can be helpful, since professionals will be able to suggest ways to cope.

Nappy rash (Ammoniacal dermatitis)

Because babies wear nappies urine is often in contact with their skin. Fresh urine causes no harm, but normal skin bacteria may break down the urea it contains to ammonia. You will often notice an ammoniacal smell when you change a nappy that has been on overnight.

Ammonia is irritant to the skin, and causes reddening and inflammation. If mild, the rash is localized around the genitalia and may take the form of discrete spots, but if more severe, redness may extend over the whole nappy area. Although the skin is inflamed, mild nappy rash is not painful, but there may be secondary infection with either bacteria or thrush (see page 29).

Prevention is all-important. It helps to protect the skin with a barrier ointment such as zinc and castor oil cream, applied to the nappy area every time the baby is changed; making sure the baby is changed regularly is also important. If any soreness does develop it will soon heal if the skin is left exposed, so that any urine dries immediately rather than being broken down to ammonia. If it is impossible to leave the area uncovered, liberal amounts of barrier cream should be applied. If the rash is severe or infected consult your doctor, as an antibiotic ointment may be indicated.

CHAPTER

5

EMOTIONAL DEVELOPMENT IN EARLY CHILDHOOD

This chapter will discuss some of the issues that children face when growing up and the coping strategies that they need to acquire to negotiate the different stages of their lives. At the outset it is important to recognize that there is more than just one way to ensure that children develop into emotionally mature adults. This will depend on the family of which they are part, and on the culture, religion and society in which they live. Given the limitations of space, most of this chapter will be related to children and families who have adopted Westernized styles of family life.

FORMING ATTACHMENTS

The scene is set for the emotional development of children long before they are born. Much will depend on the parents' views and expectations for the child, whether he is arriving into a secure adult relationship or has been conceived in an attempt to ensure that the relationship lasts a little longer.

This variation in parental attitude will have a marked effect on the newborn baby and his subsequent attachment to his mother and father, and vice versa. The baby at this time is totally dependent on the person(s) taking care of him for every aspect of his survival. Infants have been shown to respond in various ways and in doing so influence the

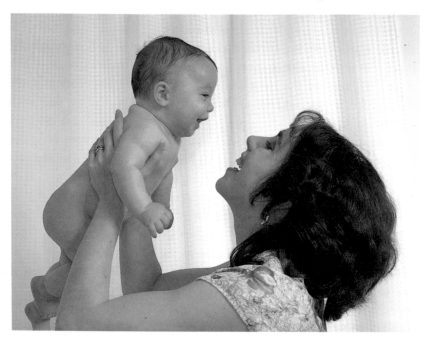

The relationship between parent and child is continuously reinforced by them doing things together and learning different ways to communicate.

behaviour of those who look after them. Researchers in America, for example, have demonstrated that children show various behavioural styles, which can be categorized into 'temperamental' differences. The defining characteristics include:

- activity level
- rhythmicity of biological function (sleeping, eating, and so on)
- adaptability
- approach or withdrawal in new situations
- intensity of emotional reaction (to pleasant and unpleasant situations)
- reactions threshold (the ease with which a child copes with changed circumstances)
- quality of mood
- distractability and attention persistence.

How a child and his care-taker cope with new developments and day-to-day living depends very much on the interaction between the child's behavioural style and the parents' own temperaments, expectations, and experiences of being parented. The match between the styles of parents and children is important: it should be considerably easier, for example, for a parent who is active and quick by temperament to cope with a child who also fits into this model, rather than with a child who sleeps for long periods and only wakes for meals. In turn, the child could find his parents' constant attempts at waking him difficult to tolerate, with the result that both parties will be fretful and potentially have a less rewarding, emotionally unstable relationship.

A common problem for mothers before or after the birth of their baby can be depression or feeling emotionally low. Many women have transient feelings of depression in the week or two following the birth. Around 10–20 per cent of women experience more severe depression which may last one or two years, and a smaller number – 1 per cent – experience severe mental illness. The situation can be made worse if partners are unsupportive or fail to take on some of the demands of child care. Sleepless nights and worry often do not help. Depression can cause a usually active, well-organized individual to feel totally out of her depth, and to experience an overwhelming sense of failure that she has let down not only herself but also the baby, as she cannot function competently. Depression can also emphasize a difference in behavioural and temperamental styles between a parent and child.

It is common for too much emphasis to be placed on these early moments as far as establishing attachment and bonding is concerned. Research has demonstrated that before 6 months, babies do not show a specific preference for particular people, and will not show distress if they are left with someone other than a natural parent as long as they are well cared for. By about 6 months most babies will have established attachments with the people who take care of them, and this shows in their behaviour: babies seek to be close to their care-takers and become distressed by their absence. They will seek them out for comfort, show confidence in their presence, and enjoy new situations without being unduly fearful.

Shortly after developing attachments, children of about 7 months become increasingly wary of strangers, who find it considerably more difficult to comfort them; this suggests that infants are sensitive to unaccustomed appearances and behaviour and to the difference between familiar and unfamiliar people.

Attachment is developed not just by parents spending considerable amounts of time with a child but, more importantly, by the quality of time spent together. Babies are thought to become attached to people who are sensitive to their individual needs and therefore do not over- or understimulate them, but rather ensure that the infant takes part in satisfying social interactions. Not surprisingly, this means that a child could become attached to a number of people who fulfil his needs, and not necessarily only to those who ensure that his physical needs are met. The attachment could be to a grandparent, a nanny or any one of the baby's care-takers.

A few years ago it was believed that if children did not become 'attached' during infancy they would develop a myriad of emotional difficulties, being insecure and unable to maintain relationships in adult life. There is, however, no evidence to suggest that what happens in the first few hours or days of life is crucial to later development. Relationships between care-taker and child develop over time and in various places, and any disturbances that do occur have the potential to be rectified. If the child receives no emotional help from his parents, then he could grow up with a variety of personality problems. Some children who have protracted periods of unsatisfactory care, because of physical or emotional abuse, can be reluctant to trust adults and to form relationships both with other adults and with children. However, if these children are provided with positive experiences of parenting and trustworthy relationships, the early deficit can be compensated for.

Attachment to siblings

Most children look forward to the birth of a new brother or sister eagerly, and are greatly excited when they first see the baby. This period of anticipation and excitement is followed by a time in which the family routine changes and many activities become centred around the baby. This can be a difficult period for an older child. Familiar routines are disrupted, the baby seems to receive maximum attention, and older brothers and sisters may perceive that they are out of favour with their parents and feel insecure.

An insecure child may become demanding and attention-seeking, and parents may find this difficult to cope with, on top of looking after the new baby. It is important that time is found for older children in the family as well as for the new baby in the first few weeks after the birth. Involving an older child in aspects of baby care such as bathing and changing can be useful. It is even more important for parents to find plenty of time to talk individually with their other children not only about the baby but also about their own activities, and to listen properly and share their thoughts and feelings.

The sibling may initially feel threatened by, as well as interested in, the baby, but with familiarity and reassurance the newcomer will be accepted. Strong relationships will develop between all the children in the family, and although rivalry and competitiveness may occasionally feature, brothers and sisters usually become very close and mutually caring.

STIMULATION

All children need to be provided with stimulation appropriate to their age, and to have a wide range of experiences. This has been found to be an important element in determining a child's intellectual and language development. In essence this means providing a child with sufficient parental contact. As with attachment, this need not necessarily be for hours at a time but should be of a high quality: there should be time to talk and play in a manner appropriate to the child's age.

Most children are adequately stimulated; these tend to be the ones who are loved and wanted, but not necessarily so. A child can be loved but if a parent has his or her own

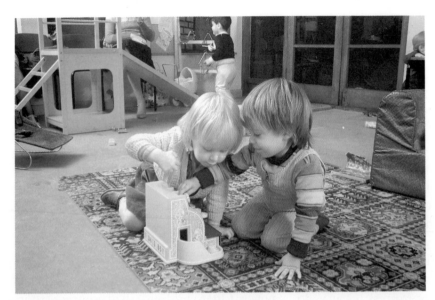

The development of social skills begins during the toddler period when cooperation with others of the same age occurs through play. Toddler groups such as this one provide ample opportunity for this necessary part of the socialization process.

problems, the child's needs may not be met. Alternatively, parents can be very young and may simply not know what is required of them, being inadvertently neglectful as a result. Lack of personal contact and play can result in a child failing to develop speech and language skills, as well as becoming emotionally detached.

In the early stages of neglect a child may attempt to form rapid attachments to, and relationships with, any new adult that enters his life, becoming very distressed when the new person leaves. A case has been described of one little girl who was so lacking in stimulation that she was found at home in her play-pen with her arms raised, as if for lifting, and her eyes dilated, looking but unseeing. She was able to stand like that for three hours at a time. Eventually this girl's mother agreed that her daughter should go into voluntary foster care because she could not cope. The mother was then given help to provide an appropriate environment for her other child. This example paints a very extreme picture of how a child who has not been played with will show very disturbed and regressed behaviour.

Previously, institutions such as state nurseries were thought not to provide adequate stimulation for children. Today, however, there is a wide variety of very good nursery provision which offers both residential and day care, and can give back-up and support to parents, ensuring that children have enough toys to experiment with, as well as receiving adult attention and reinforcement for each new activity. Recent research which examines residential nurseries has found that they are providing all the stimulation necessary to ensure that a child reaches optimal intellectual development; unfortunately it has to be recognized that a shortage of places exists.

Acknowledging that there are problems at home can clearly be difficult for parents, who have many expectations placed upon them by society. It is, however, important for parents to recognize the times when they are not coping and to seek some professional help so as to prevent the relationship with their child becoming so fraught that both sides want to give up. Instead they can be helped to find alternative ways to enjoy each other's company, such as going on outings or sharing an enjoyable activity. If this alternative is not found it may result in both parties suffering some longer-term emotional disturbance and, in the child's case, possibly delayed development in one or several areas.

THE IMPORTANCE OF PLAY

Play has an important role in children's lives for a number of reasons. It enables them to learn about relationships between individuals and to communicate with both children and adults. It also facilitates learning about physical aspects of the world and play with an adult can broaden children's experience. As young children have a limited vocabulary, play enables them to express clearly to another child or adult what they are thinking about and what they make of the world. Through play they can demonstrate both positive and negative feelings, as well as how they would like their world to be. We often see children attempting to be Superman or Superwoman: in doing so, they are re-organizing themselves and their friends in a way that suits them. Children's interpretations of their world are often seen as more frightening than is actually the case: for example, children sometimes play at being very strict teachers or parents, shouting and giving out beatings. It is, however, through this stylized play behaviour that children deal with their anxiety about punishment and power. Often children will play out an activity or event before verbalizing it. This is a

A child playing alone with dolls or toys will often act out situations and take different roles. Such activity reflects the child's growing understanding of the world around her.

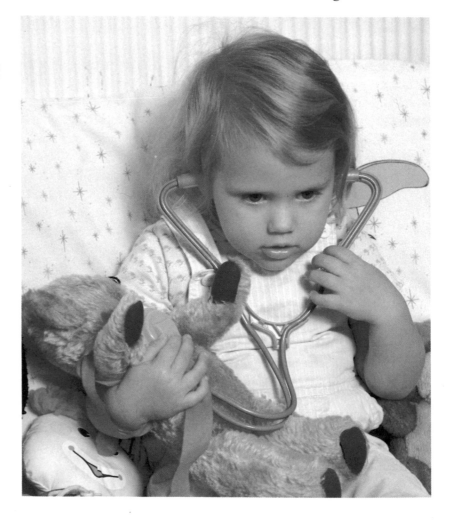

common occurrence if, for example, a family member is ill and the child is worried about the outcome. Young children who have been physically or sexually abused may well express their fears through play; in a safe environment such as a nursery school or friend's house, they can demonstrate what has been happening to them. These problems are discussed further on pages 249 and 298.

Play inevitably changes as children grow and develop, and different activities occupy their thoughts. They learn how to behave in a socially acceptable way – otherwise no-one will play with them. They also learn about the rules of chance and probability. Hopefully they also learn that it is not the end of the world if they lose a game! Next time it might be different. At this early stage children also can learn through play about how to cope with temporary setbacks and frustrations.

Play is initially based on a child's exploration of people and inanimate objects. Children will use their senses – namely, sight, taste, touch, hearing and smell – to gain a greater understanding of an object. At a later stage children will learn that objects can be used together to provide a variety of simple or complex structures or sounds. They also learn that play equipment can be used with other people to produce turn-taking games, an essential ingredient in inter-relating with others.

Children also develop an understanding of language through play, vocalizing and enjoying producing sounds of different pitch and volume, and then watching the observer's response. Children will repeat words and phrases, often not because they do not understand but rather because they enjoy making the sound and the rhythm of the words. Older children can be heard to make patterns with words, perhaps forming as many words that end in 'at' – cat, mat, fat, rat, and so on – as they can. In addition they

may introduce a whole range of nonsense words and have fun saying them to exasperated parents.

Children who are emotionally disturbed can sometimes be identified by their reluctance to play these games and wariness of the intrusions of other children or adults. Such children often prefer to keep a silent watchfulness, and are quite different to children who prefer to sit on the sidelines and participate from this distance. If you are unsure, contact your doctor or health visitor and seek his or her advice.

Children also enjoy playing symbolic games (pretend play) with dolls. At about 10 months most children will brush a doll's hair or 'feed' a soft, cuddly teddy bear. A little later they may play a much more involved game, inventing dinner parties or schools. They will provide inanimate toy cars with noises and supply voices for the drivers. They will also provide noises for farm animals and a variety of voices for the dolls in a dolls' house. In doing so they are demonstrating that they have discovered that people have different personalities and ways of talking, are temperamentally diverse, and respond to others in a variety of ways.

As children grow older they are keen to have more equipment to play with. They enjoy inventing people and making up stories in which these people have scripts. It is not uncommon to find children raiding parents' wardrobes, make-up boxes and tool kits to ensure that the story has a greater degree of realism. The use of an imaginary friend is quite normal and parents should not be concerned at their child's keenness to spend part of the time in a fantasy world. However, if this 'friend' becomes very intrusive to the extent that the child is reluctant to form friendships with peers, then professional help may be needed.

Watching children at play can provide

parents with a great deal of information about their offspring: how well they mix with other children, whether they can adapt and share when new people become involved in a game, whether they can cope with rules and tolerate frustration, and how great their powers of concentration are. It will also provide some idea about children's developmental level and whether they can organize themselves or require others to do this for them; how they use their speech and language skills to communicate; what their emotional state is and whether they are happy or miserable; and finally, how advanced their fine and gross motor skills are – for example, can they hold a crayon and scribble, or ride a bike with stabilizers? Skills are expected to be acquired at certain times in a child's life and if he does not have them by an appropriate stage, then it suggests either that he has not been given the opportunity to develop them or perhaps that he has a difficulty with them;

professional help should be sought if there is concern.

All children differ in their ability to play certain types of games. Some are exceptionally good with constructional toys but are not so good at language-based games, and vice versa. Within limits, this is not a cause for concern, but should a child not be able to do a variety of tasks in either area well after the expected time then it would be appropriate to seek professional help. Developmental skills in infancy are discussed in Chapter 4.

SOCIAL SKILLS

This term describes the ability to understand yourself in the situation you are in, and to determine what other individuals might be thinking and feeling about the same situation and about you. This is normally carried out at an unconscious level.

Children learn the fundamentals about

As well as developing physical and social skills, playing together provides excitement and fun and so contributes to the general well-being of the child.

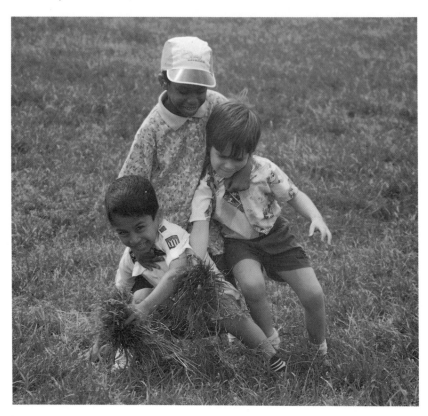

social skills within the family context. A child is more likely to form relationships with other children if he has a positive image of himself. Families can provide the right atmosphere for the child by being relaxed, confident, outgoing and able to demonstrate the emotions of love and affection. The child thus develops a positive attitude towards himself and is then more able to get on with others. If, however, the child is used to being undermined and criticized, it is more likely that he will feel inferior and lack confidence, with the result that he might well become very anxious and withdrawn. In the latter case it is not surprising that a child would find it difficult to form relationships, as others may well not be able to see him as an interesting, exciting person to know.

Children respond in several ways if they lack confidence in themselves. One such response is for a child to become very aggressive to ensure that he is able to play with a toy that another individual is playing with. However, while the child might find this a reasonably good solution in the short term, the longer-term outcome is that other children will avoid the aggressive child because of the frustration he has caused; he may then become even more aggressive and lose more friends. Other children will adopt a role, such as that of a clown, in an attempt to hide their inhibitions. Unfortunately this can result in other children not communicating with them, especially if they stop 'performing', with the result that they become stuck in this role long after it is helpful.

If parents are concerned, they should know that it is possible to teach certain social skills to a child. A first step is to help the child understand the principle of give and take. A child who takes all the time will not keep friends for very long. Grasping this fact is difficult for young children, who can be very 'egocentric', seeing things only from their own point of view and being unable to perceive that anyone else could want to have the world organized in a different way.

A second way of helping is to encourage children by praising them when they make a social contact on their own; in receiving this praise, children will hopefully increase their efforts, especially when they find them rewarding.

Parents may also act as models on which the child can base his own social behaviour. The child is physically able to watch exactly what is done and learn when to smile and nod, where to stand, and so on. A similar method is to give directions while an activity is being carried out. For example, one child may ask for another's last sweet. An anxious child, attempting to please, may give in and hand it over, and then regret it. A parent could help the child to say 'no' and suggest where the friend could buy some sweets of his own. In this example the parent is helping the child to say 'no' firmly and with conviction, then politely provide an alternative solution.

In addition to these flexible techniques there is also the more formal coaching method. In this instance, examples are role-played, and parents or professionals and children work on finding appropriate alternatives, both verbal and non-verbal.

SEPARATION AND DIVORCE

Divorce has become an increasingly common event in many children's lives. One child in three can expect to experience his parents separating or divorcing during his childhood. In families who are going through the process of divorce each member will experience the event in different ways, depending on age and previous life experience. If, for example, it is your own parents that are separating, you may apportion blame quite differently from the way in which the spouse who is leaving the family home sees the situation.

The decision to separate means that children's worlds have to be re-organized and that parents have to adapt new and different roles. This can result in periods of uncertainty for the children involved, as the old rules no longer exist and new ones have not yet been formalized. How adults handle the process of divorce will have a profound effect on how the children cope and adapt. Many parents are sensitive to their children's needs and will endeavour to understand what the divorce means to each of them personally; the result is that the children adapt positively to the change in circumstances.

In addition to making role changes, parents have to attempt to come to terms with the emotional turmoil. Not surprisingly, even the best-intentioned parents find themselves putting their own needs before the children's on occasion. It is important to recognize that divorce is not just a single event but rather a process that takes place over a long time, and children may be exposed to distress and torn loyalties over and over again. It is bound to be a difficult time, but it can offer a positive future; all too often, however, children have to experience a period of uncertainty while their parents are attempting to organize their own lives.

By the time their parents separate, children will have already seen them argue, and will have experienced a negative emotional climate. However well adults may think that they have hidden their differences from the children, the latter are in fact very sensitive to their parent's moods and will have picked up the feeling of tension; they will keep these perceptions to themselves unless specifically questioned. When the separation comes, it may provoke periods of

sadness, loss, laughter, tension and yet more confusion; all of these are normal reactions to a change in circumstances.

In the aftermath of the agreement to separate, children can find themselves in a tug-of-war situation. Each parent wants the child on his or her side, and at the time the adults rarely see that making children choose sides is upsetting. Rather they prefer to have confirmation that they were right, and to believe that if this were not so, the child would not have joined them. If this continues, unhelpful alliances can be formed whereby one parent feels that he or she has the child's total support; this situation can be used to one parent's advantage so often that the child loses his relationship with the other parent or with his brothers and sisters.

A parent may become over-protective and find it difficult to let the child carry out age-appropriate activities. This can stem from the fact that the parent has become very concerned about his or her role and ability to shoulder day-to-day responsibilities for the child. In addition, over-protectiveness can be the result of disputes over access and of one parent feeling that the other is not trustworthy or is unable to cope.

When a parent loses adult companionship, it can result in a child being promoted to the missing adult's position. Occasionally this can be fun for the child but if it continues then it is likely that he will be forced to grow up too quickly in an attempt to cope with new situations and with the new demands being placed upon him.

Talking about divorce

Telling your child about divorce can prove a very difficult task, as adult emotions can all too easily become entangled. Adults should keep the reasons and responsibilities for the divorce between themselves, so that the children do not become involved in the hostility. There is no perfect way to break bad news to a child but there are ways of telling him that make sense of the situation. The best way is certainly for both parents to break the news to the children together, so the latter are aware of their two responsible parents continuing to care for them and making appropriate joint decisions about their future. In a less than ideal world, however, that is frequently not possible, and the task is left to one parent. Nevertheless, it should be possible to help the child to understand that it is the adult's decision to separate and that he did not play a role in the separation. Children often become confused about why their parents are divorcing and will occasionally think that they are the cause of their parents' break up.

It is important not to break the news of an imminent separation too far in advance of the event. Young children have a different perception of time and in telling them too early it is possible to increase their anxiety levels; this will make it difficult for them to grasp the practical, reassuring details.

It is also important not to rush into anything until everyone is prepared to listen and share his or her thoughts. A child who has previously been running around may take a few minutes to calm down sufficiently to be able to hear what you want to say. Other children will become distressed when they know something important is about to happen and will either start to cry or distract themselves by carrying out another activity. Again it is a matter of being patient and waiting. This demonstrates to the children that you are able to put their needs first and can keep your own requirements in perspective. It is useful to remember that children absorb and understand information not only by what you say but by how you say it.

It is unhelpful to use abstraction, metaphors, vagueness or euphemisms as children all too easily misunderstand what is happening. Telling a child that 'Dad has had to go away' might lead him to believe that his father has died, because his friend's mother used a similar phrase to tell her son about his father's death. It is much better to use clear, direct, factual statements about what has happened and what will happen. It is particularly important that the information is given to young children in short phrases that are easily understandable. With older children the complexity of language and length of information should match their level of understanding of the world and events.

Children generally want to be loyal to both parents and so decisions about where the children should live and who will look after them need to be taken by both adults; the children should then be told of their parents' joint decision. Obviously there will need to be some negotiation if the child is a teenager, and if staying with one or other parent may have an effect on college or education, but the decision should rest with the parents.

Children need to know practical details, such as the length of time that will be involved between, for example, hearing the news and a house move, or when and how frequently they will see the parent who will no longer be part of the household. At times of increased anxiety it can be difficult for children to remember important facts, and it may be necessary to repeat the information several times. It can be useful for the child to act out what is happening with toys and for a parent to be around to ensure that he has the correct facts in the appropriate sequence.

Initially it is common for children to feel inhibited about discussing or acting out the events at home because of conflicts of loyalty and misunderstandings. They may, however, discuss them at school or nursery, and so it is important that schools should be notified of the situation.

The after-effects

Children will show anxiety and distress about their parents divorcing in a number of ways and to some extent this will depend on their developmental level.

For some young children development can be slowed down, interrupted or even temporarily stopped. This is most common in the areas of language and play. Skills can also be lost, most often those that have just been learnt – for example, daytime dryness; the child may start to wet himself again. Another common reaction is for young children to search for a comforter such as an old discarded dummy or a piece of blanket, or to suck a finger. If parents are not careful, they may fail to recognize this behaviour as the child's way of demonstrating that he is not coping very well with the stressful situation. Instead they can compound the problem by becoming cross and punishing him. This can lead to a negative spiral of events, the child experiencing less and less support from his parents and therefore feeling more and more insecure. Further behavioural problems may result.

Given the child's ability to show distress and frustration in a variety of ways, it is important to think about how your child is acting, and whether he is doing anything different, for better or for worse. There are several major areas that should be considered:

- increased illness
- increased aggression
- management problems
- anxiety
- regression
- failure to thrive.

It is common to see children experiencing prolonged periods of stress and becoming ill. For example, a child with diabetes may suddenly become uncontrolled, whereas previously his medication resulted in him being in control. This is because other events have superseded the medication in importance, for both child and parent.

Aggression is a common behavioural symptom in children whose parents are divorcing. A child may want to be very angry with the parent who has left, but being unable to do this, he will either become angry with the remaining parent or become aggressive with other children or adults. For example, at school a teacher may ask the child to help another pupil; instead of doing so he might become verbally quite abusive to the teacher about being given this extra task.

Children can demonstrate a wide range of management problems following their parents' separation. For example, they may refuse to eat properly, to sit at the table, or to go to bed at night unless they sleep with the parent. These problems can arise because the separated parents have different rules and expectations, and this can result in the children becoming very confused, especially if they are still quite young. Slightly older children often begin to see ways to manipulate their parents because of these inconsistencies and will attempt to play one parent off against the other.

Anxious children demonstrate their concerns in a number of ways, including becoming 'clingy' and needing close physical contact with their parent. Children may also become quite obsessional and as a result may spend time putting the house in order, becoming quite upset if items are moved. When children behave in this way it is often an attempt at gaining some control over their lives, which they feel have lost all sense of predictability. Parents can help by providing some practical reassurance.

In a small number of cases children may refuse to eat for a short time; others will become increasingly fussy about the foods they eat. If children do start to lose weight or fail to gain the appropriate amount for their years, it is important to establish why. It may be that a parent has become emotionally detached or incapacitated and is finding it difficult to think of the children's needs. In some cases a parent may be unable to provide the necessary and appropriate care.

BEING A SINGLE PARENT

Being a single parent poses some special problems for both parent and children; these need to be overcome if the family is to function at its best. Many of the problems are logistic difficulties: combining being a parent, making adequate child care arrangements when absent, working for a living,

and making sure that the child does not miss out on the opportunities that other children have can be quite a challenge.

Single parents often worry about whether their children are missing out in some way by not living with both a mother and father. This is usually an unnecessary anxiety; provided the children's home is loving and caring, they are unlikely to be adversely affected. The parent is more likely to be the one who is missing out, lacking adult companionship and someone to talk to about everyday problems and the particular difficulties that arise from time to time in caring for and bringing up children.

The child can be adversely affected if the arrangements for his care are tenuous or

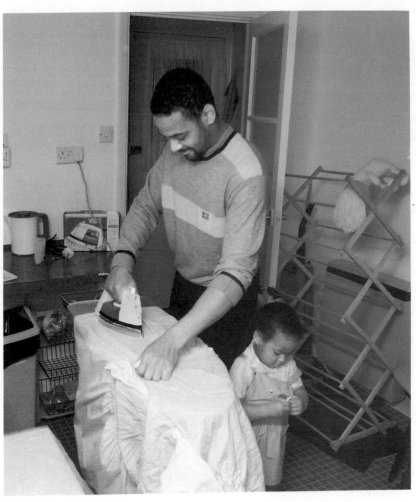

Being a single parent can pose special problems as he or she tries to strike a balance between caring for the child, wage earning and doing the domestic chores.

complex. If he is being cared for in different places by different people, and this has become a way of life, he may feel insecure; if it is only a short-term expedient, it is unlikely to cause any lasting problems.

From time to time single mothers may be anxious that children feel the lack of a man in the family; single fathers feel similarly about the children's need for a woman's presence. These thoughts are more likely to surface as puberty approaches. As almost all children get to know adults of both sexes, either within the extended family, or at school or a youth group, not having adults of both sexes in the home is not of overwhelming importance to normal development.

The child may, however, react strongly if his parent forms a new relationship. Children of single parents are likely to be very close and dependent on their parent, and anxiety and jealousy can arise if he or she seems to be making friends with someone outside the family. The situation needs sensitive handling, and the child should be reassured by the parent's actions that the parent still loves him just as much, and that there is no threat in the new relationship. The situation evolves with time, and any problems need to be worked through until a stage is reached that is acceptable to all those involved.

FOSTERING AND ADOPTION

Children who enter foster care can do so on either a voluntary or a statutory basis. There are numerous reasons for a child going into care: for example, a parent who is about to have another baby but who has no family support may require help from the social services, or a child might have become out of control and parents feel unable to cope. It is rare for a child to be given up for adoption without first going into foster care, although occasionally parents will decide before a baby is born that they are unable or not prepared to look after the child.

One of the specific problems associated with fostering is children's confusion about their relationship with their family of origin, as well as with their foster family. Children frequently develop all kinds of myths to explain why they have been placed in care; sometimes these serve as good short-term coping strategies but they can be quite detrimental in the longer term, when the reality becomes apparent and they have no resources to deal with it. The temporary nature of foster placements can create great insecurity. This can be particularly true if the child has been placed in care on a voluntary basis. In such cases parents have been known to remove the child from the placement and then return him a couple of days later. Not surprisingly such children tend to show their distress by becoming aggressive and opposing anyone in authority.

Children who have been adopted 'enter' families which resemble ordinary ones in many respects. They do differ, however, in some important ways. Firstly, the family may be childless, perhaps because of infertility, and therefore may have decided to adopt because they cannot have their own child. Couples will have to come to terms with the psychological impact of infertility and accept that they will not experience the joys and worries of pregnancy and childbirth. Another major difference is that the child joins an already established family, who will previously have generated their own rules, beliefs and ways of interacting which the 'new child' will have to learn. Both the child and adoptive family will initially need to be flexible and to adjust to each other's ways until a new negotiated set of principles can be agreed.

Pregnancy gives people time to prepare themselves for the changes that will occur in family structure, and this is very important in helping couples adjust to their new roles. Research has shown that couples who foster or adopt do not experience the same preparation time, because the formalities often mean that they are uncertain as to whether they will be accepted or not. When it has been decided that they are suitable foster or adoptive parents, the waiting time is very variable. Frequently there will be several meetings with the child before the couple decide whether they will accept him.

The emotional development of adopted children is determined by several factors. Important influences include the emotional atmosphere within the adopted family home, the models new parents provide for coping with difficult situations and dealing with frustration, and the mutual relationship between the child and his family members — how he becomes 'attached' to the family and how they become 'attached' to him.

Overall, children who are adopted are much more at risk of showing disturbed behaviour. There are several reasons for this: the child may already have experienced a very disrupted life — entering children's homes, forming relationships with care staff who then leave, and having to adapt to different adults. A further factor that may be relevant is the extent to which children who are adopted or fostered experience greater over-protection and over-indulgence. (Children living with their biological parents are also sometimes over-indulged.) The parents may also have their own feelings and uncertainties about bringing up a child.

Research does not suggest that fostering or adoption is a major source of difficulty in itself but rather that it can be a complicating factor for some parents and children. It has been shown to be a source of stress in adolescence, when developmentally the young person is being confronted with issues concerning identity and security, and can result in argument and controversy. At these times myths about biological parents can be drawn into the argument or used as a refuge.

Social workers try to place children in families who have the same cultural background, so that they are aware of their cultural origins. Previously children from all racial and religious backgrounds were placed predominantly with white families, but this caused a number of problems as the children were not a part of their new parents' culture and did not identify themselves with their cultural and religious heritage. Attempting to place children with appropriate families can mean that they have to wait considerably longer in temporary child-care placements which are less than satisfactory from a psychological point of view.

The age at which children are moved from foster homes to adoptive homes is important. Children who are moved between the ages of 6 months and 1 year have been found to show considerably more immediate and long-term difficulties in comparison with infants who were transferred under the age of 6 months. Overall, research has shown that the various styles and patterns of care in fostering and adoptive families do not matter but that the quality of care is paramount.

When it comes to telling children that they were fostered or adopted, there appears to be no agreement about method or timing. This is perhaps not surprising, given the individual variations between not only the children but also the rest of the family members. In fact the only consistent factor appears to be the need for children to be told in a sensitive and sympathetic way that is appropriate to their needs and to their stage of development and understanding. Most experts feel, however, that children should know before they go to school, so that they are told in a caring and controlled way and do not find out by overhearing a remark in the playground. Other authorities are concerned that children may be emotionally damaged if they are told that they were chosen by their adoptive families, as some children may feel rejected as a consequence by their natural parents. This could lead to feelings of being unloved and unwanted. Although telling a child can be a difficult experience, not doing so can be more damaging in the longer term. The secrecy that can develop around such issues can be very stressful and often children harbour fantasies about why certain topics appear to be taboo, invariably believing that they are somehow to blame. Although the issue of how to approach the topic is difficult, providing security while the child comes to terms with the information is clearly of help.

HYPERACTIVITY

Children vary enormously in their activity levels; some never seem to be still, while others are almost entirely sedentary and resist efforts to make them take more exercise. It is difficult to distinguish between normal healthy exuberance and hyperactivity, as there is no definite activity level which indicates the latter. However, professionals agree that there are a small number of children who are clearly beyond the normal range. This judgment is based not only on activity levels, but also takes into account associated behaviours, which include:

- a short attention span
- poor concentration
- an inability to cope with frustration
- impulsive behaviour
- mood swings
- aggressive behaviour
- socially disinhibited behaviour
- a poor sleep-pattern.

When a number of these behaviours are present, the child is considered to have the hyperkinetic syndrome.

This disorder can be accompanied by developmental delay of one kind or another. In almost all cases the children have educa-

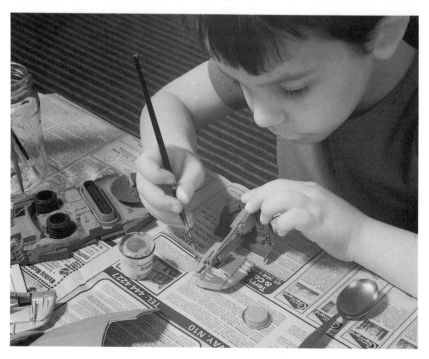

Left and right: Children vary widely in their activity levels. One child may enjoy quiet pursuits that demand skill and patience while another will prefer being outdoors and always seem to have energy to spare.

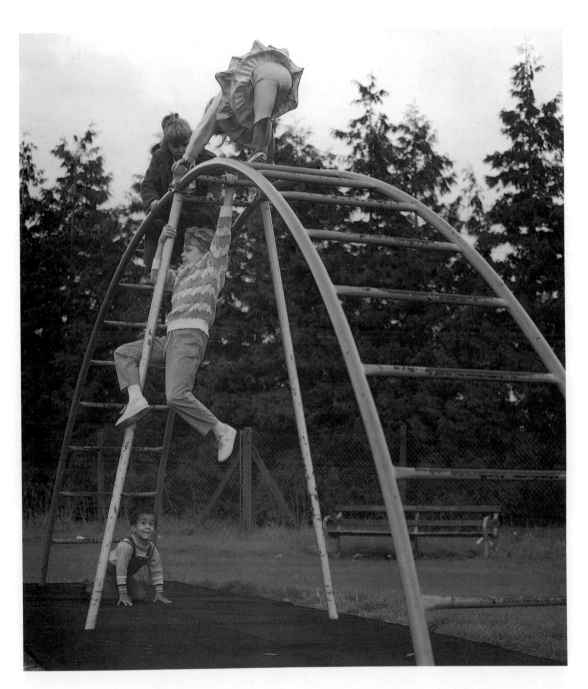

tional difficulties. Additionally some are intellectually below average or may have a mild mental handicap.

Many parents become worried that their child has the hyperactivity syndrome and so it is important to be able to distinguish hyperactivity from restlessness and boisterousness. Children who are hyperactive demonstrate problems at an early age. There will also be clear evidence that the child has poor concentration, which results in him changing activity very frequently and becoming easily frustrated. Over-activity usually shows itself by 3 or 4 years of age. Children with hyperkinetic syndrome require months of very structured behaviour modification to effect a change in everyday behaviour, whereas active normal children will respond to firm handling.

There are thought to be a variety of causes which may result in a child having the hyperkinetic syndrome. In a majority of cases there can be underlying brain damage. Temperamental factors are considered to be important. All children are born with a cluster of inherent tendencies which shape how they will behave. These interact with parental handling techniques. Children whose parents provide clear rules and limits for their behaviour are less likely to become over-active and aggressive, as there is no reinforcement for behaving in such a way. Parents who are rather more passive, and who only respond to their child when he attracts attention by being either very disruptive or very active, will in fact encourage this behaviour. The child learns that the only way to ensure his parents' attention is to behave in such a way that they have to intervene to protect other people or property.

Children who have been brought up by a large number of people may show this behaviour to a greater extent, as potentially there are as many sets of rules as there are adults. Too many varied rules can lead to confusion, as children are not sure of their limits and will exploit any loopholes.

Diet has also been considered an important factor in some children's elevated levels of activity. Large numbers of parents have indicated that when the child's diet has been altered, his behaviour has improved, but when parents decide to change the diet, other factors in the child's life may also be altered. For example, if parents spend more time with their child to ensure that he adheres to the new diet, there may be more opportunities to carry out activities together. Parents have to be very firm about issues related to food and as a result may then feel more able to

be firm about other matters. Consequently it is not easy to be certain whether behavioural changes are primarily due to diet.

Although the main problem appears to be difficulty in keeping the attention focused for very long, over-activity can lead to children having difficulty in forming relationships with other children because they are perceived to be aggressive and disruptive. Unfortunately a downward spiral can develop as the child attempts to make friends by aggressive and vindictive means. This often results in the child being actively avoided.

There are a number of ways to help these children to behave appropriately. Parents and other adults who come into contact with them can be taught behavioural techniques to encourage appropriate behaviour as well as discourage undesirable behaviour. The general aim is to reinforce the child's attempts at behaving appropriately and either to ignore the undesirable behaviour or, if it is inappropriate to do so, to have a set of consistent strategies that can be implemented.

It can also be important to focus on both environment and routines. Do either of these require some adjustment? For example, breakable objects could be removed to lessen the chance of accidents happening. In terms of routines, an active child may benefit from going swimming to use up surplus energy so that the evening period would be easier for the rest of the family.

If none of the above strategies works then you may need professional help and should discuss the problems with your family doctor.

Other aspects of children's emotional development are discussed elsewhere in this book. See Chapter 4 for information on social skills; Chapter 6 on puberty; Chapter 10 on sickness; Chapter 11 on disability; and Chapter 12 on death and dying.

CHAPTER

6

PUBERTY AND ADOLESCENCE

Puberty is the period of transition between childhood and sexual maturity. Although the primary alterations it involves are in the sexual organs, they are accompanied by profound physical, mental and emotional changes affecting nearly every aspect of an adolescent's life.

Trying to understand and come to terms with their own and other people's sexuality, and at the same time shedding their dependence on parents and becoming more self-reliant, makes puberty a stressful time for young people. It is sometimes a time of crisis within the family, too, as young people often question established attitudes and values in their bid for independence.

PHYSICAL CHANGES

The changes in external appearance that come with puberty are readily apparent. They include an increase in height, the growth of pubic and underarm hair in both sexes, together with the enlargement of the genitalia, beard and body hair growth and deepening of the voice in boys, and development of the breasts in girls. These changes are the result of processes that start much earlier.

Puberty begins when the pituitary gland, situated just underneath the brain, starts to produce a hormone called gonadotrophin, which circulates in the blood and causes

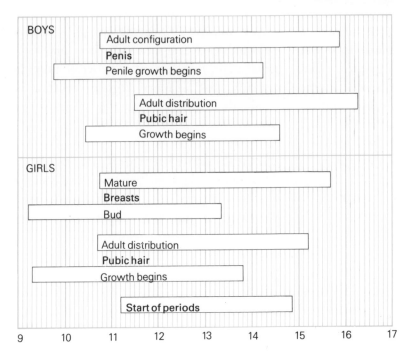

There is wide variation in the age at which puberty begins. This is true of both sexes, although as a group girls enter puberty before boys. The chart shows the age range in which most normal children reach various puberty milestones.

growth of the gonads (the testicles or ovaries). Production of gonadotrophin may start as early as 7 years of age, the amount gradually increasing. The factors which initiate gonadotrophin production are not fully understood, but include, amongst others, genetic make-up, nutritional state and body weight.

The gonads gradually increase in size and develop in structure, maturing into the adult form. As well as being organs for the production of eggs or sperm, the gonads produce hormones. The ovaries produce the female sex hormones known as oestrogens, which circulate in the blood and promote the growth of the uterus (womb) and vagina, the breasts and the pubic hair. The testicles produce male hormones, androgens, which cause growth of the scrotum and penis, and of pubic and body hair.

In boys the enlargement of the testicles at the beginning of puberty is apparent; in girls similar growth occurs in the ovaries, but cannot be seen. In both sexes the most noticeable indications that puberty has begun are the changes in the external genitalia which gradually assume an adult configuration, and the growth of pubic hair. In girls the breasts gradually enlarge, usually at the same time as the changes in the external genitalia, but sometimes earlier. The sequence of the various changes which take place during puberty vary from individual to individual, but typical patterns for girls and boys are shown in the table on the preceding page.

The puberty growth spurt

The sex hormones cause an acceleration in bone growth, too. The bones mature so that, when the puberty growth spurt is over, the final adult height will have been attained and there will be no further potential for height increase. In girls the growth spurt starts in early puberty, and in general is largely over

by the time menstruation begins. In boys the period of rapid growth is towards the end of puberty. The increase in stature associated with the growth spurt cannot happen unless there is an adequate intake of food. The appetite becomes almost insatiable at the time of most rapid growth, as building new body tissue requires a lot of food energy.

As well as growth in stature, puberty also witnesses a broadening of the body frame, and the difference in body shape between the sexes becomes more marked: boys become more muscular and girls develop a wider pelvis, with increased fat deposition on buttocks and thighs.

Menstruation

Menarche is the term used for the onset of menstruation. It is one of the last stages of puberty and periods are not likely to begin until the breasts and pubic hair are well developed and approaching an adult configuration. A girl needs to be given information and practical hints by an older person early in puberty about menstruation and its management so that when her first period does start she is fully prepared.

It is unusual for a regular monthly cycle to be established straight away. There may well be two or three months between periods initially, but a more regular rhythm is gradually established over the first couple of years.

Breast development in boys

During puberty some boys experience slight breast enlargement; a bud of breast tissue develops behind the nipple, and sometimes some excess fat is deposited. This is known as gynaecomastia and is a variant of normal puberty. It occurs because males produce small amounts of female hormones as well as a lot of male hormones, and sometimes the female hormones are enough to

CHAPTER 6 PUBERTY AND ADOLESCENCE

cause breast enlargement. As puberty progresses the breast tissue gradually shrinks, and after a couple of years returns to normal.

Although gynaecomastia is of no medical significance, it causes the affected boy great distress. He is concerned about the way his own sexual development differs from other people's, and he will also be teased by the boys at school. In some cases cosmetic surgery is indicated, so if the enlargement is marked or causing much suffering, it is worth consulting the doctor.

THE AGE OF PUBERTY

The onset of puberty is usually earlier in girls than in boys, but varies greatly in both sexes. In girls the first visible signs are the beginnings of breast development and the growth of pubic hairs between the thighs. In about 10 per cent of girls this stage is reached by the age of 10; the average age for this stage is about 11½ years; and 5–10 per cent have not reached this stage by the age of 13. The comparable stage of development in boys, the growth of the first pubic hairs, occurs before the age of 11 years in 8 per cent; the average is around 12½ years; and 10 per cent have not attained this stage by the age of 14.

The duration of puberty also differs widely between individuals. Occasionally all the visible physical stages from onset to completion only take a matter of months, but in most take around two years, and in some even longer.

Early onset of puberty

Although most girls have no features of puberty before the age of 10, some experience changes earlier than this. When puberty starts in girls of 9 or over, there is not usually any underlying abnormality; their 'biological clock', which regulates growth and development, simply seems to

run a bit faster than that of most other people. They may go on to achieve physical maturity early, or they may have a rather gradual progression of puberty and achieve maturity at the same time as their peer group. Children who are obese often have an early start. If puberty changes begin early, and certainly if they start before the age of 9 in girls, you should consult your doctor in case they are caused by an imbalance or excess production of hormones.

In some girls early breast development begins without corresponding growth of pubic hair or the appearance of other features of puberty. This seems to be because the breast tissue responds to quite low levels of circulating oestrogen produced as the ovaries start to grow. The levels of oestrogen produced are initially too low to cause other changes, but in due course these changes will occur when the production of oestrogens is stepped up.

Precocious puberty is less common in boys than girls, and it is rare for there to be signs of puberty in boys before the age of 10.

Children who develop any signs of puberty before others in their class may become very self-conscious. They need understanding and support from their parents, particularly if they are subjected to teasing at school.

Delayed puberty

Considerable anxiety can be caused if a child has not started puberty when the rest of his peer group are obviously pubertal. Late-developing boys are particularly prone to be upset, as classmates grow very much taller and can be cruel in their teasing about lack of sexual development.

One of the factors governing the onset of puberty is body weight, and children who have been slow-growing, either for constitutional reasons or because of chronic illness, are often late. In some cases this is familial. Although a father may not remember exactly when he started puberty, he may recall that he had not stopped growing by the time he left school, growth being another indicator of slow bodily maturation.

If you or your child are concerned about the late onset of puberty it is worth consulting the doctor. He or she will want to measure height and weight, as slow growth may explain the delay. In boys the earliest sign of puberty is an increase in the size of the testicles, and the doctor may be able to reassure you that puberty has started before it is signalled by the start of pubic hair growth. Only in very few children is delay due to hormonal abnormalities or any failure of the gonads, but if the cause is not apparent the doctor may want to do further investigations. In some situations hormone treatment is used to initiate puberty.

EMOTIONAL DEVELOPMENT

Although emotional development occurs throughout the growing period and beyond, the teenage years are notable for the changes that take place in emotional maturity and outlook. Various separate factors come together at this stage of life. They include an increasing ability to look after oneself compared with childhood, growing knowledge, the development of special interests and aptitudes, a greater sense of identity with the peer group, adjustment to the changes of puberty, and increasing independence from the family.

Parents always have a vital role in providing love and support, and this continues to be very important throughout adolescence. Such encouragement should foster maturity and self-reliance, but at the same time set limits.

Young children tend to be active rather than reflective, and only consider events from a personal viewpoint. They do not often think about how they are regarded by others. This outlook changes with age, and concern about personal appearance, clothes and other people's opinion is an important feature of the teens. There is an increasing wish both to be in fashion and to merge with the peer group, rather than to be seen to be different. Both boys and girls are very insecure about their appearance and attractiveness, and may be shy or awkward in social contacts.

Worrying about school performance may add to the anxieties of adolescence. Most parents and many other adults stress the importance of doing well. Young people can only measure how they are doing by the comments of parents and teachers, and by comparison with their peer group. Often they do not realize that all of the group is making satisfactory progress, and that learning is not or should not be a matter of competition. Anxiety as to what career to choose, whether they will pass the right exams and whether they will 'succeed' in life are common.

You should try to help your child with subject choices at school, and with thinking about a career. It is worth pointing out that there is a lot of flexibility in choosing jobs, and that many people do not decide what they want to do until after leaving school or college. You should be prepared to seek out information and discuss possible future careers, but you should not force children in the direction of any particular one; neither should you pressurize them into making choices before there is a need to do so.

Parents must see their role as providing guidance and support during this stage. The child suffers much indecision, and many anxieties and self-doubts. Parents should try not to exert undue influence on decision-making, and should beware of always being critical of appearance, behaviour or school performance. Instead, recognize that the pressures on teenagers give rise to many insecurities. Calmness and support from parents are all-important.

The physical and emotional changes associated with puberty affect the whole personality. The individual observes these bodily changes with a mixture of interest, speculation and apprehension. The significance of sexuality begins to intrude more and more on the consciousness. Intitially, an adolescent is interested in his or her own development, then that of others of the same age and sex, and then of the opposite sex.

Teenagers need to be accepted as part of a group, and membership of such a group provides the opportunity for non-threatening social interaction between the sexes. With further maturity special relationships may develop between boy and girl; the sharing of thoughts and feelings, and interest in and discovery of another's personality is an important stage in social development. Parents often worry about such a relationship becoming too serious or too physical. If you have imparted acceptable standards of behaviour by example and precept while the child was younger, these are likely to prevail.

If your children are to have your help

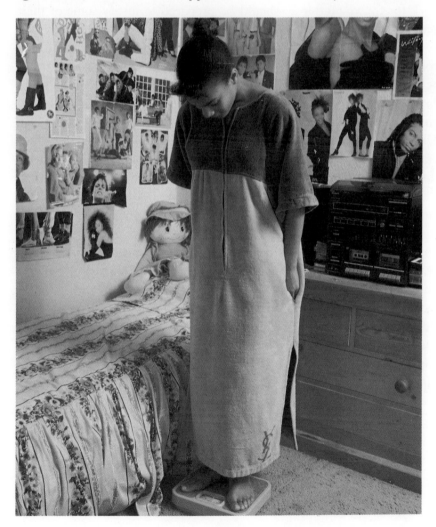

At around the time of puberty all teenagers become interested in the changes occurring in their bodies. Some degree of anxiety about facial or bodily appearance is almost universal.

during adolescence, they need and expect you to set limits: on behaviour, on how often they go out with their friends, on what time they come in and go to bed, and on many other aspects of life. They will argue about the restrictions and there has to be some negotiation and compromise on both sides. A frequently cited reason for disputing the rules is that 'everyone else is allowed to do it'. This usually means that one or two in the group are permitted to, so it is often worth ascertaining if 'everyone' really is allowed or not. If only a few are, it probably indicates which parents are not good at setting limits in their domestic relationships.

The boundaries that you establish help to provide a safe framework for the youngster to gain new experience, to mature and to begin to become independent.

Adolescents gain confidence, acceptance and social skills by belonging to a group. However, membership creates its own pressures. It may highlight anxieties about appearance, family background or abilities. All of these, and many other personal characteristics, are compared to those of others in the group and found wanting. When the group is together, however, it provides reassurance for each of its members that he or she is acceptable after all. Members also exert pressure on each other to move on to adopt behaviour which is seen either as more adult or as a rejection of 'boring' parental attitudes and values. This peer group pressure is one of the factors which propels the child towards greater maturity and independence and as such is important; parental guidance is needed as a regulating force so that individuals can control their own progress, only moving on to the next stage of development when they feel ready and confident to do so.

In adolescence many adult and especially parental values may be rejected, providing grounds for endless arguments. This is an indication that the teenager is thinking for herself, and as such is a sign of increasing maturity. This can be a difficult time for the family. The teenager is trying to assert independence by rejecting the values of family and adult society. There is nothing new about this. The Greek poet Hesiod, in 720 BC, wrote 'I no longer have any hope for the future of our country if today's youth should ever become the rulers of tomorrow, because this youth is unbearable, reckless – just terrible.'

Questioning parental authority is a necessary part of growing up and may take the form of defiance or disobedience. Parents should be prepared to justify some of their standards and explain why they feel as they do. They should be prepared to admit that some of their attitudes are determined by habit rather than insisting that theirs is the only way of considering an issue. Parents should try to keep calm, although that is not always easy; remember that this is a phase which will pass and that, in spite of what might be said and the impression that might be given, your child is still relying heavily on you for example and support.

Inevitably, in learning to do things for themselves, young people will make errors and misjudgments, as these are an essential part of achievement. As a parent it can be difficult to know when to give advice, and when to stand back and let a child learn by experience.

At times the young person's behaviour, within or outside the home, may be unacceptable. Antisocial behaviour, drunkenness, vandalism, smoking and substance abuse are all features of teenage activity, and young people may get caught up in them. Parents should take an interest in who their children are going out with, where they are going and what they are doing, without being too inquisitive or disapproving. Sensible advice given by parents at an early stage rather than later may prevent some of the wilder excesses of behaviour.

If your child is found to be involved in antisocial or illegal behaviour you must not reject the child, only the action. Your support, love and guidance can often be crucial factors in getting through this period and keeping family relationships intact. It is likely to be a trying time and the family may need outside advice and help. The family doctor, priest or a social worker may be useful to talk to, and may be able to put you in touch with someone who can help.

In *The Prophet* the Middle Eastern poet Kahlil Gibran summed up parenthood when he said of children, 'You may give them your love, but not your thoughts, for they have their own thoughts. You may strive to be like them, but seek not to make them like you. For life goes not backward nor tarries with yesterday.'

SEXUAL BEHAVIOUR

Young people become sexually mature during adolescence, grow increasingly aware of their own sexuality, and feel attraction to and interest in members of the opposite sex. Parents may first become aware of this when they find bedrooms covered in pin-ups, or see popular magazines appear. At first, interest in the opposite sex may be directed towards a remote being such as a pop star or other media figure. Such people are

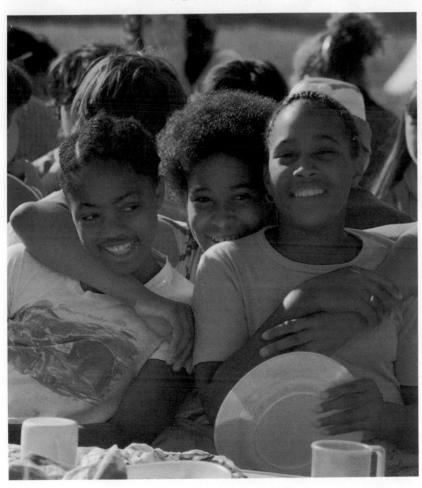

Being part of a peer group is an important aspect of teenage development. The initial reassurance of acceptability encourages members of the group to adopt more adult behaviour and to move towards greater maturity and independence.

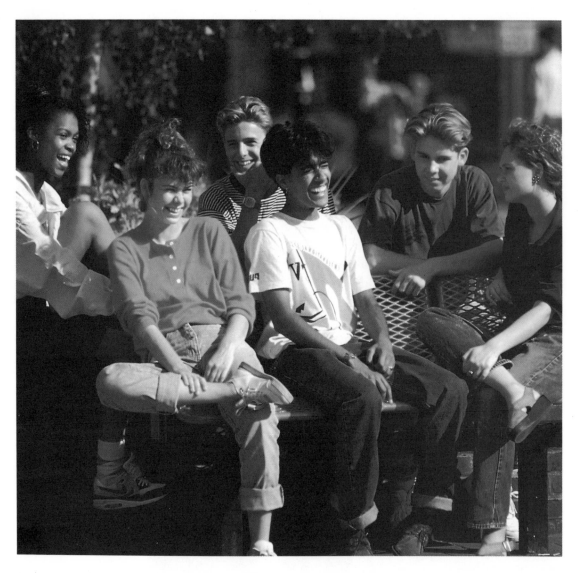

Getting to know members of the opposite sex can be accomplished more easily from within the relaxed atmosphere of a mixed group.

glamorous, are often portrayed as having a dream lifestyle and, because they are remote, are non-threatening. Sometimes young adolescents may show an interest in members of their own sex; this is quite normal and should not be a cause for concern.

Masturbation is a normal phase of developing sexuality and is common in both males and females. Parents are only likely to discover it by accident, provided their child is discreet. By recognizing their child's right

to privacy (for example, by making a point of always asking permission before entering his or her bedroom or the bathroom), parents can usually avoid any potential embarrassment on this score.

The importance of belonging to a group is discussed on page 85, and social mixing of the sexes is likely to be a group activity at first. At some stage during adolescence teenagers may pair up and start a special relationship. Almost all young people believe that sex should not be isolated from a loving and caring relationship, and first relationships with the opposite sex are initially likely to be almost or completely non-physical. If the bond continues to deepen a physical aspect will obviously develop.

Parents should recognize that young people will choose their own friends, and will determine for themselves the extent of any relationship. Parents may give guidance, but the autonomy of the adolescent has to be respected. There are often stresses for young people in forming romantic attachments and parents can continue their invaluable supporting and caring role if they do it without criticism.

In the last twenty years society has changed. More young people are sexually active, and often at an earlier age than their parents. By the late teens many young people will have had at least one sexual relationship. Parents need to recognize that life nowadays is somewhat different, and that their children are growing up in and are influenced by today's society. The differences, however, are fewer than the similarities. Most young people wish to form loving, lasting and caring friendships, of which the sexual aspect, although very important, represents only one part.

Sex education

Learning about sexual matters should be a gradual process that continues through childhood. If you have a close relationship with your child various aspects of sex and reproduction will have been talked about naturally from time to time, at a level he or she can comprehend. There are several good books for younger children on the physical and emotional aspects of reproduction; these are assimilated in an unemotional manner at this stage, and provide a useful foundation for later learning.

In the years approaching puberty and during puberty itself, children should learn how their own bodies function, about the anatomy and physiology of the opposite sex, and about adult behaviour. Talk at school amongst peers will cover all of these areas and it is important that the child is given accurate information rather than speculative or fantasized accounts from friends.

It is important that the emotional and ethical aspects of sex are emphasized as well as the physical ones, and this can best be done at home. Children coming to terms with their own sexuality need guidance on respect for members of the opposite sex, and should know what are acceptable standards of behaviour in their personal relationships.

Many parents find the discussion of sexual topics with their children difficult. It is important to be as natural as possible, and to be prepared to talk about sexual matters when they come into the conversation. Choosing a good explanatory book written for teenagers can be a help. It needs to be informative on the whole range of sexual and reproductive topics, including subjects like masturbation and contraception. Young people around the age of puberty are much more interested in sexuality than they are in where babies come from, and books which concentrate only on the reproductive aspects of sex, or do not answer the questions they ask, are unlikely to appeal to them.

A general explanation of contraception should be part of early sex education, and it should be an acceptable subject for occasional conversation in a general context within the family. In this way the concept of contraception becomes familiar to the young person. With this sort of grounding the individual is likely to find out more, and obtain contraceptive help at a time when he or she is thinking about the possibility of moving into a sexual relationship.

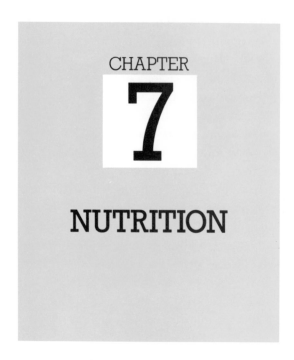

CHAPTER
7

NUTRITION

Children and parents need frequent opportunities to eat together in a relaxed manner, to ensure good relationships and easy communication between all members of the family.

The low childhood mortality that has been achieved over the last fifty years and the present good health of most children in developed countries owe much more to adequate nutrition than to medical advances. In many parts of the world malnutrition is regrettably still common; in these places disease and disability are due to a shortage of food.

The current interest in healthy eating and concern over the composition of the diet need to be seen against the background of the great health benefits that have stemmed in the Western world from the ready availability of adequate food in good condition.

Only when children have certain diseases is diet likely to make a major difference to their health; for most children varying the types of food eaten will have little effect. There is, however, some evidence that dietary factors can play a part in the development of certain adult problems, such as coronary heart disease. Some of the recommendations that are made for children's diets are put forward with the aim of establishing an eating

All parents want their children to be well nourished and healthy. If adults are choosing a healthy and prudent diet for themselves it is likely to be ideal for their children. In thinking about nutrition and children it is important to remember that preparation and presentation are just as important as the type and amount of food. Eating, as well as being a necessity, is also an important social activity.

Family meal times should be a time for communication and socialization as well as for eating. Special meals like parties and picnics provide the opportunity for fostering family relationships.

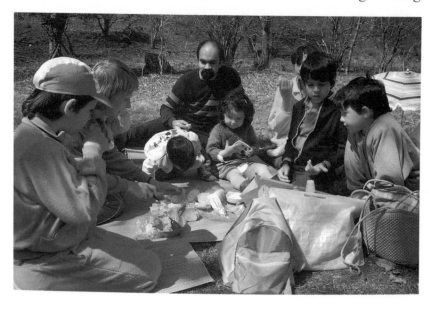

pattern which, if carried into adult life, will confer benefits then.

Advice as to what constitutes a healthy diet is often confusing, and sometimes conflicting. Understanding the basics of nutrition and the background to the various dietary recommendations will help to clarify the various issues. This will enable you to choose, for yourself and your family, attractive and appetizing food that also provides a balanced and wholesome diet.

THE COMPOSITION OF FOODS

All foods are composed of one or more of the major nutrients: proteins, carbohydrates and fats. They may also contain vitamins, minerals and fibre. An adequate diet consists of a mixture of all three of the major nutrients (providing enough energy for growth and an active life), together with sufficient amounts of the essential vitamins, minerals and fibre.

Proteins

Proteins form the structure of many of the cells of the body, and are essential for life and growth. Although the body can turn one form of protein into another, proteins cannot be synthesized from carbohydrates or fats. Proteins occur in animal and plant foods: meat, fish, milk, cheese and eggs are rich sources, as are many other foods such as beans, flour and vegetables.

If dietary protein intake is inadequate, health fails, and malnutrition supervenes. Fortunately this is not a concern for healthy children in developed countries as the ready availability of protein-containing foods means that a normal diet provides much more protein than is needed. The body uses any excess protein in the diet as a source of energy. In short periods of illness where the appetite

may be depressed there is no likelihood of protein deficiency, but in prolonged illness it is important to make sure intake is adequate.

Carbohydrates

Carbohydrates are used by the body to provide much of the energy necessary for movement and for the vital body processes. There are two main types of carbohydrate that occur in foods: starch and sugars.

Green plants have the ability to synthesize sugars and then to convert them into starch for the storage of energy. Many seeds, such as cereal grains, peas and beans, are good sources of starch, as are potatoes and other tubers. Animals, including humans, are only able to store small amounts of carbohydrate, and any carbohydrate eaten in excess of immediate requirements is converted to fat for storage.

Sugars in the diet occur naturally in many fruits and in honey, and sugar is added in the preparation of many dishes, especially cakes and biscuits. Most sweets and confectionery are almost entirely composed of sugar. Most children like sweets and sweetened foods; excessive consumption, however, leads rapidly to dental caries. An important aspect of positive dental care is to make sure that the intake of sugar is restricted, not only by limiting consumption of sweets, but also by avoiding too many sugar-containing foods. (see Part Two Chapter 7).

When we eat starches they are digested in the intestine to form sugars before they can be absorbed into the body. Starchy foods are absorbed more slowly than sugars and give more sustained satisfaction.

Fats

From a nutritional viewpoint fats comprise both solid types, such as butter and margarine, and also vegetable oils used in cooking and food preparation, as their chemical structure is similar. Fats in the diet are a source of energy, and if not immediately needed can be stored as body fat.

Many of the more tasty foods contain fat. Children's favourites, like chips, crisps, sausages and other fried foods, have a high fat content, as do biscuits, cream, meat and some cheeses. With the gradual improvement in standards of living, the proportion of fat in the average diet has grown bigger. This has led to concern that the increasing incidence of coronary heart disease in adults could be related to the high and rising dietary fat intake. High consumption of ordinary fat causes a rise in the level of blood cholesterol (fatty substance that is present in the blood and is an essential constituent of cell membranes) and it is a high blood cholesterol level that is thought to be harmful. Many different factors play a part in the development of heart disease in adults, but the evidence that dietary fat is significant among these is sufficiently strong for various health bodies throughout the developed world to have made recommendations on limiting its intake.

Dietary fats may be divided into two types which have different chemical structures: saturated and polyunsaturated fat. Most fat from ordinary sources is saturated. Thus meat fat, butter, ordinary margarine, the fat in cheese, and ordinary vegetable oil for cooking are mainly saturated. Polyunsaturated fats occur in fish and chicken, and in corn, sunflower and safflower oils and products made from them. Saturated fats tend to raise the blood cholesterol; polyunsaturated fats have no effect. Cholesterol itself also occurs in the diet, principally in eggs and liver, but the amounts of cholesterol in the average diet have little effect on the level in the blood. Furthermore a low saturated fat diet will also be low in cholesterol.

The current recommendations suggest that not more than 35 per cent of calories should come from fat, and within that limit foods high in saturated fat should be partially replaced by foods high in polyunsaturated fats.

Involving children in the preparation of food is a good way of getting them interested in what they eat and of introducing them gradually to a broad range of ingredients.

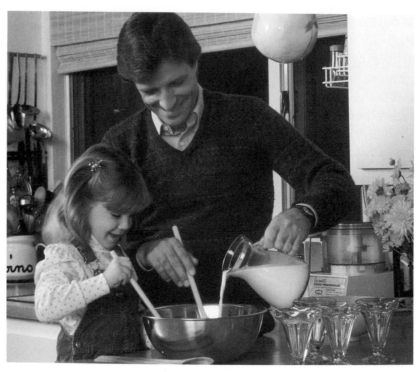

The major vitamins

As well as the major nutrients – proteins, carbohydrates and fats – there are various other dietary substances, called vitamins, which are necessary for health. They are needed only in very small amounts, often only a few milligrams a day or even less.

Vitamin A

This is present in liver, milk, butter, fortified margarine and eggs. It can also be made by the body from caroteinoid pigments that occur in carrots and some other vegetables. It is essential for night vision, and for the health of the skin. Deficiency does not occur in children eating normal Western diets.

Vitamin B

There are several B complex vitamins, including thiamine (B_1), riboflavin (B_2), folic acid, nicotinamide, pyridoxine (B_6) and vitamin B_{12}. They play a part in many body processes and are needed for the health of the skin, nerves and blood. There are a variety of good dietary sources for these various compounds. Most occur in liver, meat and fish and some are also found in yeast, green vegetables, cereals and wheatgerm. Deficiency diseases, such as pellagra and beriberi, do not occur in children on mixed Western diets.

Vitamin C

Vitamin C or ascorbic acid is present in fresh fruit, particularly oranges and tomatoes. The vitamin is important to strengthen small blood vessels. It is destroyed by cooking. Severe deficiency gives rise to scurvy, which is now extremely rare, but lesser degrees of deficiency are common in children who do not eat much fresh fruit. It is uncertain whether these partial shortages are important, but they may predispose to minor infections.

Vitamin D

Vitamin D occurs in butter, milk and meat, and can also be synthesized in the skin if it is exposed to sunlight or another source of ultraviolet light. Vitamin D is necessary for the absorption of calcium from the intestine and for the deposition of calcium in the bones and teeth (see page 188). Deficiency results in a softness and deformity of the bones known as rickets, and also affects the teeth. Many diets do not contain enough vitamin D for a child's needs during a period of rapid growth, such as infancy or puberty, when a large amount of calcium is needed for the bones. Provided the child goes out in the sun any dietary shortfall is compensated for by production of the vitamin in the skin, but climatic or cultural factors may prevent this.

Vitamin E

Vitamin E occurs in leafy vegetables, nuts and seed oils and plays a part in neuro-muscular function. Deficiencies have been described in premature babies and in some disease states, but probably never occur in otherwise healthy children on normal diets.

Vitamin K

This vitamin can be made by bacteria in the intestine, so deficiency states only occur in the newborn period, before the gut has been colonized by bacteria, or in malabsorption states. Vitamin K plays an important role in blood clotting.

If children are eating a mixed Western diet they are likely to be taking in all vitamins in adequate amounts. All manufactured baby milks have vitamins added to prevent any deficiency developing, and margarine is fortified with vitamins A and D to make it resemble butter. For infants and toddlers who are no longer taking manufactured baby milk it is recommended that they be given supplemental vitamins A, B, C and D up until the age of 2. They have a high requirement as they are growing rapidly, and supplementation is a precautionary measure as they may not be taking a sufficiently varied diet.

There is no need to give additional vitamins to other children unless recommended to do so by a doctor. Vitamins are sometimes given when a child is run down or is prone to frequent infections, but there is no evidence that they are of any benefit in this situation. If certain vitamins are given in excess they may cause ill health, so vitamins in general must never be given in doses greater than the recommended daily requirements.

Minerals and trace elements

As well as the major nutrients and the vitamins the diet must contain some minerals if the individual is to remain healthy. Sodium and potassium salts are two minerals that are present in most foods in adequate quantities, so are never deficient.

A small amount of dietary iron is needed to prevent anaemia (see page 149). At birth there are iron stores in the body which provide adequate amounts for the first few months of life; this is important as milk contains almost no iron. Babies born before term do not have adequate iron stores so they are given iron supplements. Beyond the first few months iron needs to be present in the diet. The major sources are liver and red meat; some is also found in egg yolk and green vegetables. Some toddlers are reluctant to eat meat and may become anaemic, but iron deficiency is not otherwise common in childhood.

Calcium is needed for the growth of bones. It is present in high quantities in milk and in bread, and also occurs in many other foods. A dietary deficiency of calcium is very rare, but the body cannot absorb it if there is a deficiency of vitamin D.

Other minerals, including zinc and copper, are also necessary for health but are only required in trace amounts; a mixed diet provides adequate amounts of them all.

Dietary fibre

Not all of the food we eat is absorbed into the body; the unabsorbed residue is known as fibre or roughage. Fibre derived from seed husks and plant cell walls is important for providing bulk to the intestinal contents, aiding their propulsion along the bowel. In the large intestine water is absorbed from the intestinal contents so that they become solid. Fibre prevents too much water being reabsorbed which would lead the stools to become hard.

It has been shown that a high-fibre diet can prevent constipation. Other benefits have also been attributed to dietary fibre, including the prevention of obesity, but these are speculative. The food industry has responded to the realization that adequate fibre in the diet is important by modifying its practices. High-fibre breakfast cereals, wholemeal bread, and bread with extra fibre are now readily available. If the diet is mixed and includes vegetables or wholemeal bread it will contain enough fibre.

Intestinal gas is increased with a high-fibre diet, and this can occasionally cause abdominal pain in children who eat high-fibre foods such as muesli or beans.

DIETARY DEFICIENCIES

Various disease states are known to be due to dietary deficiency. Inadequate amounts of the major nutrients give rise to protein calorie malnutrition, marasmus and kwashiorkor, but are fortunately not seen in industrialized societies. Deficiencies of various vitamins can also cause diseases; these conditions are not generally seen in countries where there is adequate food and a varied diet is eaten.

The only dietary deficiencies seen in otherwise healthy children in Westernized societies are iron deficiency anaemia (see page 280) in the toddler who does not eat much meat, and very occasionally rickets due to vitamin D deficiency, where the traditional family diet is low in foods containing the vitamin, and the cultural pattern of the family makes it unlikely that the child will get into the sunlight to synthesize it.

Normal children over the age of 2 who are eating a varied diet do not need to have supplementary vitamins or minerals.

Children with poor appetites due to chronic (long-term) illness, and those on exclusion diets to remove various foods, are prone to dietary deficiencies. Vegetarian diets, diets avoiding food additives and antiallergic diets are by their nature restrictive, and can give rise to dietary deficiency if they are not supervised by a dietitian, and if necessary supplemented by vitamins and minerals.

FOOD ADDITIVES

Various substances may be added to food in its preparation to improve one of the properties of the product. There are thousands of such additives and flavourings; many are derived from natural sources, but some are synthetic. All additives have to be not harmful to health, and new ones have to undergo rigorous testing before they are approved for use.

In view of this testing and the widespread use of additives, it is highly unlikely that they represent a significant health risk for most people. It is possible that a small number of individuals may develop adverse reactions to a particular food additive, in the same way that some people develop reactions to natural foods that others take without harm.

Certain additives have been implicated in hyperactive behaviour in some children (see page 78). Some scientists have found that other food additives may cause various allergic conditions or migraine in some people. The widespread condemnation of all additives as unnatural and therefore by implication bad for you is irrational.

The growth of modern food technology has done much to improve nutritional standards for everyone by ensuring that food is available in adequate amounts, is wholesome and free from micro-organisms that could cause disease, and is not wasted because it is rotting or attacked by pests. Additives are important in various ways of improving the quality of manufactured foods.

The main categories of additive are preservatives, anti-oxidants, emulsifiers and stabilizers, sweeteners and flavour enhancers, and colourings, but there are others, including acids, bases and buffers, flour bleachers, anti-caking agents, and raising and glazing agents. Flavouring agents are also widely used in food preparation, but in quantities much smaller than for other additives. Many flavourings are traditional and they have not all been subjected to the same rigorous testing as have additives.

Food additives have produced great benefits in food preparation. They are carefully controlled, and study of their uses and effects is continuing. Legislation requiring the contents of processed food to be stated on the label makes it easier to know which additives have been included. The European

Community has harmonized the categories and substances approved for use, and designates E numbers to different food additives once they have been fully scrutinized. Patients with allergic or other diseases whose symptoms may be related to a particular additive can avoid those foods which contain it but there is no general reason to remove food additives from the diet.

The function of the main categories of additive are as follows.

Preservatives

These are added to help food keep longer. This prevents wastage through spoiling, gives a longer shelf life, and enables foods to be available out of season. Preservatives also help to prevent some forms of food poisoning by inhibiting the growth of bacteria.

Some preservatives, like salt for meat and sugar in jam, have been in use for centuries, and because they are foods do not count as additives. Other preservatives have been introduced more recently, and include such things as potassium nitrate (saltpetre), sorbic acid, benzoic acid and sulphur dioxide. Almost all foods that keep indefinitely or have a long shelf life will contain preservatives. Such foods include cured and tinned meat, dried and packet foods, bottled foods and many drinks.

Anti-oxidants

These are added to foods made with oils and fats to delay deterioration due to the fat becoming rancid. Ascorbic acid (vitamin C) is a natural anti-oxidant and is sometimes used; there are also synthetic anti-oxidants like butylated hydroxytoluene.

Emulsifiers and stabilizers

Emulsifiers help in the mixing together of fats and watery solutions, and stabilizers prevent them separating again. There are natural emulsifiers in foods like butter, cream and eggs, and most of the emulsifiers and stabilizers used in food production come from natural sources. They include alginates, pectins, gums and cellulose.

Sweeteners and flavour enhancers

Saccharine is an extremely sweet substance so only small amounts are needed to add sweetness to foods and drinks. Mannitol, sorbitol and aspartame are other sweeteners often used in food production. Monosodium glutamate is the main flavour enhancer. It does not have its own flavour, but adds to the taste of the food to which it is added.

Colourings

These improve the appearance of manufactured foods. Many colourings are natural products, such as caramel, curcumin and carotene. There are some permitted artificial colours, and tartrazine, a synthetic orange azo-dye, is one of the most widely used of these. It has been implicated in hyperactive behaviour in some children (see page 78) and there are case reports of a marked improvement in behaviour following its withdrawal. Manufacturers do not use colourings in the preparation of baby foods.

CHOOSING THE RIGHT DIET FOR CHILDREN

The various aspects of a healthy diet are covered in this chapter. Provided that meals are varied, there is no likelihood of dietary deficiencies, and if the variety extends to different types of foods it is unlikely that the consumption of any particular one will be excessive. Children in the home mainly eat the same food as their parents, so a careful diet has benefits for everyone.

It is unnecessary to be obsessional about exactly what is eaten, and if a few simple rules are remembered the detail of the diet can be left to choice. It is important to avoid excess consumption of sugar, as this is the major cause of dental caries, so restriction of children's intake of sweets, cakes and biscuits

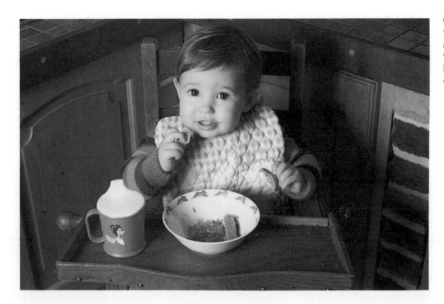

Children begin to express their food preferences at an early age. They need a varied and balanced diet but should be allowed to express some choice.

is wise. Eating too much saturated fat is also probably unhealthy in the long run; the intake of foods containing fat, like meat, cheese and crisps, should be moderate, and frying is best done in polyunsaturated oil. Avoidance of fat and sugar also helps to prevent obesity.

Provided the diet is mixed and includes plenty of fruit and vegetables, fibre intake is likely to be adequate; many breakfast cereals and fibre-enriched bread provide a palatable way of increasing fibre intake if this is thought necessary.

VEGETARIAN DIETS

Eating meat is not necessary for health, and children can stay fit and grow well on a vegetarian diet. However, because the diet is more restricted, the possibility of deficiencies could arise if it is not well balanced nutritionally. Vegetarian diets can be divided into those that avoid meat and fish, but not milk and its products (butter, cheese, and so on). This is sometimes referred to as a lacto-vegetarian diet. If, in addition to this, eggs are also eaten, the diet can be referred to as lacto-ovo-vegetarian. A strictly vegetarian diet, with no meat, fish or animal products, is known as a vegan diet.

Meat is a concentrated source of protein and of calories, both of which are important to the growing child. Milk, cheese and eggs are good alternative sources of protein and calories, and lacto-vegetarian or lacto-ovo-vegetarian diets are perfectly adequate for children. Meat is also an important source of iron, and if the diet is not to be deficient the alternative dietary sources – egg yolk and green vegetables – need to be included.

Vegan, macrobiotic and other diets in which the range of foods eaten is severely restricted pose health threats to young children. A nutritionally planned vegan diet can provide all the necessary nutrients except vitamin B_{12}. While eating a very mixed diet is a protection against dietary deficiencies, any severely restricted diet increases the possibility of deficiency, either of specific nutrients or of total energy content.

The diet may be deficient in available calories. Beans, peas and whole grains are not easy for a young child to digest, and some of the calories consumed pass through the body without being absorbed. Many vegetables and fruits do not contain concentrated

Establishing a healthy pattern of eating early on and avoiding foods with a high sugar or fat content will confer benefits in later life.

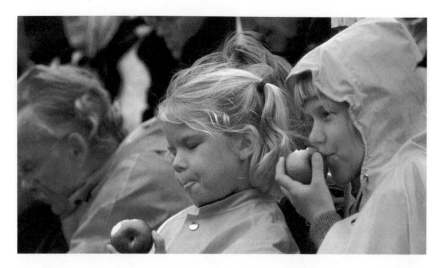

calories, having a high fibre and water content, and therefore large amounts have to be consumed to obtain adequate calories. Children's appetites may be satiated before they have taken in enough calories for adequate growth. Growth is at its most rapid in the first two years of life, and all children on restricted diets should have their height and weight measured regularly to ensure that growth is proceeding normally.

If parents want their child to follow a vegan diet they should ensure that it is adequate for his needs. Advice should be taken from a trained dietitian or the national vegetarian society about what to eat, and whether vitamin supplements are required. Parents may be concerned when an older child decides to become a vegetarian. The child's choice should be respected and parents should help in providing attractive alternatives to meat. Provided cheese and milk are still part of the diet it is likely to be perfectly adequate in nutritional terms.

OBESITY

Food that is eaten but not needed immediately by the body is stored to be used during illness when the appetite is depressed, or in periods of food shortage. Most of this extra food is stored as fat. Obesity means an excess amount of body fat. Whether or not obesity is present can be reliably judged by appearance: if children look fat it is likely that they are obese. There are various scientific definitions of obesity. The simplest is when an individual is more than 20 per cent over ideal weight for height. The range of 10–20 per cent over ideal weight for height is referred to as overweight.

Babies born before 36 weeks of gestation have very little body fat. During infancy there is a gradual increase in the amount of fat, so that the face and body become more rounded, and at around 1 year of age many toddlers are obese. A change in body shape occurs during the pre-school years, with children becoming leaner and more muscular. During this time obesity is less common. This pattern persists until puberty, when in all girls there is a general increase in body fat as well as fat deposition around the breasts and hips; there is no general increase in body fat with puberty in boys. Obesity is more common during adolescence than in mid-childhood and more likely in girls than boys.

Obesity in childhood can cause a variety of problems. In very overweight babies the extra fat around the trunk causes some restriction of chest movement. They are prone to attacks of respiratory infection, and may develop wheezing with them.

At all ages obesity impedes movement. The extra weight means that obese children tire more quickly when walking long distances, run more slowly than non-obese children, and become breathless sooner. The physical bulk of the limbs and body may make performing some movements difficult, and obese children may be clumsy.

One of the biggest problems of obesity for children is that they are teased and made fun of by their peers. For many of them this leads to great unhappiness, and as obesity is difficult to treat, this may be ongoing.

Obesity that starts in childhood often persists throughout life. The problems of mobility remain; for some the condition brings social isolation, and in later adult life obesity predisposes to difficulties with the joints and the locomotor system, which enables us to move around, and with blood pressure.

There is no full explanation as to why children may become obese. Some definitely overeat, but others do not obviously eat more than lean children of the same age. Differences in body metabolism may account for why some are more prone to obesity. Children vary in how active they are, and those who are relatively inactive may not use up as much food energy as others. Children of obese parents often become obese themselves and genetic factors may also play a part.

Even though obesity is not fully understood, parents have an important role in its prevention. Obesity occurs because more food is being taken in than the body needs for daily energy. Attention should be paid both to the amount and to the types of food in the diet.

For babies, starting solid foods early has been shown to be associated with an increased incidence of obesity. There is never a need for solids before 3 months and for most babies 5 or 6 months is the best age to begin (see page 47).

Meals given to children should be filling but they do not need to be excessive. Three meals in the day are adequate, and if tea or an evening meal has been eaten there is no need for a supper before bed. Eating between meals is to be discouraged.

Although adequate calories are needed to satisfy appetite, bulk is important too. Sweets, which are almost pure sugar, provide a lot of calories but are not filling as they only have a small bulk. Other foods with a high calorie concentration but little bulk can also lead to excess consumption: examples are very sugary foods, fried foods and crisps, which are fattening if eaten frequently. Conversely, many vegetables like carrots, beans and other green vegetables have a high bulk for the calories they contain.

It is important for children to eat a mixed and balanced diet, and some foods should be given only as occasional treats.

Treating obesity is difficult, and the aim should be to establish a more healthy pattern of eating and lifestyle rather than to achieve rapid weight loss. Even after a period of dieting the pounds will be rapidly regained if children then return to their previous pattern of eating.

The quantity of food energy (calories) eaten has to be significantly reduced, and this is likely to be best achieved by the avoidance of foods with a high sugar or fat content, cutting out snacks between meals, and the adoption of a more active lifestyle. Children should not be started on a reducing diet without professional guidance, and if you are worried about your child's weight you should consult your family doctor.

Sticking to a reducing diet requires high motivation on the part of both child and parents. This is often lacking in young children who are not much concerned by their own appearance, and attempts to restrict their diet are almost doomed to failure. If a child is on a restricted diet other family members must eat similar food.

POOR APPETITE

A sudden loss of appetite may well signal the beginning of an illness or be the result of an emotional upset. If the cause is not soon apparent parents need to consult the doctor to try to find out the reason.

More of a problem are those children who cause their parents longstanding concern because they do not seem to eat enough. It is important to distinguish children who dislike certain foods but who will eat plenty of the things they like, from those who never seem to eat well. A child whose favourite foods are fish fingers, sausages, baked beans and chips and who is reluctant to eat other meat and vegetables may seem a problem to his parents, but if he is left within limits to choose his own diet, and the whole family does not have to conform to eating only what he likes, then it is probably better to accept the situation than to make it a cause of tension or friction. People's tastes vary as they grow older. Many small children do not like meat because it requires a lot of chewing but will very happily eat processed or minced meat. As children mature, savoury flavours are likely to have greater appeal, and the range of foods eaten will be extended.

Children who always have a small appetite and never seem to eat enough can be a worry. Mealtimes are often dreaded on both sides, parents coaxing or forcing food on the child, and the child slow and reluctant to eat anything. Such a situation needs to be defused. Children with small appetites will not eat more just because they are pressured.

They are more likely to eat less, as emotional tension takes away the appetite.

When a parent feels a child is eating poorly the first essential is to find out whether the child's food intake is adequate. There is a great variation between the amounts different children need: some are always hungry, while others eat very little. If growth is normal and the child has plenty of energy, then food intake overall is adequate, no matter how small it seems at times.

Satisfying a hungry child's demand for food strengthens the bond between parent and child. If a child is reluctant to eat and rejects food his parents can feel rejected too. Insecurity can fuel a parent's anxiety over a child who has a small appetite. The healthy child with a small appetite is still dependent on his parents' care and love, and so the situation should be accepted and not perceived in emotive terms.

If a child has a poor appetite and is not growing as well as he should there may be an underlying cause that is not apparent, and the doctor should be consulted.

Recommended calorie requirements for children

Age in years	Calories per kg body weight per day	Average calories per day for age group
Girls		
		Wide variation with
Under 1	100–130	age and weight
1–3	100	1,300
3–6	90	1,600
6–9	85	2,100
9–12	65	2,200
12–15	55	2,500
15–18	45	2,300
Boys		
		Wide variation with
Under 1	100–130	age and weight
1–3	100	1,300
3–6	90	1,600
6–9	85	2,100
9–12	75	2,400
12–15	65	3,000
15–18	45	3,400

GENETICS AND INHERITANCE

Heredity – that is, the transmission of physical or behavioural characteristics from parent to child – has always been a source of mystery and fascination. The developments that have occurred in genetics and molecular biology over the last thirty years have led to an enormous increase in understanding how genetic information is passed from parent to offspring, and how genes bring about growth and development from a fertilized egg into a complete human being. As more is

understood about the mechanism of heredity, interest and wonder have increased.

The physical and physiological similarities between every member of the human species are genetically determined, as are many of the variations between individuals. Such things as physical appearance and intellectual ability are largely inherent, and other characteristics, such as aptitudes and personality, have a genetic element.

There are also some diseases which are genetically determined, or which have a strong genetic component. As diseases due to infection and dietary deficiencies are becoming less common in childhood in the Western world, genetic diseases are assuming a greater importance. It is estimated that around 20 per cent of hospital admissions for children are for diseases which are partly or wholly genetic, and genetic disease is a major factor in about half of all childhood deaths.

THE PRINCIPLES OF INHERITANCE

Each cell of the body has a nucleus which contains chromosomes. There are normally forty-six chromosomes, arranged in twenty-three pairs. When viewed through a micro-

Chromosomes from a single cell, as seen through the microscope when prepared for analysis. Each strand-like chromosome is made up of numerous genes.

scope, each chromosome can be identified by its length and physical characteristics. Each consists of hundreds of genes joined together to form a thread made up of a material called DNA, or deoxyribonucleic acid. Because the chromosomes are paired, each gene also has a pair. A single pair of genes is concerned with the inheritance of one of an individual's characteristics. The gene is thus the basic unit of inheritance.

A gene pair may determine the structure of a particular protein, or an enzyme, or eye colour, or may influence the shape of the nose or the number of fingers. As there are so many different characteristics involved in an individual's make-up, there are many thousands of different genes.

For many inherited characteristics the genes in a pair will be identical, but the make-up of some genes does vary; this variation is the basis of the inherited differences between individuals. When an individual has a pair of genes that are different they may both have an equal influence in determining a particular characteristic, or the effect of one of them may predominate. In comparing a child's physical appearance to that of her parents, some features will resemble one parent more than the other, others will be a mixture between the two, and yet others will be unique to the child and not present in either parent, even though that feature might have been determined by genes passed on from each parent.

Some characteristics, such as skin colour, height and intellectual potential, are not the product of a single gene pair, but are influenced by the interaction of several different pairs of genes.

Although body cells normally contain twenty-three pairs of chromosomes, these pairs split in the formation of the germ cells — ova (eggs) and sperms — so that the nucleus of each sperm and ovum contains twenty-three

single chromosomes. At the moment of conception, when a sperm fertilizes an ovum, the chromosomes from the father and the chromosomes from the mother join together, so that the fertilized ovum has forty-six chromosomes. From this will develop all the other body cells. The genetic material in the fertilized ovum comes equally from both parents and is blended together in a combination which is unique. This fertilized ovum has the potential to grow first into an embryo, then a fetus, then a baby, and so on through all the stages of life.

The genes that are inherited at the moment of conception control and influence the development, growth, intelligence, character and health of individuals throughout the whole of their lives. A person's genetic make-up is therefore of fundamental importance. There has been great progress in understanding how genes work over the last few years and along with this new knowledge have come new insights into the roles played by genes in the causation of some diseases. Genetic diseases can result from an abnormality affecting a chromosome, or a single gene pair, or sometimes several genes together.

CHROMOSOMAL DISORDERS

Each body cell normally contains twenty-three pairs of chromosomes, and each ovum and sperm contains twenty-three unpaired chromosomes. Sometimes there are errors in the cell division that leads to the formation of the ova or the sperms, so that instead of containing twenty-three chromosomes they may either have some extra chromosomal material or some may be missing. If such an ovum becomes fertilized, or such a sperm fertilizes an ovum, the resultant fertilized ovum will have an abnormal chromosomal comple-

How a child's sex is determined

The chromosomes are arranged in twenty-three pairs, and for twenty-two of these the genes carried on each of the pair control the same factors. Each of these chromosomes is separately identifiable through a microscope, and they are numbered from 1 to 22. The remaining pair of chromosomes, known as the sex chromosomes, is special. The sex chromosomes determine the child's sex, and there are two sorts, known as X and Y. There may be two X-chromosomes, in which case the individual is female. Alternatively, if there is one X-chromosome and one Y-chromosome, the individual will be male. For the sex chromosomes, therefore, the genes will be paired in the female, who has two X-chromosomes (usually written as XX); in the male, who has one X- and one Y-chromosome (written XY), the genes on the sex chromosomes are unpaired.

As a female has a pair of X-chromosomes and no Y-chromosomes, her ova will contain all X-chromosomes. Sperms, however, will either contain an X- or a Y-chromosome. If an X-containing sperm fertilizes an ovum, the resulting individual will have two X-chromosomes and will be female, whereas if a Y-containing sperm fertilizes the ovum the resulting individual will have one X- and one Y-chromosome and will be male.

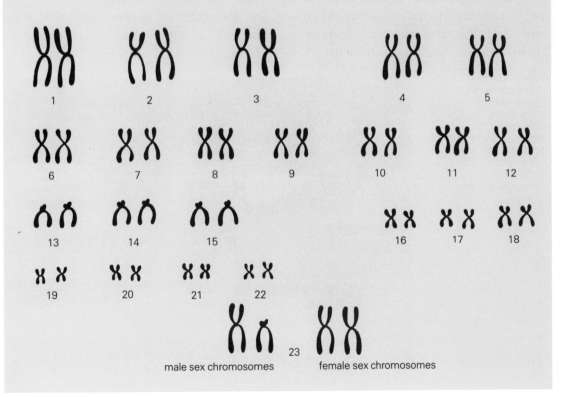

male sex chromosomes   23   female sex chromosomes

ment, and this is likely to have serious effects.

Many chromosomal abnormalities interfere with the normal development of the embryo, and as a result the embryo dies and there is a miscarriage. Some chromosomal disorders are compatible with life, but the affected individual is likely to have some abnormalities; as a chromosome contains many different genes, the abnormalities may be very severe. Down's syndrome was the first disease that was found to be due to a chromosomal abnormality, but as the techniques for looking at chromosomes have improved, many other chromosomal disorders have been discovered.

Down's syndrome

People with Down's syndrome have extra chromosome material from chromosome 21 in all their body cells. Usually they have three chromosome 21s, instead of two, and this condition is known as trisomy 21. In a few patients there is a normal pair of chromosome 21s, but also an extra part of a 21-chromosome joined on to one of the other chromosomes, usually chromosome 14. This is known as a translocation.

When ova or sperms are formed in the ovary or testis by the division of precursor cells, all the chromosome pairs in the precursor cell split so that normally twenty-three single chromosomes go into each germ cell. If, instead of the 21-pair separating, both go into one germ cell, that cell will have an extra 21-chromosome. If such a cell fuses in fertilization with another germ cell that has twenty-three chromosomes as normal, the chromosomal make-up of the fertilized ovum will be a trisomy 21, with a total of forty-seven chromosomes in each cell, instead of forty-six.

We do not know what goes wrong when the chromosome 21 pair stay together and both go into a single germ cell instead of separating; nor do we know why trisomy 21 is more common in the offspring of older mothers. The overall incidence of Down's syndrome is about 1 in every 700 births, the incidence in mothers aged 20 being about 1 in every 2,000 births, and in mothers aged 40 about 1 in 100 births. The

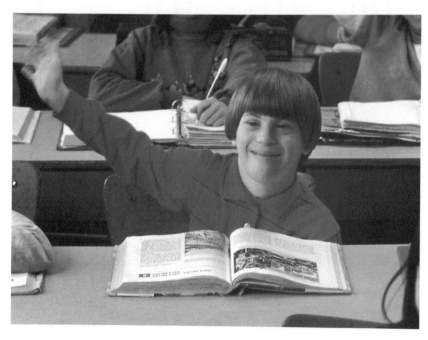

In Down's syndrome each cell in the body has an extra chromosome 21 which causes developmental problems. Down's syndrome children need extra stimulation and encouragement to help improve their developmental progress.

risk of having a baby with Down's syndrome remains low for mothers throughout their twenties and early thirties, but rises rapidly above the age of 35. Down's syndrome can be detected by performing chorionic villus sampling or amniocentesis in early pregnancy (see page 15), and in many antenatal centres this service is offered to all mothers over the age of 35. If the fetus is found to be affected an abortion can be performed, if the mother wishes.

Although the other type of Down's syndrome, known as a translocation, only occurs in about 5 per cent of people with Down's syndrome it is important that it is recognized. A parent of a child with a translocation Down's syndrome may himself or herself have a chromosomal translocation, with one of the 21-chromosomes attached to chromosome 14. If there is only one other chromosome 21 there is no excess chromosomal material and the translocation is said to be balanced; the individual will be normal. People with balanced translocations are at very high risk of having children with Down's syndrome.

Chromosomes are studied in all children born with Down's syndrome, and if a translocation is found the parents' chromosomes are also checked. They can then be advised whether or not they have a balanced translocation, and whether there is a high risk of recurrence of Down's syndrome in a further pregnancy.

The features of Down's syndrome are described on page 259.

Other chromosomal diseases

In Down's syndrome there is an extra chromosome in each cell, and this causes widespread effects in the body. Trisomies of other chromosomes may also occur, but most are incompatible with life, and the pregnancy ends in a miscarriage. Trisomies of chromo-

somes 13 and 18 do crop up, but are fortunately rare as the children have multiple problems and do not survive for very long after birth.

In some uncommon conditions there is an extra part of a chromosome in each cell. This has effects on various organs and parts of the body, often causing an unusual appearance and some degree of mental handicap.

Some diseases are due to chromosomal deletions, missing chromosomal material, as opposed to extra material. Errors in cell division in the formation of the germ cell, or in very early embryonic development, give rise to these problems. The absence of a complete chromosome usually causes such major abnormalities that the pregnancy ends early in a miscarriage.

The exception is a condition of girls where the X-chromosome is missing, which is known as Turner's syndrome. Because the X-chromosome contains a relatively small number of genes, the abnormalities due to the absence of one X-chromosome in a girl are compatible with life; sometimes the associated abnormalities are not even apparent in early life. Short stature and failure to develop proper ovaries are constant features of the syndrome, and there may also be associated congenital heart disease. Other features are relatively minor. Turner's syndrome is often only diagnosed when investigations are undertaken for short stature, or for delayed or incomplete puberty.

Other chromosomal deletions affecting only part of a chromosome also occur. Apart from Down's syndrome and Turner's syndrome, chromosomal diseases are individually rare. However, as there are forty-six chromosomes in which abnormalities can occur, the group of chromosomal disorders is correspondingly large.

Chromosomes are often examined in children who have multiple congenital abnormalities or unexplained mental handicap, because chromosomal abnormalities can sometimes account for such conditions.

GENETIC DISEASES

The genes are the basic units of inheritance. Each pair of genes in an individual is responsible for a single inherited characteristic, and the genes in a pair may be identical or may be different. Genetic variation explains why every individual is different at birth. Characteristics such as facial features, intellectual potential, and eye or skin colour are largely genetically determined.

Where the genes in a gene pair are different, the effect of one may predominate over the other, or they may both have equal effect. There is a single gene pair that determines eye colour, and there are different genes for brown and for blue eyes. An individual with two 'brown-eye' genes will have brown eyes, and one with two 'blue-eye' genes will have blue eyes. Somebody with one 'brown-eye' and one 'blue-eye' gene will have brown eyes. The 'brown-eye' gene is said to be dominant, and the 'blue-eye' gene is recessive.

An individual with brown eyes may have either one or two 'brown-eye' genes, but an individual with blue eyes must have two 'blue-eye' genes. Thus for dominant features

Members of the same family share many of the same genes. This often shows in facial resemblance, but may also lead to similarities in body configuration and metabolism.

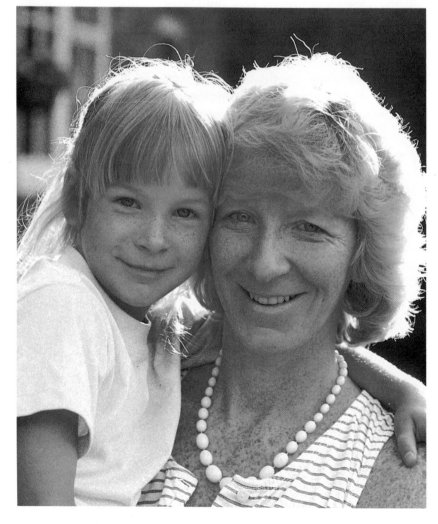

or conditions it is only necessary to have one causal gene, inherited from one parent, while for recessive characteristics two causal genes are needed, one from each parent.

Genetic variation for such things as facial appearance or skin colour leads to individuals being different, but does not affect health. Some genes, however, can have effects that cause disease. Such harmful genes may be either dominant or recessive. Where a harmful recessive gene is carried on the X-chromosome in the female it will have a dominant normal gene as its pair on the other X-chromosome. In the male, however, as there is only one X-chromosome, a single harmful recessive gene on the X-chromosome will exert its effect. Genetic diseases are therefore divided into dominant, recessive and sex-linked conditions, depending on their mode of inheritance.

Genes are passed down from parent to offspring from generation to generation, and usually remain unchanged themselves. From time to time, however, a gene may be altered, and have a different effect. This is known as a mutation. Once a mutation has occurred, it can then be transmitted to future generations.

Dominantly inherited diseases

Diseases inherited in a dominant manner are caused by an individual having a single harmful dominant gene, which was passed from one of the parents or, less commonly, which arose in that individual because of a new mutation. Many dominantly inherited diseases do not manifest their effect until adult life.

When a parent has a dominantly inherited condition there is a 50 per cent risk of passing it on to each child; the child inherits one of the pair of genes concerned, which may be either the dominant, disease-causing gene or the recessive, normal gene.

The most common serious dominant disease is familial hypercholesterolaemia (see page 265), affecting about 1 in every 300 of the population. A biochemical abnormality is inherited, so that affected individuals have a very high blood cholesterol (cholesterol is a fatty substance present in the blood); this persists throughout life. As adults, affected individuals are prone to the development of premature coronary heart disease, and in many a heart attack is the first sign that they have a problem.

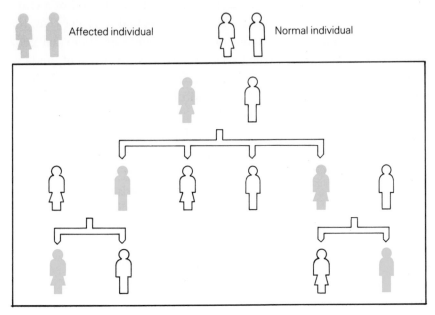

Affected individual   Normal individual

In dominantly inherited conditions individuals with one abnormal gene have the disease and are likely to pass it on to about 50 per cent of their offspring.

Other dominantly inherited diseases include Huntington's disease or chorea (see page 276), neurofibromatosis, myotonic dystrophy and Friedreich's ataxia, which are all rare neurological conditions in which symptoms usually do not develop until adulthood.

If a dominant disease has serious effects in childhood, affected individuals are less likely to have children of their own when they grow up. The condition would therefore tend to die out after a few generations, and in such cases there is often a high mutation rate. Achondroplasia is a form of short-limbed short stature which is dominantly inherited (see page 229). People affected by it may have children, of whom half on average will also have achondroplasia. In practice affected individuals often do not have children, and new mutations account for a significant number of new cases of achondroplasia.

Recessively inherited diseases

Recessively inherited disorders only occur in individuals who have two affected genes, one inherited from each parent. People with a single harmful recessive gene will not have the disease, and probably will not know that they are carrying the gene. As the gene is recessive, a normal gene present as one of the gene pair has the dominant effect, and the individual develops normally.

It is estimated that most people probably carry some genes from recessive disorders, but the risk of them marrying someone carrying the same gene is normally small, unless the marriage is consanguineous (between blood relatives). The most common serious recessive disease is cystic fibrosis (see page 255), and only in about 1 in 500 couples do both individuals carry the harmful gene. A couple do not usually know that they are both carriers of a harmful gene until they have an affected child.

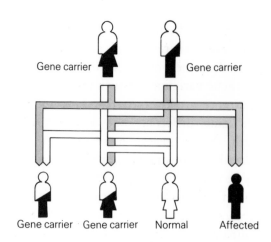

Gene carrier — Gene carrier

Gene carrier — Gene carrier — Normal — Affected

In recessively inherited diseases affected individuals have a pair of abnormal genes, one inherited from the father and one from the mother.

Individuals with only a single abnormal gene are carriers for the condition but are themselves unaffected.

Where a couple are both carriers, the risk of having a child affected by the disease is 25 per cent, or 1 in 4. Half of the ova of the mother and half of the sperms of the father will carry the harmful gene, and so the possible combinations in the resulting offspring are as follows: children may have a normal gene from each parent; one normal and one abnormal gene; or an affected gene from each parent. The likelihood of a child having both genes normal is 25 per cent; for having one normal and one abnormal gene (the carrier state) it is 50 per cent; and, as stated above, the risk of both genes being abnormal and of the child being affected is 25 per cent.

If a couple have already had one affected child, the likelihood of the condition recurring in further offspring is thus very high. The couple should take advice from a paediatrician or genetic counsellor about what the risks are, and whether they can be modified.

Sex-linked disorders

Sex-linked disorders are due to abnormal recessive genes carried on the X-chromo-

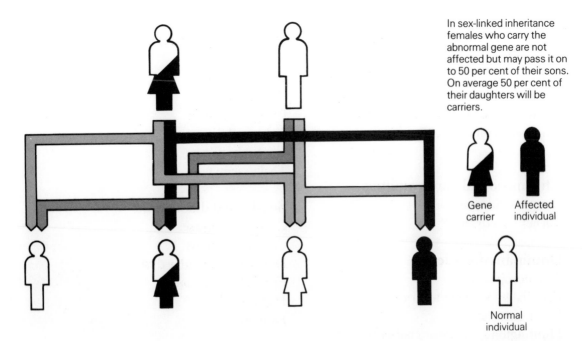

In sex-linked inheritance females who carry the abnormal gene are not affected but may pass it on to 50 per cent of their sons. On average 50 per cent of their daughters will be carriers.

Gene carrier

Affected individual

Normal individual

some. In women the effect of this gene is cancelled by a normal gene on the other X-chromosome, but in males, who have only one X-chromosome, the action of the abnormal gene is unopposed and causes the disease. Haemophilia, Duchenne muscular dystrophy (see pages 271 and 287), and a form of severe mental deficiency called fragile-X syndrome are inherited in this way.

If a woman is a carrier for the condition, there is a 50 per cent risk that a son will have the disease, as she can pass on either the normal or the abnormal gene. Similarly, 50 per cent of her daughters will be carriers for the condition.

A woman may know she is likely to be a carrier if she has had a brother affected with one of the sex-linked diseases, and for several of the X-chromosome-linked conditions it is possible to test for the carrier status. Sometimes sex-linked recessive disorders arise because of new mutations.

Polygenic disorders
Dominant, recessive and sex-linked patterns of inheritance apply for characteristics which are determined by a single gene pair. Other conditions may run in families, but do not follow one of these patterns, as the characteristic depends on more than one gene pair.

Skin colour is a characteristic which is influenced by several pairs of genes, so that instead of there just being black and white, all shades of skin colour can be seen.

Diseases in which several gene pairs play a part are known as polygenic disorders. For such disorders an individual will inherit a tendency to develop the condition which may be weak or strong. If the tendency is strong the disease will occur. This pattern of inheritance applies to atopic asthma, congenital pyloric stenosis and to cleft palate (see pages 153, 164 and 251). In some polygenic diseases the inherited tendency only gives rise to the disease if there are also adverse environmental factors. For example, spina bifida, a failure of fusion of the lower spine (see page 301), in many cases seems to be due to a genetic predisposition together with nutritional deficiencies of the mother in early pregnancy.

Some common genetic diseases

The disorders not described in this chapter can be found in the A-Z section, which starts on page 228.

Chromosomal abnormalities
Down's syndrome
Turner's syndrome

Dominant disorders
Achondroplasia
Familial hypercholesterolaemia
Friedreich's ataxia
Huntington's disease or chorea
Marfan's syndrome
Myotonic dystrophy
Neurofibromatosis
Polycystic kidneys (some forms)

Recessive disorders
Albinism
Cystic fibrosis
Galactosaemia
Phenylketonuria
Sickle cell disease
Tay-Sachs disease
Thalassaemia

Sex-linked disorders
Christmas disease
Colour blindness
Duchenne muscular dystrophy
Fragile-X syndrome
Haemophilia
Icthyosis

Polygenic disorders
Cleft palate
Congenital pyloric stenosis
Spina bifida

Treating genetic disease

In the future it may be possible in some conditions to implant normal genes into the body to replace defective ones. This cannot yet be done, although with present-day advances in molecular biology it could be feasible in the near future. Already organ and marrow transplants have been used experimentally to try to correct some inherited disorders of body chemistry.

Even though it is not yet possible to replace defective genes, many genetic disorders can be treated. The commonest genetic disorder, familial hypercholesterolaemia (see page 265), is diagnosable in childhood in affected families, and the child can be put on cholesterol-lowering treatment which, if continued, will delay the onset of coronary heart disease in adult life. Newborn screening for phenylketonuria (see page 291) is carried out because, if this condition is diagnosed early, the patient can be given dietary treatment: even though the defective enzyme persists, the build-up of the amino acid phenylalanine in the blood is prevented, and the child does not develop a severe mental handicap. Cystic fibrosis (see page 255) used to be characterized by death in early childhood. Nowadays, with good treatment of the lung and digestive problems available, many patients are surviving into adult life.

Both the severity of a genetic condition and whether it is treatable are important aspects to be considered in making decisions about planning a family when there is the possibility of genetic disease; these are some of the factors that a paediatrician or genetic counsellor (see next page) will be able to discuss with you.

CONGENITAL ABNORMALITIES

A baby may be born with abnormalities that are not due to chromosomal disorders or to defective genes. Problems can occur in the development of the embryo or the fetus that give rise to congenital abnormalities.

The factors known to be potentially harmful to the growing embryo in early pregnancy include dietary deficiencies, some infections (particularly rubella or German measles), alcohol, other toxins, medications and ionizing radiation (X-rays), as discussed on page 8. Such harmful influences at the time the major organs of the body are being formed may cause significant developmental abnormalities, producing effects such as congenital heart disease, cleft palate (see pages 146 and 251) and neurological mal-development. Even after twelve weeks, when the major organs are formed and the embryo becomes a fetus, adverse events can affect growth and development. Infections, alcohol and irradiation are still amongst the hazards.

For many congenital abnormalities there is as yet no indication of what goes wrong in pregnancy; the conditions are not obviously inherited, and none of the known hazardous risks seems to apply. Parents with a handicapped baby want to know why it happened. A geneticist will be happy to discuss this and may be able to find a cause, but in many cases the reason remains unknown.

Congenital abnormalities are described individually in the A-Z section, which begins on page 228.

GENETIC COUNSELLING

With any pregnancy there is a risk of producing a child who has a genetic disorder or congenital abnormality. Between 1 and 2 per cent of babies have a genetic or congenital disorder, which is a relatively small proportion but not insignificant. In some situations however, the risk may be very much higher. Where a couple feel that they may be at an increased risk of having a child with a serious disorder of this kind, they may benefit from discussing their situation with a genetic counsellor.

Genetic counselling should be available for any couple who have had a child with a genetic disease or congenital abnormality, or where there is a family history of such problems, or where either prospective parent has such a disease. Couples who are blood relatives, such as cousins, and who are contemplating starting a family may also want to seek advice.

The aim of genetic counselling is to inform an individual or a couple of the likelihood of a genetic disease occurring in their children or the offspring of other family members. They also need to be advised about the particular disease and its severity, and whether there are effective treatments. Where there is a high risk of a couple having a child with a significant abnormality it may be possible to reduce the risk, and this will also need to be talked over. The counsellor will then discuss all this information with the couple to help them to understand and come to terms with it, so that they can then make their own informed decisions as to whether to embark on a pregnancy.

An accurate diagnosis has to precede genetic counselling, so it will be necessary for the counsellor to obtain a full family history, with as many medical details as possible of any congenital or genetic disease in the family, and medical information on any relatives who died of disease in childhood, including the results of an autopsy if it was carried out.

Reducing the risks

The desire to have children of one's own is often very strong, and many couples will decide to go ahead even when they know the risk of problems is high and the potential disease is serious. In many situations there are ways that the risk can be lowered. The options available depend both on the disease itself, and on the form of inheritance. Some of the choices that are technically available will not be acceptable to all couples on personal or ethical grounds.

For an increasing number of genetic diseases it is possible to determine early in pregnancy whether a particular fetus is affected by a particular disease, either by studying fetal tissue obtained by chorionic villus sampling or amniocentesis, or by using ultrasound (see pages 13 and 15). Of the relatively common conditions this can be done for chromosomal disorders, spina bifida, sickle cell disease, thalassaemia and muscular dystrophy, but there are also very many other conditions in which these techniques can be used. If a serious disorder is detected early in pregnancy abortion is an option which many couples would find preferable to having a child with a severe handicap.

Where both partners are the carriers of a serious recessive gene, the risk of having an affected child is 1 in 4, and when the father carries a harmful dominant gene the risk is 1 in 2. These are very high odds, and some couples will feel that artificial insemination of the woman by an anonymous donor would be a better alternative than either childlessness or the risk of having an affected child.

As already discussed, it may soon be possible, with the advances that are taking place in genetics, to insert a normal gene into a fetus in place of a defective one, and thus to treat the underlying condition. Genetic advances are currently very rapid, and couples who need genetic advice should ask the family doctor to refer them to a specialized geneticist to make sure the information they are given is up to date.

Genetic counselling is always tailored to individuals, as every couple's situation is unique. Clinical geneticists have both the technical knowledge to inform the couple and the sensitivity to deal with the anxieties and needs of those seeking advice. They are there to support people and help them to make their own decisions and not to advise on any particular course of action.

COUSIN MARRIAGE

Cousin marriages, and other marriages between relatives, carry an increased risk of producing children with genetic disorders. The reason for this is that cousins have many identical genes, as they have each inherited some of their genes from the pair of grandparents they have in common.

With recessively inherited conditions both parents are themselves healthy, but both carry a single harmful gene. Most recessive disorders are rare, and being a carrier for the disorder is also uncommon, so that the chance of both partners having the same harmful gene is unlikely unless they are related. In marriages between first cousins, where there is no family history of an inherited condition, the risk of having a child with a recessive disorder is not high, but is higher than for the general population. However, in cultures where consanguineous marriage has been common for generations, cousins will have even more genes in common with each other than do cousins in families where there has not been previous intermarriage, and the danger will be somewhat greater.

Related couples who are thinking of having children may wish to talk over with a geneticist whether there are significantly increased risks in their particular case.

CHAPTER

9

INFECTIOUS DISEASES AND THEIR PREVENTION

Children today are much healthier, and childhood mortality is much lower, than fifty years ago. The reductions in the frequency and severity of serious infection are largely due to the introduction of immunizations and antibiotics, and to improvements in public health and nutrition.

The resulting improvement in health can lead to complacency about the need to prevent infection. Infections are still a major cause of illness in childhood, and the threat of serious infection is always present. Parents can help to protect their children from infection by having them fully immunized and bringing them up in a home where hygiene is a way of life, and by keeping them away from infectious diseases where possible. This chapter is about these important measures; information about the diseases themselves can be found in the A-Z section, which starts on page 228.

Infections are due to the invasion of the body by disease-causing micro-organisms. The common micro-organisms are bacteria and viruses, but infections are also caused by

fungi, or by protozoa (microscopic animals). Not all microbial organisms are harmful. The mouth, nose, intestines and skin all harbour bacteria which normally cause no harm; these are known as the normal flora for that part of the body.

Infections may spread in food and drink, through wounds or by direct or indirect contact with a person who has an infection. Straightforward measures can lessen the likelihood of children developing infection in each of these ways, and immunization can reduce the susceptibility of the individual to specific infections.

IMMUNIZATIONS IN CHILDHOOD

Individuals can acquire immunity to certain infectious diseases by being inoculated with live but harmless strains of particular micro-organisms, or by extracts of killed bacteria. As a result of this inoculation the body produces specific antibodies against the organism, and the person is protected from catching that particular infection. This immunity is long-lasting, provided the full course of injections is given. Because such immunizations prime the body to make its own antibodies whenever there is exposure to the infection, the procedure is known as active immunization.

Passive immunity to certain diseases can be induced for a few weeks by injecting antibodies themselves. This is used to protect against specific exposure to a serious infection. Gamma globulin is the fraction of the blood that contains antibodies, and gamma globulin injections may be used to give passive protection against hepatitis, or to children with immune deficiencies when they are exposed to chickenpox or measles.

Immunizing children protects them from specific infections. If enough children in the

Immunization against polio, using drops of the vaccine into the mouth.

Doses are given at intervals between the ages of 2 months and 18 years.

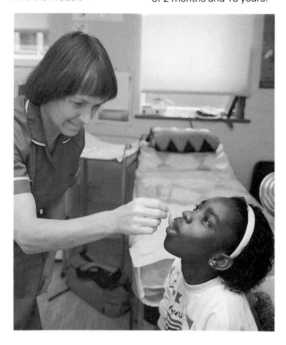

population are immunized, the chances of an epidemic developing are reduced, because epidemic spread occurs only when there are a large number of susceptible individuals in the population. It follows that if most people are immunized, even the unimmunized get some protection.

In many parts of the world, the recommended immunizations to be given to all children (unless there are specific contra-indications – see next page) protect against poliomyelitis, diphtheria, measles, mumps, whooping cough (pertussis), tetanus, rubella (German measles) and tuberculosis.

Poliomyelitis and diphtheria used to cause much death and disability in childhood and fortunately have now been almost entirely eradicated from developed countries. They could, however, become serious health risks again if immunization rates dropped. Furthermore, with increasing affluence more people are holidaying in parts of the world which have poor preventative health services, and

where poliomyelitis or diphtheria still pose a major risk for the unimmunized, whether child or adult.

Measles, mumps and whooping cough remain serious and unpleasant infections. Although recovery is usually complete, some children are left with permanent after-effects, and each year there are a small number of deaths.

Tetanus is a potentially fatal disease that damages the nervous system and provokes muscle spasms; it is caused by wound contamination by dirt or soil containing the tetanus bacterium. As dirt is introduced into wounds in many accidents, and as accidents are unpredictable, all individuals should have a course of tetanus immunizations; a booster injection after accidents in later life then gives full immunity.

Rubella (German measles) is a trivial infection, except to the developing embryo. When mothers are infected with rubella in early pregnancy the fetus may sustain damage to the brain, eyes, ears or heart, and the baby may be born seriously handicapped. When rubella immunization was first introduced it was only given to females, as rubella caused no direct harm to males. The policy has been changed and boys and girls are now both immunized, as it is considered preferable to try to eradicate rubella completely. Previously the unimmunized males enabled rubella to spread, and unprotected pregnant women were still giving birth to rubella-damaged babies.

The BCG (bacille Calmette-Guérin) vaccine used to safeguard against tuberculosis gives some protection against infection, but this protection is not complete. It does, however, alter the body's immune system so that if tuberculosis is contracted later the bacteria are likely to remain localized in one part of the body and not to spread to cause meningitis and other disease elsewhere.

Many of the immunizations are given together, to reduce the number of attendances needed to give full protection. Immunization schedules usually start at 3 months of age, as before that the infant does not have a full protective response to the vaccine. Courses can begin later than the ages recommended in the schedule on page 116.

Contra-indications

Live vaccines (polio, BCG, measles, rubella) should not be given to children who are on high-dose steroid treatment, or who have an immune deficiency disease, or who are having treatment for leukaemia or any other malignant disease which might suppress their immunity.

Allergy is not a contra-indication to immunization, but a previous violent reaction to egg is a contra-indication to measles and mumps vaccine.

A serious reaction to a previous dose of the same vaccine is a contra-indication; mild reactions are not. You should discuss any reaction with the doctor, and ask advice on whether the course should continue.

Whooping cough immunization is occasionally contra-indicated in children with brain damage, or who have had convulsions, or where there is a strong family history of epilepsy (see page 262). Each case should be considered individually by the doctor. Although the risk of immunization may be slightly higher in such patients, the effect of the disease itself is also likely to be more severe.

Immunization should be postponed if a child is suffering from any acute illness, but should be carried out as soon as he has recovered.

Reactions

All injected vaccines are likely to cause the limb injected to be slightly sore. A small hard lump may be noted in the area of the injection for a few days, and occasionally it will be red and swollen. Only if this is severe is it necessary to consult your doctor.

A mild fever on the night following an immunization is not uncommon, and may be accompanied by slight malaise (a general feeling of being unwell). This does not require treatment, and soon improves. Measles immunization is an attenuated form of the virus, and may give rise to minor symptoms including malaise, fever and a rash 5–10 days after immunization. This is much less severe than natural measles and

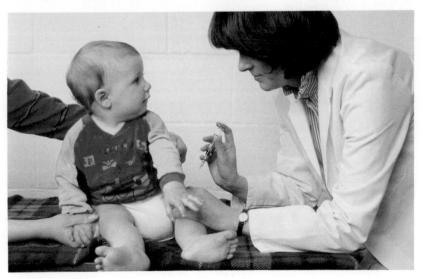

Routine immunization protects children against many common serious diseases. It is important that the full course is given, otherwise the effectiveness of the vaccine is undermined.

The common childhood infections

Disease	Incubation	Contagious period
Chickenpox	11–21 days	From 24 hours before onset of spots until all spots are scabbed, usually about a week after onset of the rash
Gastro-enteritis	2–36 hours	Variable depending on causative micro-organism
Infectious hepatitis (jaundice)	2–6 weeks	From a few days before to seven days after the onset of jaundice
Measles	10–15 days	From a few days before to five days after onset of rash
Mumps	14–26 days	From a few days before the onset of symptoms until swelling subsides
Rubella (German measles)	14–21 days	From just before to four days after onset
Scarlet fever	2–5 days	Until antibiotic treatment is started
Whooping cough (pertussis)	7–10 days	From one week after exposure to three weeks after onset of the cough

The recommended immunization schedule

Vaccine	Age given	Comments
DPT: Injection (Diphtheria/tetanus/whooping cough)	1st dose 2 months 2nd dose 3 months 3rd dose 4 months	If whooping cough is prevalent DPT can be given at 3, 4 and 5 months
Poliomyelitis: Oral	1st dose 2 months 2nd dose 3 months 3rd dose 4 months	Can be given at same visit as DPT
MMR: Injection (Measles/mumps/rubella)	12–18 months	Only one dose needed
DT: Injection (Diphtheria/tetanus)	4–5 years	Pre-school booster
Poliomyelitis: Oral	4–5 years	Pre-school booster
BCG: Injection (TB)	10–14 years	
Tetanus: Injection	15-18 years	School-leaving booster
Poliomyelitis: Oral	15-18 years	School-leaving booster

does not usually require treatment. Very occasionally, in children prone to febrile convulsions (see page 265), the fever following an immunization may precipitate an attack. A tendency to febrile convulsions is not a contra-indication to immunization, as convulsions are much more likely after the natural disease.

Apart from the above, other reactions are very uncommon. A doctor should be consulted if significant illness follows immunization.

HYGIENE IN THE HOME

Infections occur when a pathogenic or disease-causing micro-organism infects a susceptible individual. Hygienic measures are designed to lessen the risk of contact between such germs and such people. As it is impossible to predict when pathogenic organisms are going to appear and spread, hygienic measures, to be fully effective, must become a routine that is always followed. Routines can easily become upset on holiday and at times of domestic crisis, and a special effort is needed in these periods to ensure that safe standards are maintained.

Not every contact with pathogenic micro-organisms does cause disease. Even in susceptible individuals there is some degree of natural resistance. These natural defences are not well developed in babies, who are therefore particularly prone to infections, and there may be reduced immunity in children of any age who are debilitated through illness.

Food preparation

Gastro-intestinal infections commonly arise from infected food and drink and contaminated food can cause other infections. Such complaints are always unpleasant, and in babies the dehydration caused by gastro-enteritis can threaten life (see page 266).

Foodstuffs may be contaminated when purchased, may become contaminated by the cook in preparation, or may become infected if not eaten when freshly prepared. Food should only be prepared in clean surroundings. The food itself should be thoroughly cleaned; poultry is often contaminated with salmonella (bacteria which cause gastro-enteritis) and must be thoroughly cooked, and cooks must wash their hands carefully after the preparation. Once prepared, food should be eaten fresh or properly stored in a freezer. Routines of food preparation and storage should be so well established that they are automatic.

For pre-packaged food the instructions with regard to freezing, cooking and expiry date should be followed. Listeria is an uncommon infection becoming commoner. It grows on pre-cooked food that is stored at low temperatures that would prevent the spread of other organisms. It does not grow at freezer temperatures, but can grow in an ordinary refrigerator.

Many episodes of food poisoning due to the consumption of infected food or drink occur because of infection carried by the cook. People with or recovering from diarrhoea should not be involved in food preparation.

Preventing wound infections

The intact skin is one of the body's defences against infection; wounds which break the skin may allow infection into the body. Micro-organisms from the skin may invade a wound, or the wound may be caused by a dirty or bacterially contaminated implement. All grazes and cuts need to be properly cleaned, and protected by a dressing until they are healed (see page 223). Deep wounds are difficult to clean, and will require medical attention.

Tetanus spores are commonly found in manure and in the soil in agricultural areas. If a wound is sustained that introduces these spores into the body tetanus may develop, unless the individual has been immunized.

CONTACT WITH INFECTED PEOPLE

The importance of preventing infection by avoiding contact with individuals who have infectious diseases appears obvious. Nevertheless it may be neglected in situations where the potential risks are not appreciated.

Babies have little resistance to infection, and may become seriously ill as a result of respiratory infections that only cause trivial illness in an older child or an adult. Such respiratory infections are spread by droplets (from coughs and sneezes) and by viruses in the air around an infected person.

Most people enjoy picking up and cuddling babies, but the more people that handle them, the more likely they are to develop respiratory infections. Parents should try to limit the number of people that handle their baby unnecessarily, and should discourage those with coughs and colds coming near unless there is no alternative. Similarly, in crowded places babies may well contract potentially serious infections from apparently healthy people, so crowds should be avoided where possible.

The severity of an infection can vary with the degree of exposure. This is often apparent in children with chickenpox or measles. Those who develop the infection from casual contact may well have mild disease. The child who catches chickenpox from a sibling often develops much more extensive disease because of prolonged contact, and therefore invasion of the body by a larger number of viruses.

Parents know that if one child in the family has an infection it is likely that any others will also develop it, so they do not take steps to separate the children from each other. Separation may not prevent infection if it does not take place until the infection is recognized, but avoidance of close and prolonged contact may result in a milder disease.

FOREIGN TRAVEL

Going on holiday and travelling increase the risks of contracting infection. The change of environment, break in routine and unfamiliar foods may all make it more difficult to maintain personal hygiene. Going abroad, particularly to less developed parts of the world, further increases the risk of contracting infection. Diseases that have been largely eradicated in the Western world may still occur and pose a risk to the traveller. Furthermore, in some places water purity, drainage and hygiene may not be of an adequate standard.

When travelling abroad with children parents should bear these factors in mind, and make preparations before departure. The steps to be taken depend on which part of the world is being visited. Some countries require international certificates of vaccination against yellow fever. You may need immunizations against typhoid and cholera, and as poliomyelitis and diphtheria still occur in underdeveloped countries, basic immunizations also need to be up to date. Your family doctor or travel agent will be able to advise on what immunizations you need for travel to individual countries.

Malaria is also a hazard in many parts of the world, and travellers should take preventative treatment. Different types of malaria are prevalent in different regions, and so travellers need to take the appropriate anti-malarial drug for the area they are visiting. This is something you should consult your doctor about. Anti-malarial treatment should start one week before travelling and be continued for four weeks after return for complete protection.

Malaria poses a particular risk for individuals brought up in malarial areas and for their families when they return there, even if only for a holiday. In many parts of Asia and Africa the inhabitants do not take anti-malarial treatment, and develop a resistance after repeated infections in childhood. This resistance is not long-lasting, and if they leave the area for a year or more, they may lose their immunity and be at risk of a serious malarial infection on returning home. Furthermore, people living in such areas do not perceive malaria as a risk because of their own acquired immunity. Children born in the developed world and taken back to visit relatives may not be given anti-malarials, and are at high risk.

If going abroad with small children it is also important to think about the possibility of gastro-intestinal upset from water or local food. If there is uncertainty about supply, adequate amounts of baby milk need to be taken for bottle-fed infants, and the water used to make up feeds should ideally be boiled. Breast feeding has obvious advantages.

It may be better for older children (and indeed adults) to drink mineral water rather than local tap water. Pepsi and Coca Cola are almost universally available and provide a guarantee of bacteriological purity.

Recommended vaccinations for travellers overseas

Area	Malaria	Cholera	Typhoid	Polio	Yellow Fever*
Europe and USSR	—	—	—	—	E (some countries)
West Indies	—	—	R	R	E (some countries)
Central and South America	R (some countries)	—	R	R	R or E (some countries)
North Africa	R (some countries)	R (some countries)	R	R	E (some countries)
Sub-Saharan Africa	R	R (some countries)	R	R	E or R (some countries)
Middle East	R (some countries)	R or E (some countries)	R	R	E (some countries)
Indian subcontinent	R	R	R	R	E (some countries)
South-East Asia	R (some countries)	R (some countries)	R	R	E (some countries)
Australia, New Zealand USA and Canada	—	—	—	—	—

NOTE This table should be used as a rough area guide only. Your doctor or travel agent should be consulted for specific and up-to-date regulations. *Children under 1 year of age should not normally be vaccinated against yellow fever.
KEY: E = essential if arriving from an infected area; R = recommended.

CHAPTER
10

CARING FOR THE SICK CHILD

There are many different aspects to caring for a child who becomes unwell. Initially parents will be concerned as to the cause, will be sorry for the child who is feeling poorly, will be trying to make her feel more comfortable, and will be wondering whether to call the doctor. The child may be cared for at home or may need to be admitted to hospital. In either case she is going to feel anxious and need a lot of support, and parents will have to organize life around her needs while continuing with other essential activities and caring for other family members.

CONSULTING THE DOCTOR

Parents should consider themselves in partnership with the doctor in providing health care for their child. Much of the time this will consist of routine health checks and immunizations (see Chapter 9) in the child health clinic, where parent and doctor will have the opportunity to discuss the child's

health and well-being, and to consider any anxieties the parents may have.

Whenever a baby is ill parents should think about consulting the doctor. Infants have little resistance and infections are often more serious than in older children. Fevers, coughing, difficulty in breathing, vomiting and diarrhoea are symptoms that in babies may all indicate significant infection. Without treatment the illness may become serious.

The doctor does not have to be consulted every time older children are ill, provided parents know that the problem is self-limiting and the child does not seem particularly unwell. However, the doctor should be seen if the child appears unwell or if parents are at all worried. If you are in any doubt about whether or not the doctor should be consulted, it is always better to be cautious and seek advice.

Symptoms such as unexplained fever, noisy or difficult breathing, persistent vomiting, and severe or persistent abdominal pain or earache will normally warrant a prompt medical opinion. Doctors usually prefer to see sick children in their surgery or office rather than in the home, as all the facilities are available there for a full examination and the taking of specimens and other tests, but parents should not wait until the surgery is open if they are concerned about sudden illness in a baby or child.

Many disorders of childhood are not emergencies. A child may develop a symptom such as a cough or recurrent headaches or tummy aches, or a parent may be concerned over growth, development or behaviour. A routine appointment should be made so that the problem can be discussed.

Do not put off going to the doctor because you are unsure whether or not anything is wrong. If you are worried about some aspect of your child's health it is best to consult the doctor. All doctors experienced in looking after children accept that a significant part of their work is going to be checking that they are healthy, and relieving parental anxiety. Parents often find it difficult to remember what they wanted to ask the doctor, perhaps because they are concerned that he or she is busy and they do not want to take up too much time or burden him or her with trivia. Often they will not mention psychological or social concerns because they think the doctor might only be interested in physical difficulties. Sometimes questions are forgotten because of the anxiety the situation causes, or answers may not be heard properly. Lack of time may also be a factor. It is vital, however, that parents' questions are answered if the family as a whole is not to be bewildered by the sequence of events that may follow.

NURSING A SICK CHILD AT HOME

When a parent is caring for a sick child at home there will be many extra duties to perform. The child may be feeling poorly

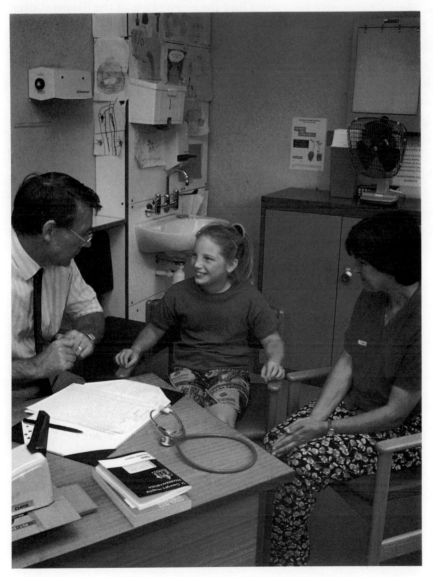

Children should see the doctor for regular health checks and immunizations. If a child is ill or parents are worried about the child's health or development the doctor should be consulted.

or insecure, and will need comfort and support, or may become bored and need distraction or entertainment. Some children who are feeling weak or ill may want to be in bed, but there is no medical advantage to insisting on it. Others often prefer to be sitting up reading, watching TV or playing rather than confined to bed, and if the child wants to walk around or play on the floor this should be permitted.

If the invalid is not eating and drinking as much as usual it is worth encouraging fluid intake by offering favourite drinks. When a child is reluctant to eat it may be better to concentrate on nourishing drinks such as milk and thick soups rather than to try to persuade her to eat.

A temperature can usually be lowered by giving paracetamol liquid in doses appropriate to the child's age. In addition, it may help to make sure that the child is not wearing too many clothes or sleeping under too much bedding when her temperature is high. If a child complains of feeling hot she may feel more comfortable after having her face and trunk bathed with a cool flannel.

Giving medicines can be a problem with small children. In general liquids are easier than tablets and usually the child will take them from a spoon. With babies and infants squirting the medicine slowly into the mouth with a syringe is sometimes helpful. Tablets can be swallowed whole, or may need to be crushed between two spoons and mixed with food or fluid.

Children who are ill often sleep fitfully at night and wake frequently. They may be reassured by having someone sleeping in the same room while they are feeling unwell.

Once the acute phase of the illness is over, frustration and boredom are likely to set in. The parents again have to show versatility in trying to keep the child occupied. Provided the weather is not too bad and the child is adequately clad, trips outside may be very beneficial and help the convalescence.

Children who have frequent bouts of illness and miss a lot of school may find themselves getting behind with their school-work and abandoned by friends who have found new playmates. Parents need to be sensitive to the potential problems on the

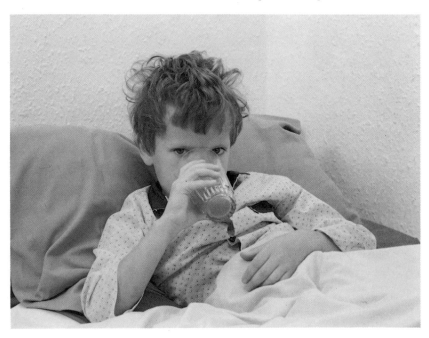

When children are ill they often want to stay in bed. However, they should not be confined to bed if they would be happier sitting out or playing indoors.

child's return to school and should be prepared to give extra attention and support until reintegration has been achieved.

REFERRAL TO HOSPITAL

The family doctor will often wish to refer a child to hospital, either as an emergency or for a routine visit. This is usually because the hospital has facilities that are not available in primary care or because a specialist opinion is required. Children may be referred to all sorts of different specialists. The box on page 124 describes the most common specialties concerned with children.

The child is likely to be apprehensive about a hospital visit and parents should endeavour to explain each stage and help the child not to be worried about the experience. This is not always easy to do as sometimes parents themselves are also anxious about the visit, confused as to what is going on, and worried about the outcome. They should always ask about anything they do not understand and may find it helpful to consider what

arrangements they need to make, what they are going to say to the doctor or nurse, and how they are going to cope from both a practical and emotional perspective if their child has to be admitted to hospital.

Children should only go into hospital when it is vital and necessary, and the medical and nursing professions are keen for children to be discharged as soon as medically appropriate, and when parents feel able to take charge of the child's after-care.

Preparing a child for admission

Going into hospital can be a worrying time for children and parents. Frequently it is the first time that a parent has been back to hospital since the child was born, and if parents are unable to be resident with their child it may be their first experience of separation.

When it is known in advance that a child is due for hospital admission she can be prepared for the event so that she understands what is going to happen. Most

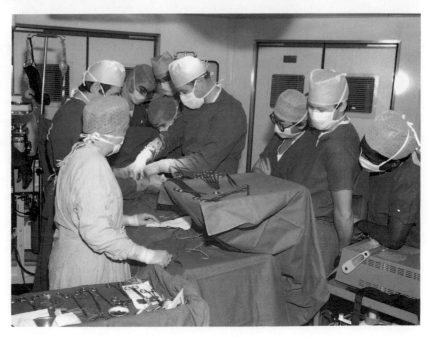

An operation in progress. Operating on children requires special training and experience. Newborns, infants, and children requiring specialized procedures are usually treated by paediatric surgeons in special centres. Other children may be cared for in district hospitals by a surgeon with special interest and experience in working with children.

Medical specialties concerned with children

Audiology Audiologists are physicians who have training in testing hearing in children, and in the management of hearing disorders.

Child psychiatry Most behavioural disorders in childhood are bound up with other problems within the family. Psychiatrists who work with children therefore tend to become involved with the whole family so that they can work towards understanding and helping not only the child but also other family members.

Developmental assessment Assessment clinics and child development centres are involved with the appraisal and help of children whose development is causing some concern. As well as the developmental paediatrician, other professionals may be involved, including psychologists, physio- and speech therapists, and social workers.

Ear, nose and throat (ENT, Otorhinolaryngology) This specialty is concerned with diseases of these parts of the body. Because children often suffer from ear infections and glue ear, recurrent tonsillitis and nosebleeds, much of the work of ENT surgeons is concerned with children.

Genetics Clinical geneticists are trained in the diagnosis and counselling of families where there is a condition which is, or may be, genetic or chromosomal in origin.

Ophthalmology This specialty is concerned with eyes and includes visual defects and squints.

Orthopaedics This specialty is concerned with fractures and deformities which affect bones and joints, and the muscles that move them.

Paediatrics This is the medical care of children; as well as knowing about diseases, paediatricians have training and experience of normal child growth and development and the special needs of children. In large centres some paediatricians may have sub-specialty interests, including neonatology (care of the newborn), neurology (nervous system), child development, and so on.

Paediatric surgery Children who need operations may be seen by surgeons who also treat adults; these surgeons often specialize in one system or part of the body. There are also paediatric surgeons who limit their work to children. They have more specialized expertise, and are also trained in the particular needs of children in hospital. Paediatric surgeons usually only work in special centres.

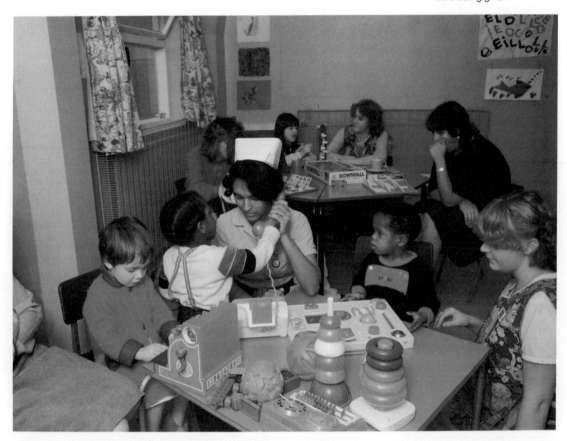

Hospital wards for children should welcome parents at all times. Your child will be happier if you are around frequently and help in the care being given.

children's wards are very happy for the child to visit beforehand so she can see what the ward is like and form an idea of where she will be staying. Mothers of young children should find out whether they can be resident and, if possible, should make arrangements to stay with the child. If the mother cannot be with the child all the time, another relative may be able to stay. A number of studies have found that children whose mothers stayed with them were better adjusted and showed less emotional disturbance after discharge. If other commitments mean that a parent cannot be resident, it is easier for children to cope if they know what the visiting routine

will be. It is important that children should not feel let down, otherwise they begin to feel insecure.

Children should be told about going to hospital and why it is necessary at a level and in language that they will understand. There are several books available that explain about hospitals, and parents can buy or borrow these to help prepare the child for the admission. The child also needs reassurance that the hospital visit will not last any longer than necessary, and that afterwards she will be coming home again.

The hospital may be able to help in preparing the child for what is to happen. This does not mean the child will be totally relaxed, but rather that she will be aware of hospital procedures. Some degree of worrying may be an important preparation: this is one way in which a child's coping strategies are put into action in order to lessen the impact of the trauma. Some children may not benefit from this approach, however, and will be more distressed beforehand than they are during the event itself. Seeing other children who are going through the same procedure and finding ways to cope can be very helpful. This may be done with a book with photographs, a video film, or acting out a procedure with a puppet. The way in which the child views these procedures will be very much affected by her parents' interpretation and presentation of them.

In hospital

Parents may have had a chance to prepare themselves and their child for hospital admission, but many children are admitted to hospital as an emergency without warning.

Children who go into hospital may be worried about the same things as adults or by different things. The way of showing their anxiety about something new and strange varies from child to child.

Parents should endeavour to remain with their child as long as possible immediately after admission. In this way both child and parents will be aware of what is going on, and will have the opportunity of talking about what is happening and going to happen between themselves and with the medical and nursing staff. Although babies in the first few months of life usually settle into hospital with little upset, toddlers and young children find the experience bewildering and frightening. The staff are trained to help them, but the presence of a parent day and night is much more effective in relieving anxiety, and means that the child is unlikely to become depressed or disturbed by the admission.

On or shortly after admission the doctor will come and take details about the child and the illness, and perform an examination. He or she should then explain what is planned and may order blood tests, X-rays or other investigations. Once a diagnosis is established, appropriate treatment can be planned and started. If an operation is needed the parents will be told what the arrangements are and the procedure should be fully explained to them.

Parents who are visiting or staying in hospital with their children should share in the care of them. As well as the child's medical needs, feeding, washing and changing still have to be carried out, and parents should participate with the nursing staff in all of these activities.

The organization of a child's stay in hospital is an important element in decreasing emotional disturbance. Many hospitals have a school attached which children can attend for the duration of their stay. It provides some structure to the day, and is a familiar activity. It can also act as a forum for the child to discuss what is happening to her with a person who is not a member of the family and therefore not emotionally involved.

Coming home

Children coming home after a stay in hospital may well be subdued or more clingy than usual, or may act out some of their feelings and become rather difficult to manage. These are all natural reactions to an experience that is likely to have been bewildering and maybe frightening too. Gentle handling and extra attention for a few days will go a long way towards restoring normality. Handled properly, the experience of having coped with a hospital admission adds to children's understanding of themselves and of life, and heightens their maturity.

CHAPTER
11

DISABILITY IN CHILDHOOD

Childhood disability is present when some aspect of the child's body or mind fails to develop adequately or is disrupted by disease, illness or accident. The presence of a disability may jeopardize the development of skills and independence. If the child's potential is limited by disability he may then be described as handicapped.

Childhood disability may occur at any time throughout pre-natal life, infancy, childhood or adolescence. It may be the result of a genetic malformation, illness, infection or accident, or stem from unknown causes. The extent and nature of the problems may be immediately apparent or gradually evolve over a period of time. Problems may be confined to one particular aspect – for example, the absence of a finger or the presence of an extra toe – or be extensive and affect the child's abilities to move, speak and learn.

At some time during pregnancy, many couples fear the possibility of their child being 'less than perfect'. At the birth many parents' first question is, 'Is she all right?' or 'Has he got all of his fingers and toes?' What if the answer to either of these questions is 'no'? What does this mean to the child and the family and what are the repercussions for the future?

HEARING THE NEWS

No family wishes to be told that its child is disabled. If the presence of a disabling condition is apparent at birth this news will come at a time when the family is very vulnerable, emotionally very reactive and not well equipped to absorb such information. Often the birth will have taken place in hospital and the new parents will be on unfamiliar territory, with little privacy and surrounded by other young parents delighted with their new family member. If the disability is the result of accident or illness the news may be received by parents who are already exhausted and anxious. If the problems have evolved over months or years the family may still be shocked and bewildered when their suspicions are confirmed and the future holds even more uncertainties.

Doctors who are experienced at delivering unwelcome news develop an awareness of parents' needs. They will attempt to be honest, factual and constructive. They know that it is difficult, if not impossible, for parents to take in more than a minimum amount of information at the time that they first hear of their child's difficulties. Doctors will frequently offer to see the family again very soon after the first interview. They will be prepared to repeat what was said, to answer a host of questions, to interpret information, to share a family's anger and frustration, or just sit with a family who can do nothing but feel sad.

Hearing the news is just a beginning. Over the next days, months and often years the family will move in and out of feelings of grief, anger, disbelief and aggression, searching for reasons why or maybe a person to blame. These are steps towards a reasoned understanding of their child and his strengths, weaknesses and needs, and a search for how best to help him and plan for the future of the family and the individuals within it.

NAMING THE DISABILITY

Disability can come in many guises. When the same sort of problems repeatedly cluster together in different people, giving rise to similar disabilities, this may be called a 'syndrome'. The most common syndrome to occur in infants is Down's syndrome (about 1 in 700 births). This condition is caused by an abnormality of a chromosome and can be confirmed by a blood test from the infant (see also pages 104 and 259). Other disabilities are given more descriptive names – for example, visual handicap, hearing loss, spina bifida – which indicate where the problems occur.

There is considerable controversy as to whether naming a child's problems is helpful or just a way of 'labelling' him as handicapped. Many people find that the 'shorthand' of a name for the condition can be useful when describing the problem to family members, neighbours and friends. It is, however, important that this shorthand can be expanded to an articulate description of the specific child and his needs and abilities, so that his individuality is not masked by preconceived ideas – for example, 'all Down's syndrome children are placid and happy'. Anyone who has met a group of children with Down's syndrome will know that a full range of personalities and a considerable range of skills will be found within such a group. Each child is a unique person.

THE CAUSES OF DISABILITY

Despite dramatic progress in techniques used in diagnosis, the precise cause of many conditions remains unknown. It may be possible to describe what has gone wrong but not to ascertain why. Frequently, it is not even possible to locate precisely what has gone wrong and the nearest we can get is to describe the things that we see in the child – the 'signs and symptoms'. This inadequacy is the cause of much frustration to parents and medical staff alike. Knowing why may help to prevent the same problem occurring in another family member; it may not help to improve the situation for the child himself.

It is of enormous importance to establish whether the cause of a child's problems is responsive to medication, as conditions like thyroid deficiency (hypothyroidism), diabetes and some forms of epilepsy are (see pages 278, 257 and 262). It is also essential to ascertain whether there is a risk of the condition recurring within a family unit or with other relatives.

Where human error is suspected of being part of the cause it is important that the family talks to an unbiased person. To do this it may be necessary to arrange a second opinion through the paediatrician or family doctor.

OBTAINING HELP

The child with a disability is part of a family. In order to be effective, any assistance given to that child must take account of the needs of the family as a whole and of the individuals within it. If the parents are worn out the children will suffer. If all family life revolves around the disabled member the whole family will suffer, including the disabled child. The child needs to feel that he is a valued member of the family unit, and that implies the opportunity to contribute and share as well as to be the recipient.

It is important to remember that although the child's disability may have been diagnosed by a medical team, the ramifications of disability and potential handicap spread into all areas of life. The family will need social, educational, emotional and financial support as well as good medical care. This help may come from many sources, including other parents, young people with similar conditions, support groups, relatives, friends, voluntary organizations, and professional health, education and social service agencies.

Meeting other parents

Any new member of a family brings challenges to the parents. If all is well with the baby most parents develop confidence in their own judgment and in their ability to cope with this young infant and his childhood. There are places to go for advice, and family, friends and neighbours who have had children are happy to support and advise. When a baby is born with a disability the parents' trust in their ability to meet their child's needs is often shaken. They feel that

they are on their own and do not know who to turn to for advice. Which of their friends or neighbours knows about children with spina bifida, for example? Parents often find it helpful to meet up with other people who have had the same experience, to be able to share feelings, fears and fantasies as well as practical advice and mutual support.

Meeting other children

This can be helpful to some parents, especially if the child is able to talk with the new parents about himself and his interests. A very real concern for the parents of a child growing up with a disability is 'How will he feel about himself?' 'Will she feel frustrated by her limitations?' Great care should be taken to ensure that the young person with a disability does not feel 'on show' or 'under interrogation', but with skilful handling such meetings can be very reassuring to new parents and give the older child a sense of contributing something useful.

Voluntary groups

These will vary from area to area: some are very small, others are large, perhaps with national organizations; some cater for

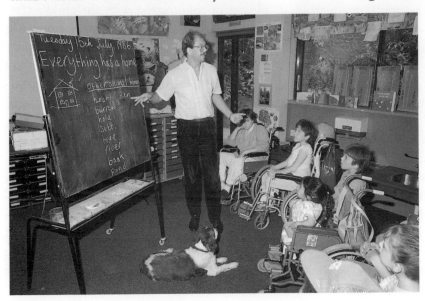

The needs of children with disabilities may most closely be met by a special school such as this.

specific disabilities, others for children and families with a wide range of problems. Their activities vary from social meetings for parents, through children's clubs, to holiday play schemes and workshops to enable parents to learn new skills to help their child with 'special needs'. Many of the groups are run by parents and are able to respond to local needs in the activities they choose to do.

Professional help

This may be divided according to its source into health, social services and education.

Children with disabilities may receive help from specialist doctors working with child development teams in addition to the assistance available to them through the health services. Therapists with special skills in child development and disability may offer assistance. They will work with and through the parents to find the most effective ways to help the child make the best possible progress in movement, communication and independence. Other team members may have particular knowledge of local services and activities and of special help that is available for the child and family with a disability. Teams may include an occupational therapist, paediatrician, physiotherapist, psychiatrist, psychologist, social worker and speech therapist. How services are organized will vary from locality to locality but they will usually involve a mixture of visits to hospital departments and home visits by the professionals concerned.

The social services will give help to the family in their home. This may be by making adaptations to the home – providing bath rails, for example – or in the provision of special equipment to help the child in his daily life – perhaps a chair to help the child eat with the family. Some social service departments make special provision for the nursery care of children with special needs.

Social workers may give support to the family as it adjusts to the child's disabilities.

The education service aims to help each child develop skills to reach his full potential. Where disability is present the child's potential for developing physical skills and learning skills may be greatly affected because he is disadvantaged by a limitation of movement or a reduced ability to understand. Each child is an individual and in order to meet his education needs it is critical that a picture of his strengths, weaknesses and consequent needs is established. Parents and other people who know the child well will have a major contribution to make in forming this profile. The next step is to consider where these needs can most closely be met. It may be that a local 'mainstream' school can provide all that the child requires in terms of access, resources, teaching skills and the total educational environment. However, extra help may be needed for some activities – for example, extra supervision during play or a word processor to assist with written work.

Many children with a disability need a very carefully planned and implemented individual learning programme. This is frequently co-ordinated by an educational psychologist in conjunction with the child's class teacher and the various therapists who work with him. Attending the local community school has the advantage that the child mixes with neighbourhood children, and friendships established in school can easily continue after school and during the holidays. It may, however, be too difficult to provide the essential resources and environment within a mainstream school. Many special units and special schools provide excellent facilities for children with more complicated needs. Furthermore, some children find it easier to fit into the community of a special needs group where they can relate to their peers on more equal terms.

THE EARLY EFFECTS ON FAMILY LIFE

With the arrival of any new family member, changes take place. The number of people who relate to each other is increased, and the family resources are redistributed. Space is needed for this new person. Routines have to adapt to accommodate the infant's daily needs. Within the existing family there are often mixed feelings of pleasure and hostility, especially as far as other children are concerned. If disability is diagnosed or suspected this process of adjustment may be more complicated, and family life may be considerably disrupted.

Parents will be shocked and sad on hearing the unwelcome news. They will frequently experience days of feeling numb and overwhelmed, days of being unable to believe that the diagnosis is correct, days of desperately wanting the company of other people, and days of wishing to be left alone. At times they will feel joy at the young life that is part of their family, at others they will feel protective towards the young and vulnerable child, and at yet others they may wonder why they have been given this extra challenge and responsibility.

A child with a disability will have needs over and above those of any other child. He may take longer to feed or require a special diet. He may need extra stimulation, exercises or help to develop communication skills. It will often take longer than usual for the child to become independent; indeed some may never achieve total independence. Visits to the clinic or hospital may be necessary. The child may need tests which can only be carried out at a hospital, or may need to stay in hospital for longer than usual after the birth.

Other children in the family are not only making adjustments to a new family member, but also to changes within their mother and father. Even very young children will be aware of the distress and anxiety their parents are feeling. They will sense their uncertainty about the baby, and will find their changing moods confusing. They need simple but accurate explanations. Some parents talk about the baby as being 'different', 'having very special needs', 'having difficulties which will need a lot of help and patience'. There is no 'right' or 'wrong' wording. The words used need to feel right to the family and be appropriate to the understanding of the children. The brothers and sisters of the new baby will need extra reassurance that they too are special and precious to their parents, that their needs will continue to be recognized. Where possible they may be encouraged to help with their disabled brother or sister, just as they would with any other baby activities. They can help at bathtime or exercise time, and by playing with the baby for short periods. Take care that this remains fun and does not become a chore or an imposition.

Grandparents, aunts and uncles will have their own difficulties in working out how they feel about the young child and his problems. It is never easy to strike a balance between being helpful and supportive and being interfering, between offering help and being accused of taking over. They may have anxieties of their own but find it hard to express them. They may have concerns about the hereditary nature of the problems. Grandparents may search for evidence that they 'should have known this might happen' or proof 'that there is nothing like this in our family'. Aunts and uncles may be worried that the risk of their having a child with a disability is increased, or feel guilty that they have a tribe of healthy, well-developed children. Frank talking within the family can help to alleviate these anxieties. Most paediatricians will willingly answer questions from other family members and arrange for

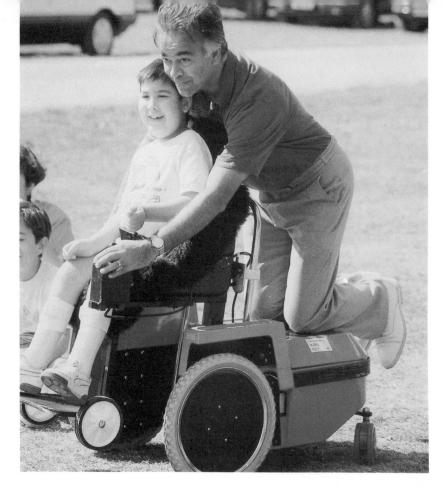

Opportunities for family outings and shared relaxation are important, even if a child is disabled.

counselling where this is necessary. The extended family can be an enormous asset to the family with a disabled child and to the child himself. Baby-sitting is invaluable, enabling the parents to have time alone together. Days out, weekends away and holidays spent with auntie and uncle can be very important introductions to the world outside the child's own home.

Neighbours and friends also have their part to play. Frequently they live closer than the extended family. Their rapport with the family is different from that of parents or brothers and sisters. They too will be shocked at the news that the expected child has a disability, or that the little one they have been getting to know has unforeseen problems. They will find it hard to know how to react. Should they be bright and jolly, and pretend nothing has happened? Or miserable and cheerless, and confirm that there is no justice in the world? Is it best to leave the family alone to get over it? Or to

rush round with copious advice and suggestions? Maybe it is helpful if friends just sit quietly with the family, helping them to move backwards and forwards between joy at the new life and sadness at the changes in expectation they are already experiencing. Perhaps they will share the parents' confusion, and allow them to be sad or angry. Friends and neighbours may also be able to offer help with the other children in the family while parents take time to adjust, or to visit specialists or clinics. They too make very reliable and trusted baby-sitters.

LATER ON

Family life is a continuous, shifting balance between the needs of the individuals that make up that family and of the group as a whole. One member may want to play the trumpet, another to become a champion swimmer: the family will need to make changes to accommodate these activities. As the child with a disability grows up there will inevitably be some effect on the pattern of family life. The needs of the individual take their place with those of the family as a whole and not to the exclusion of other members. Some needs will rate as more important than others but care should be taken that this is decided on merit and not just because of the child's disabilities.

Many disabled children will need space for their special equipment. Those with mobility problems may need large push-chairs, wheelchairs and walking aids. Being able to run a family car is even more import-ant for parents. The home may need to be extended to enable the child to live on a single level. The family may need to move to a more suitable house. All of these factors involve extra expense and disruption. There are many grants and allowances available to assist families with the financial burden. Your paediatrician or social worker will be able to help you find out more about these.

An important part of any child's develop-ment is establishing friendships and relation-ships outside the home. Many of these arise from contacts in playgroups, schools and recreational activities. From an early age children will spend an hour or two playing with friends, leading to the first adventure of 'staying the night' and eventually longer periods away with groups of friends. For the child with a disability it may appear harder for these experiences to occur. There may be very real practical difficulties. The child may not go to school in the immediate neigh-bourhood so that friends all live a distance away. It may be more difficult for parents to get to know each other because the children are taken to school by bus and regular meetings outside the school gates do not happen. The family may feel that the child is too reliant on its very attentive care to be entrusted to other people. The extra effort of working to establish a wider circle of friends and experiences for your disabled child will greatly enrich his overall development and prepare him for the independence of adult life. Once you feel that the child is in reliable hands you too will be able to enjoy a few days when you are freer to pursue your own interests. When the child returns you will all have news to share and much to talk about. Many schemes are developing to enable families to establish trusted 'respite' facili-ties, either with other families or in small homely units. Your local child development team will help you to find out more about these if you wish to do so.

GROWING UP WITH DISABILITY

For many families the early months with their disabled child will become an exciting and interesting journey. As each new skill is acquired it will be appreciated all the more for the extra effort that has gone into that piece of learning. Parents will learn to recognize the small and subtle stages that contribute to their child's development; these may have passed almost without notice in any previous children.

It is important to regard the child as a whole person and not to become preoccupied with the areas affected by disability. Areas of strength and ability need the opportunity to be developed to the full. A child with a visual problem needs encouragement to explore the world around and develop language to express himself. A child with a mobility problem needs activities to stimulate manipu-lative and imaginative play as well as every opportunity to become mobile. A child with learning difficulties needs to develop social skills and take part in creative play to enable him to build up friendships with other neighbourhood children.

Physiotherapy is given as part of the treatment programme for many types of permanent disability. It is being used here to help improve the balance of a young girl with a locomotor problem.

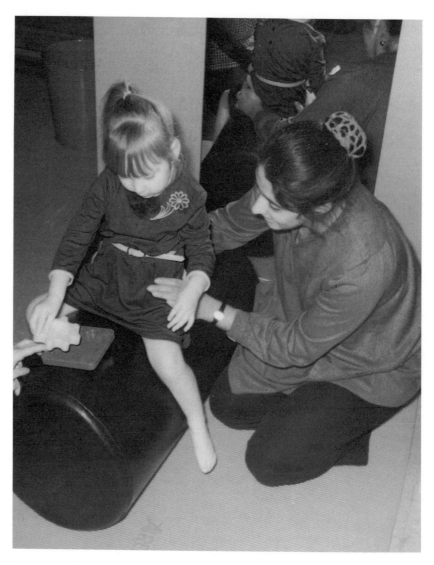

By the end of the first year of life most children are starting to mix with other little playmates, often as part of mother and toddler groups. This presents the first opportunity for the young child with a disability to establish a place in the wider world. Later, playgroup and nursery school may open the doors to meeting more children and extend the child's trust to a wider group of adults. Toddler gymnastic groups, swimming clubs, dancing classes and the like enable the child to participate in community activities and the family to establish links with other people in their area. Young children are very open in their acceptance of each other and respond to simple and practical explanations of a child's special needs. Other parents may be a little reticent to initiate conversations about the child's disabilities but will respond to the matter-of-fact lead given by his own parents. It is important that the child with a disability feels that it is acceptable to talk about disability just as it is to talk about where he went for his holiday or his favourite television programme. Whispered conversations in dark corners will do nothing to prepare the child for answering questions from his peers later.

During the formal school years it may

need an extra effort to keep the disabled child in touch with the local community, especially if it is necessary for the child to attend a special class or school some distance from home. Joining after-school clubs and holiday play schemes can help to minimize the effect of isolation from the neighbourhood. At this stage other children may become more questioning about disability. They may try to work out for themselves what it means to the individual. They are, after all, learning to make sense of many aspects of their world; disability is just one more. If they are fortunate enough to establish a rapport with a young person with special needs they have a unique opportunity to understand about that person's strengths, weaknesses and requirements. They will learn about the 'person' and not the 'problem'. It is vital that the child with a disability is encouraged to talk with confidence about himself, to contribute to the group as a whole, and to feel able to ask for help when he needs it. This is another important aspect of becoming independent.

Education does not end with the school years. Further education, college courses and adult education classes continue to develop for young people with a range of disabilities. Opportunities for work experience and recreation vary from area to area. The young people most able to benefit from these are those who throughout their lives have been enabled to develop confidence in themselves and a respect for their own abilities as well as a knowledge of their own limitations and special needs.

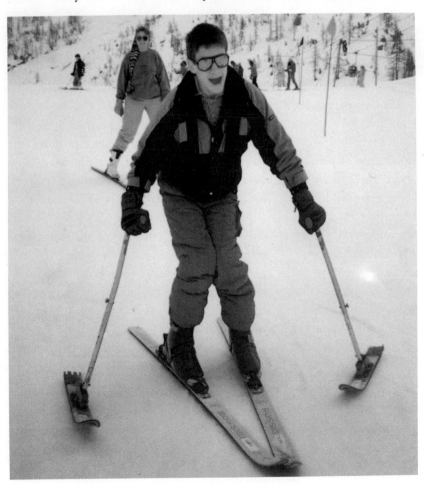

This young man is learning to ski in spite of his disability. Sport is an excellent way of encouraging disabled children to extend their range of abilities.

CHAPTER

12

LOSING A CHILD

All death is intrinsically sad, and the death of babies and children especially so. The usual expectation is that parents will grow old and die before their children. When a child dies first, parents feel that this is against the natural order, and there is a particular sense of loss.

One of the great changes in medicine over the last fifty years has been the fall in the death rate of babies and children. No longer is the death of children familiar, and many adults will not have experienced it among their families and close friends. One consequence of this is that many people do not know how to be of comfort to the bereaved as they have difficulty in coping with their own emotions. This can add to the grief of the parents and other people close to the dead child, and make it harder for them to pick up the threads of everyday life again.

Although less so now than formerly, deaths of babies and children still occur. Some babies are stillborn, or die in the newborn period of prematurity or congenital malformations. Babies can die unexpectedly,

the so-called cot death or sudden infant death syndrome. Accidents are the largest single cause of childhood deaths after the first year of life; they are always unexpected and usually kill previously healthy and active individuals. Other deaths occur after a period of illness or handicap. Putting all the causes of death together for developed countries, around 6 babies in every 1,000 are stillborn, about 10 per 1,000 die in the first year, and there are another five deaths per 1,000 before the age of 19.

STILLBORN INFANTS

Babies who are born after twenty-eight weeks of pregnancy and do not breathe or show any other signs of life are classified as stillbirths. Death usually occurs in labour but there may have been concern about the well-being of the fetus earlier in pregnancy.

For the parents the loss of the baby is no less painful because the child was not known to them as an individual. The hopes and expectations that they had built up before and during the pregnancy centred around this baby, and the loss is bitter. There is, however, often a sense of unreality about the mourning. Normally part of mourning is adjusting to life without a loved one. With a stillborn baby the process of adjustment can be much more difficult: the sense of loss is great but what has been lost is unclear, in that the stage between pregnancy and loss was not filled with caring for and loving a separate individual.

It is helpful to give the baby a name, because having a name is part of being a person, and will also make it easier later when parents want to talk about her. Not all parents want to see or hold their stillborn baby, but although distressing it is a very natural thing to do. Those parents who have had the opportunity of holding and touching the baby will have a more realistic awareness of their loss and a focus for their grief. As a result many are better able to cope with life after the loss, and to come to terms with their sadness.

On a maternity ward the mothers of still-born babies are often given individual rooms so that they can have open visiting and are not surrounded by other mothers with babies. There is a need for solitude at this time, but there is also a need for the support of loved ones and caring friends. Relatives and friends are often upset by the death them-selves and may feel that they will be intruding on the parents' grief if they visit. This is seldom the case; their distress can be shared with the parents and there is mutual support and comfort in being sad together. This sharing of sadness needs to continue after the mother has left hospital. Parents will find that their best friends over the coming months are those that are supportive and maintain close contact with them.

COT DEATH (SUDDEN INFANT DEATH SYNDROME)

Some infants die unexpectedly, and even after autopsy no definite cause can be found. This is referred to as a cot death or sudden infant death syndrome (SIDS), and affects babies in the first few months of life. The peak incidence is around 2–3 months. The overall cot death rate varies in different pop-ulations, but is between around 0.5 and 3 per thousand live births. Cot death is more common in boys than girls, more common in bottle fed than breast fed infants, more common in winter and in poorer socio-economic groups, and more common in babies who were born pre-term or of low birth weight.

Extensive research into the causes of cot death has been carried out in recent years and much is ongoing, but there is no definite answer yet. It is unlikely that all cot deaths have the same cause, and possible factors identified have included overwhelming in-fections, hypothermia, heart rhythm disturb-ances, disturbances of function of the brain, allergic reactions and apnoea (the cessation of breathing) during sleep.

Typically, when cot deaths occur the baby has previously been apparently healthy, or has only had a minor illness and did not seem particularly unwell. The baby is put down to sleep, and later when she does not wake, it is suddenly realized that she is unresponsive and not breathing. If the baby is cold, death may have happened some time before. The parent or a neighbour will usually call an ambulance and the child will be taken to a hospital emergency department. Resuscita-tion will be attempted if there is any likeli-hood of success, but is usually of no use.

Once the news has been broken, parents may want to see and hold the baby. This can be a very precious as well as agonizing few moments, and the hospital should provide privacy and as much time as the parents want to be able to express their immediate grief and say personal goodbyes to the baby.

Because cot deaths are unexpected they have to be reported to the coroner, who will usually want an autopsy performed to ascer-tain the cause of death. Once the cause is determined the coroner issues a death certifi-cate and the funeral arrangements can then be made.

For the parents the sudden and unexpected death of their baby is both a tragic loss and a great shock, and may be hard to comprehend because medical science does not yet under-stand the causes. It is known, however, that cot deaths are not related to any act or omis-sion on the part of the parents, who should not feel themselves to blame in any way.

CARING FOR THE DYING CHILD

In spite of the achievements of modern medicine there are still conditions which cannot be cured and some of them are ultimately fatal. Other people will concern themselves with the medical treatment, but the care, comfort and support of children who are dying fall largely on the parents because they are the people closest to the child, whether she is at home or in hospital.

Parents may have great difficulty in coping with their own feelings and may not know how best to help the child. When bad news is first broken it takes time to absorb and understand it. At first parents will have difficulty in carrying on with day-to-day living, but established routines provide a familiar structure which is itself helpful in enabling them to cope and is also useful to the child.

When the doctor first tells the parents of the diagnosis and its significance, death may be many years away. Although initially the fact that their child will one day die seems overwhelming, the very remoteness of the event does help in enabling the parents to carry on as normal; most will often not look too far into the future but will live life one day at a time.

There is a temptation to treat such children as special, giving them presents and treats and skimping on discipline. This is not helpful. Children need to know they are loved, but ordinary and gentle discipline helps children learn how to behave and become more mature. The more the child can be treated as normal, the better.

Children are aware of parental concerns even when these are not voiced or discussed. They should be given a simple explanation of their illness appropriate to their age. As they grow they will need to know more and will want to discuss their disease and its significance from time to time. This desire to understand is very strong, and children's anxieties about themselves are greatly increased if they are aware that something is being kept from them.

Brothers and sisters also need to have some understanding about a sick sibling, but do not need to be burdened with things that may happen in the distant future. As they get older they will want to know more about their sibling's disorder and should be given information and an explanation appropriate to their maturity.

At some stage in talking to the ill child questions about death and dying will come up and must be faced. Telling children about it gently but honestly can be harrowing, but the parent–child relationship becomes very close if there can be total honesty. If death is only a relatively short time away the child will be concerned about what dying will be like, and how her parents will be afterwards. Having the opportunity to talk with someone about such things will be helpful.

For most parents helping their child in this way will not be easy, and they will need support themselves; the child may also need someone outside the family to talk to. The family doctor or paediatrician should be able to recommend a psychologist or counsellor with experience of working with dying children and their families, who will be able to help and support.

Children of different ages have different perceptions of death. Until the age of about 5 years they really have no concept of what death is or means; as they grow, their understanding gradually increases and they are often able to be more honest and realistic about it than many adults.

Not everything that individuals want to communicate to each other needs putting into words, and being close, holding hands or putting arms round each other can say more than words ever could. Death is sad but natural, and families should try to be as natural as possible in their relations with each other, in supporting each other and in sharing their feelings.

BEREAVEMENT

When somebody very close to us dies the immediate sense of loss is catastrophic. We become unaware of our surroundings, cannot think coherently or control our feelings, and feel lost, sad and devastated. For parents who have lost a child these feelings are overwhelming. Even when the death was expected there can be no real comprehension before the event of what the effect will be, so there is little that can be done in preparation, and nothing to lessen the sense of desolation afterwards.

If a child has been handicapped or has been ill for some time there may be an element of relief that death has brought an end to her suffering, but this does little to lessen the pain that the parents feel. When a child has been severely handicapped the parents may feel that a burden has been lifted from them, which is very natural, but they may then feel unnecessarily guilty for having the thought. Furthermore, as caring for an ill or handicapped child is usually very time-consuming, it is likely that a large part of their previous lifestyle will disappear with the death of the child, and this can increase the feeling of being bereft.

Those left behind after a death always have some regrets – about things done or undone, said or unsaid, about their own actions and the actions of others – and these will recur in thinking about the person who has died and going over the circumstances of the death and the time leading up to it. Eventually situations have to be accepted as they are; nothing can change the past, even though some regrets will always linger.

All people become rather frightened when they are not in control of their own emotions, and may become embarrassed about the expression of grief. Fathers may feel that it is unmanly to weep or otherwise lose control. There should be no embarrassment. Death has taken away a very close and much-loved baby or child and there is nothing more natural than to be devastated by this loss and to weep.

Long after the significance of the death has been appreciated and accepted there will be occasions when sadness will be overwhelming and tears will flow, sometimes taking the person by surprise. Life is never going to be the same as it was before, and the sense of loss never fades entirely.

When a couple have lost a child they will both feel drained and empty, and may have difficulty in providing support for each other. This may be a problem immediately after the death or it may become so later. Each partner should try to express his or her feelings to the other honestly and constructively, for although many emotions will be common to both of them ways of coping may vary considerably. Parents must never feel inhibited in talking to each other about their lost child.

If there are other children they are likely to be a comfort. Parents should explain to them all about what is going on, and help them to express their own feelings. They will be bewildered and will not know what is expected of them; they will need help over this. They may also at times seem callous, wanting to take over the dead child's possessions or privileges. Young children do not have as much insight into the significance of death as adults, and often rapidly adjust to the altered situation. Older children will have greater understanding and deeper feelings, but may have difficulty in expressing them, and may not know how they are expected to behave. Parents, grandparents and family friends should try to help them as much as possible. This may include encouraging them to participate in all normal social and sporting activities without a sense of guilt or disloyalty to the dead sibling or the parents.

There is a temptation to try to preserve the memory of the child in an unrealistic way, leaving all clothes, toys and possessions unchanged; the alternative reaction is to have a big clear-out or move house too early, as though sad thoughts could be banished along with personal possessions. Parents will want to keep some of the child's belongings, but most important is being able to share memories of the child as he or she was, and of the things the family did together.

All parents find it difficult to adjust to the loss of a child. Sharing feelings with friends may be helpful, but not everyone has friends with the skill and experience to assume this role. Some social workers and clergy can be helpful, and there are also bereavement support groups and counsellors in many areas who may be available to help parents through this difficult time.

Friends and relatives who wish to help a parent who has lost a child need to be sensitive to his or her current mood and respond to it. No good is achieved by trying to distract bereaved parents, or by telling them to pull themselves together or 'snap out of it', or by any form of criticism. Being there, ready to listen or talk, to share tears or laughter, for as long as it takes is the caring approach. If you are the sort of friend who feels that the person 'should have got over it by now', you are unlikely to be helping the situation and may well be adding to the problems.

In adjusting to the loss of a loved one people go through different phases, sometimes feeling sad and sometimes business-like, sometimes wanting to relax and sometimes to be very busy. With a couple who have lost a child these phases may not coincide, and the general emptiness of life can make communication between them difficult. Furthermore, different people have different ways of coping with grief; some need to talk and others to internalize their feelings. In the midst of life seeming empty and meaningless it is important for the couple to hang on to each other, even though their relationship may also feel dead at times. If there are serious difficulties with the relationship itself, counselling may be helpful.

Some bereaved parents find difficulty in taking up enjoyable leisure activities again, either because they feel it might be disloyal to the memory of the dead child or they are concerned about what others might think. None of us would want our loved ones to be social outcasts after we are dead, and similarly there is no disloyalty to the memory of the dead child in going out for a meal, dancing, or to the theatre or cinema. Although the saying 'life must go on' is a cliché, it is none the less true.

When parents have lost a baby they may think of having another child fairly soon afterwards, and friends may suggest this. It is important that any new baby is wanted for itself, and not as a replacement or substitute for the baby that died. The time to start thinking about a possible new baby is when the death of the previous child has been accepted and come to terms with. For some couples this may be only a short while; others may want to wait for many months or a year or more; yet others will not want to have further children. The far-reaching decision of whether to have another child needs to be carefully taken when parents are beginning to think again about their future.

PART TWO

THE MAJOR BODY SYSTEMS

A Guide to the Body and How It Works

This section describes the purpose and workings of the various body systems, explains many of the diseases of childhood and outlines their treatment. A broad base of medical information is provided to enable those who are caring for a sick child to gain a better understanding of both the medical problem and the treatment. This information aims to supplement the advice given by the family doctor or other health professionals.

CHAPTER

1

THE HEART, CIRCULATION AND LUNGS

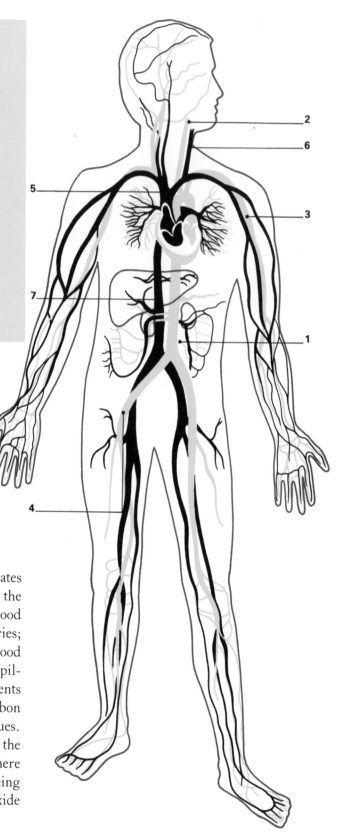

Blood is carried by the arteries (shown in brown) to all parts of the body and is returned to the heart by the veins (shown in black). The main arteries are the aorta (**1**), carotid (**2**), brachial (**3**) and femoral (**4**). The main veins are the superior vena cava (**5**), jugular (**6**) and inferior vena cava (**7**).

The heart is a living pump that circulates blood both to the lungs and throughout the body. The large blood vessels carrying blood away from the heart are known as arteries; the veins bring it back. The small blood vessels within the tissues are called capillaries. Blood transports oxygen and nutrients to all parts of the body, and removes carbon dioxide and waste products from the tissues. The blood returns from the body to the heart and is then pumped to the lungs, where gas exchange takes place, more oxygen being taken in to enrich it, and carbon dioxide being breathed out.

THE HEART

The heart is a hollow organ made of muscle which contracts with every beat, pumping out the blood that is within it. The chambers of the heart are arranged so that the left side of the heart receives blood enriched with oxygen from the lungs and pumps it around the body, and the right side receives blood back from the body and pumps it to the lungs. Four valves inside the heart make sure that, as the heart contracts, the blood is pumped forward.

The blood which comes back to the heart is collected in two thin walled chambers called atria; at the start of each contraction the atria contract and move the blood into the next pair of chambers, the ventricles. When the ventricles contract, the blood from the heart is forcefully ejected into the large blood vessels. The left ventricle sends blood into the aorta, the main artery, and thence around the body, and the right ventricle sends blood into the pulmonary artery to carry the blood to the lungs (see the illustration below).

Inasmuch as the left and right sides of the heart have different functions the heart acts like two separate pumps working together, but developmentally and in fetal life the heart functions as a single organ. Until the moment of birth there is no need for blood to be pumped around the lungs to be oxygenated, as the lungs are small and unaerated, and oxygen comes to the fetus via the placenta (see page 11).

Many of the congenital abnormalities which affect the heart and blood vessels arise from failure of part of the heart to develop and adapt to the circulatory changes that take place between embryonic life and birth.

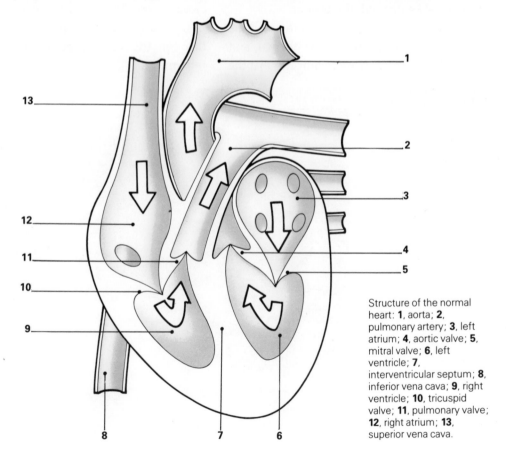

Structure of the normal heart: **1**, aorta; **2**, pulmonary artery; **3**, left atrium; **4**, aortic valve; **5**, mitral valve; **6**, left ventricle; **7**, interventricular septum; **8**, inferior vena cava; **9**, right ventricle; **10**, tricuspid valve; **11**, pulmonary valve; **12**, right atrium; **13**, superior vena cava.

EXAMINING THE HEART AND CIRCULATION

Examination of the heart and circulation is part of the child's routine medical assessment as well as part of the examination of a sick child. As well as determining how the heart is functioning at the time of the examination, the doctor has to consider whether there is any evidence of abnormality that might give rise to problems.

The child's colour can give information about the circulation. If the lips and tongue are blue this indicates that the blood has a reduced amount of oxygen; this may be due to heart or lung disease. Pallor may indicate anaemia (see page 149), or that the circulation is poor, but some children always look pale and are healthy, and all children can become pale with cold or emotion.

In feeling the pulse the doctor will be interested in whether the rate is normal, and if it can be easily felt, which indicates that the circulation is good. The doctor will also often feel a pulse in the groin or legs to make sure there is no blockage of the circulation to the lower part of the body. Blood pressure may also be measured, but this is less commonly done with children than with adults, as blood pressure problems are very uncommon in childhood.

In examining the heart itself the doctor will check the position of the heartbeat, as this gives an indication of heart size and function. With some congenital abnormalities the heart is enlarged. Listening to the heart with a stethoscope gives many pointers about how the heart is functioning. Normally the closing of the heart valves can be heard, the first pair of valves closing as the ventricles of the heart begin to contract, and the second pair closing at the end of ventricular contraction. The sounds made by valve closures are known as the first and second heart sounds. Any additional noises heard through the stethoscope are referred to as murmurs.

Listening to the heart is part of the routine medical examination. The sound of the heart valves closing can be heard, and sometimes heart murmurs are detected.

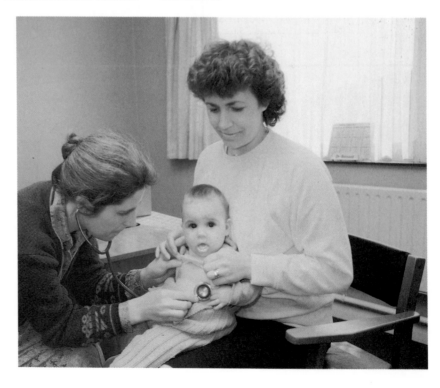

Heart murmurs

In many children with normal hearts a murmur may be heard because the blood makes a noise as it goes rapidly through the heart, rather like the sound made by swiftly flowing water. Such murmurs, called flow murmurs, are particularly likely to be noted when the child has a fever, as with a high temperature the circulation is speeded up. Flow murmurs are also called physiological or innocent murmurs to indicate that they are not due to a structural or functional disorder.

Some heart murmurs do indicate a structural abnormality of the heart or of the large blood vessels near it. If one of the heart valves is too narrow, the blood passing through will move faster and make an extra sound. Murmurs may also arise if there are holes in the partition (septum) that separates the right and left sides of the heart, so-called septal defects or 'holes in the heart'.

Sometimes murmurs do not arise from the heart itself, but from the great arteries. The aorta may have a narrowing, called a coarctation, which may first be noticed as a murmur picked up on routine examination. Another large blood vessel anomaly occasionally present is a persisting (or patent) ductus arteriosus. In fetal life the ductus arteriosus allows blood to bypass the non-functioning lungs by carrying blood from the pulmonary artery to the aorta (see page 44). Normally the ductus arteriosus closes at birth or shortly after, but sometimes it persists, and then blood will pass from the aorta to the pulmonary artery, giving rise to a continuous murmur.

If a child is found to have a heart murmur on routine examination, the cause needs to be determined. If the doctor is sure that the murmur is a physiological flow murmur, no further action is needed, but if there is any uncertainty the child may be referred to a specialist, and tests may be performed.

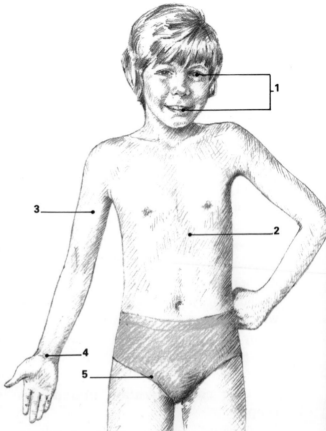

An examination of the heart and circulatory system includes feeling the pulse and measuring the blood pressure: **1**, the mouth and eyes are checked for anaemia; **2**, by listening over the heart the doctor can detect murmurs; **3**, blood pressure is tested by applying a cuff to the top of the arm; **4**, the pulse is felt at the wrist and in the groin (**5**).

INVESTIGATING THE HEART

Chest X-ray

A plain chest X-ray gives useful information about the heart. Many heart diseases are associated with a change in the shape or the size of the heart, and these may be apparent from the X-ray. Furthermore, if the child has a hole in the heart that results in extra blood flowing through the lungs, enlarged blood vessels can be seen in the lungs.

Electrocardiogram (ECG)

The electrocardiogram is a recording of the

electrical activity of the heart made by attaching electrodes to the limbs and the front of the chest. The heart rate and rhythm is shown and the ECG will also indicate if there is any enlargement of the right or left ventricle.

Echocardiography (cardiac ultrasound)

The introduction of ultrasound has revolutionized the investigation of the heart. It is now possible for a skilled cardiac ultrasonographer to examine in detail the structure of the heart and great vessels non-invasively (without entering the body) and to determine with almost complete certainty whether there is any abnormality. A good picture can be obtained even in very small babies.

Cardiac catheterization and angiography

In cardiac catheterization a very fine tube or catheter is passed along a limb artery into the various chambers of the heart under X-ray control. In small children this is performed under an anaesthetic. This catheter can be used to measure the pressure and to take blood samples to determine the amount of oxygen in the blood in different parts of the heart. This provides information about the functional disturbance caused by any cardiac abnormality. The catheter can also be used to inject dye into the heart to enable X-rays to be taken of the chambers of the heart and the major blood vessels, a technique known as angiography.

CONGENITAL HEART DISEASE

There are many different forms of congenital heart disease due to abnormalities during the development of the heart. While some of them are serious and may be life-threatening,

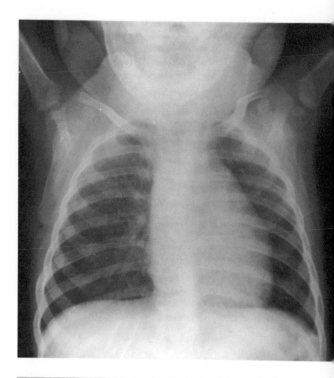

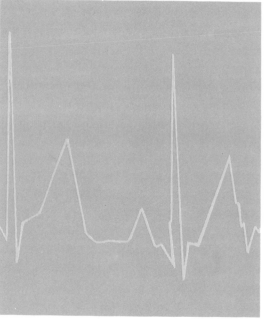

Top: A chest X-ray, such as this one of a baby, provides the doctor with important information about the heart. Changes in the size and shape of the heart are characteristic of many heart diseases and are detectable by X-ray.

Bottom: A normal ECG trace from a 15-month old baby, showing the rate and rhythm of the heart. The tall waves indicate contractions of the ventricles.

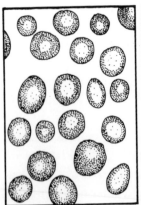
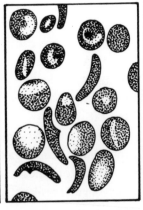
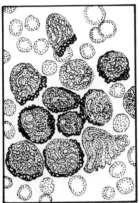

Blood tests are an essential part of investigations for many different diseases. **Far left:** Normal blood cells. **Middle:** Blood cells in sickle cell disease, in which some red cells are sickle shaped. **Left:** A cluster of abnormal cells in leukaemia.

some may never cause any problems. About 7 in every 1,000 babies have a congenital abnormality of the structure of the heart, so abnormalities are relatively common. In most cases the cause of congenital heart disease is unknown, but occasionally it is familial, and is sometimes due to maternal infection in early pregnancy.

Congenital heart disease is often suspected because a heart murmur is noted on routine examination. Not all congenital heart disease can be detected so early in life and a murmur may not be found until a school medical examination is performed, or even later. Some infants with congenital heart disease do have symptoms, however. Breathlessness, poor feeding or a blue colour may suggest congenital heart disease; if it is suspected, the child will be investigated to determine whether there is an abnormality and to decide on treatment.

The commonest forms of congenital heart disease are ventricular septal defect, atrial septal defect, aortic valve stenosis, pulmonary valve stenosis, and transposition of the great vessels. These are all described in the A–Z section, which starts on page 228.

THE BLOOD

The blood acts as a transport system which extends throughout every part of the body. It carries oxygen from the lungs to the tissues and nutrients from the alimentary tract to all the body organs. It conveys waste products to the lungs or kidneys, and has many other major transport functions, including taking white blood cells to sites of infection and hormones from the glands to their sites of action.

The blood is a very specialized tissue, and has a complex make-up. It has a cellular part, containing red blood cells, white blood cells and platelets, which makes up nearly half of the circulating volume of blood; there is also a fluid part, which contains proteins and other metabolic chemicals. The blood has a clotting mechanism so that haemorrhage (bleeding) following injury can be stopped (see illustration on page 149).

BLOOD CELLS AND BONE MARROW

There are three main types of blood cell: red blood cells, white blood cells and platelets. They all have different functions.

The red blood cells have a red, iron-containing pigment called haemoglobin, which gives blood its characteristic colour. There are large numbers of red cells; in healthy people there are around 5 million in every cubic millimetre of blood. The haemoglobin binds to oxygen as the red cells go through the lungs, and transports it around the body. The oxygen is gradually given up as the blood passes through the tissues. A deficiency of haemoglobin is known as anaemia (see next page).

There are several different sorts of white blood cell. All of these are concerned with preventing and overcoming infection, and take part in inflammatory reactions. Some white cells, the granulocytes, can actually engulf bacteria and kill them, while the lymphocyte cells and others produce antibodies and other chemicals that help to overcome infection.

The platelets are very much smaller than the red or white cells. Their role is in the initiation of the clotting process and the repair of wounds. When part of the circulatory system is damaged the platelets congregate around the wound and release substances that cause the activation of specialized blood proteins known as clotting factors. When activated these factors react together to form a clot consisting of interlocking strands of a material called fibrin, which prevents further haemorrhage and provides the framework for repair of the wound.

The red cells and platelets are formed in the bone marrow, as are many of the white cells. Some of the white cells are formed in the spleen and the thymus, lymphatic organs in other parts of the body. Inside many of the bones of the body there is a marrow cavity which is partly filled with bone marrow, and partly with fat. The bone marrow contains stem cells and precursors of red cells, which gradually develop and become haemoglobinized, and when they are mature they are released into the circulation. Red cells have a life in the circulation of around four months: all the time some are breaking down and being removed by the spleen, while others are being formed.

As well as the red cell precursor cells the marrow contains precursor cells for white cells. They are continuously producing new white cells to replace those used up. In times of infection the production can be stepped up markedly so that more cells are available to fight it.

There are also some large cells in the bone marrow called megakaryocytes. Platelets are formed from these; small parts of the megakaryocytes break off and enter the circulation as platelets.

BLOOD AND BONE MARROW TESTS

Because the blood takes part in nearly all the metabolic processes in the body it may undergo detectable changes in composition in disease; blood tests are therefore an essential part of investigation for many different diseases. The blood and the blood-forming tissues may be directly affected by disease. Some of these conditions are considered in the A-Z section, which starts on page 228.

Where the blood is thought to be involved in a disease process there are various helpful tests the doctor may perform. These include a full blood count in which the haemoglobin concentration and all the different sorts of cell in the blood are measured and counted. Other tests that are sometimes useful include analysis of the types of haemoglobin present, measurement of the levels of iron and vitamins in the blood, and studying the clotting mechanism.

Sometimes the removal of a small sample of bone marrow is helpful, so that it can be studied under the microscope. Using a local or general anaesthetic a needle is inserted into the relatively soft bone of the pelvis, and a small sample of the marrow can be sucked out with a syringe.

ANAEMIA

Anaemia is a condition where there is a reduced amount of haemoglobin in the blood. If the haemoglobin level is only slightly reduced there may be no symptoms, but more marked anaemia gives rise to problems. As the function of haemoglobin is to carry oxygen, a deficiency of haemoglobin reduces the amount of oxygen that can be carried by a given amount of blood. As a consequence, in anaemia the heart has to pump more blood round the circulation to make sure the tissues still receive adequate amounts of oxygen.

The initial symptoms of anaemia are reduced exercise tolerance and easy fatiguability. With severe anaemia the individual may be breathless at rest. Apart from the general symptoms, there may be others depending on the cause.

Anaemia may result from iron deficiency, from blood loss or from hereditary disorders of haemoglobin production or red cell formation. It can also arise in dietary deficiencies and in other chronic (long-term) diseases. It is always important to detect the cause of anaemia, so that rational treatment can be given.

Iron deficiency anaemia, sickle cell disease and thalassaemia are discussed on pages 280, 299 and 303 respectively.

BLOOD CLOTTING

One of the properties of blood is its ability to clot within a few minutes if it is outside the circulation, and this is an important protection against serious haemorrhage. It is also important that blood should not clot while it is in the blood vessels, or it will impede the circulation.

Clotting is a complex process. The factors that trigger it are present in the tissues and

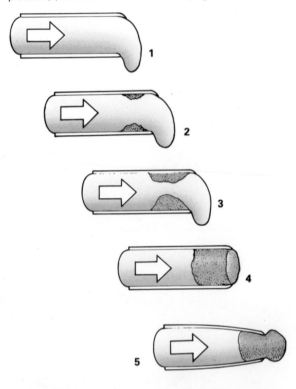

Blood coagulation. When a blood vessel is cut (**1**) the damage to the tissue activates the clotting process (**2**) and a clot forms at the surface of the cut (**3**). The clot becomes firmer and more extensive (**4**) and eventually retracts to form a plug (**5**).

circulation, but are only activated if there is injury. Clotting is started by substances called thromboplastins which are released from tissues when they are damaged, and also from blood platelets. These thromboplastins then react with other clotting factors present in the blood, until the final stage is reached, the conversion of a protein in the blood called fibrinogen to solid fibrin. Fibrin forms the basic structure of the clot, and over the few hours after clot formation the fibrin undergoes a process called polymerization which makes it even tougher. As it dries out it forms a scab which protects the wound until healing takes place.

Clotting disorders are discussed under 'Haemorrhagic disease of the newborn' and 'Haemophilia' on page 271 of the A-Z section.

THE LUNGS AND RESPIRATORY SYSTEM

The primary function of the respiratory system is to provide the body with enough oxygen to maintain the metabolism of the vital organs and to provide energy for movement. In health this happens efficiently at all times.

An adult at rest needs to breathe in about 5 litres (about 9 pints) of air per minute, and up to six times this amount with vigorous exercise. Children breathe smaller volumes than adults, but in proportion to their body

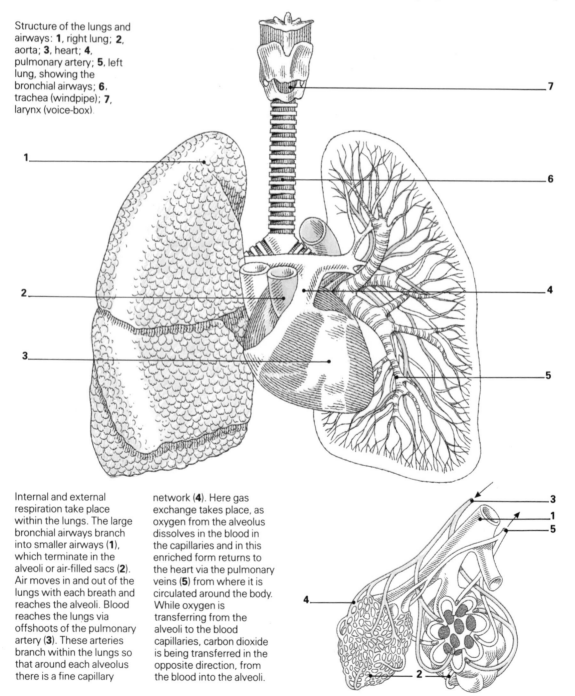

Structure of the lungs and airways: **1**, right lung; **2**, aorta; **3**, heart; **4**, pulmonary artery; **5**, left lung, showing the bronchial airways; **6**, trachea (windpipe); **7**, larynx (voice-box).

Internal and external respiration take place within the lungs. The large bronchial airways branch into smaller airways (**1**), which terminate in the alveoli or air-filled sacs (**2**). Air moves in and out of the lungs with each breath and reaches the alveoli. Blood reaches the lungs via offshoots of the pulmonary artery (**3**). These arteries branch within the lungs so that around each alveolus there is a fine capillary network (**4**). Here gas exchange takes place, as oxygen from the alveolus dissolves in the blood in the capillaries and in this enriched form returns to the heart via the pulmonary veins (**5**) from where it is circulated around the body. While oxygen is transferring from the alveoli to the blood capillaries, carbon dioxide is being transferred in the opposite direction, from the blood into the alveoli.

size they have a higher oxygen requirement.

The respiratory system is often divided into the upper and lower respiratory tracts. The upper respiratory tract consists of the nose, sinuses, mouth and pharynx, and the lower respiratory tract comprises the larynx (voice-box), trachea (windpipe), bronchi (airways) and lungs.

With each breath the upper respiratory tract filters, warms and humidifies the incoming air. Slight humidification also goes on in the lower airways. The exchange of oxygen from the inspired air to the bloodstream takes place in the alveoli, the air sacs in the substance of the lung at the end of the airways. At the same time as oxygen is taken up by the blood, carbon dioxide is trans-

ferred from the blood to the alveolar air. The air breathed out has a somewhat reduced oxygen content, and a raised concentration of carbon dioxide and water vapour.

Because large amounts of air are continually breathed in and out, the respiratory tract is repeatedly exposed to microbial organisms, many of which can cause infection. It is also exposed to toxins, dust and smoke. There are good defence mechanisms against infection in the respiratory tract, where cells of the immune system are widely found. Some of these can engulf and destroy invading bacteria, while others produce antibodies which are secreted into the mucus that lines and continually washes the respiratory tract. As well as antibodies the mucus also

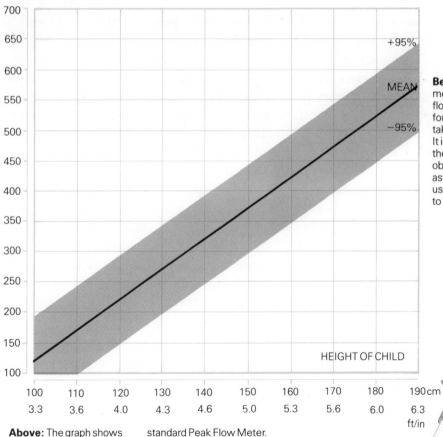

PEAK FLOW (1/Min)

Below: A Peak Flow Meter measures the maximum flow of air that a child can forcibly breathe out, after taking a deep breath in. It is useful for assessing the severity of airways obstruction in cases of asthma, and can also be used to measure response to treatment.

Above: The graph shows normal peak flow readings for children aged between 5 and 18 years, using the standard Peak Flow Meter. The peak flow rate is measured in litres per minute.

contains other substances that can inactivate or kill micro-organisms. In spite of these mechanisms infections of the upper respiratory tract are common.

The inhalation of smoke and dust also provokes protective mechanisms. The production of lung and upper respiratory tract secretions increases, and there is a reflex narrowing of the airways, which decreases the amount of toxins entering the body. Coughing forces both secretions and inhaled particles out of the lungs.

PHYSICAL FITNESS

Physical fitness consists of the ability to perform vigorous activity without distress and to recover quickly once the exercise is over. Fitness depends on being able to increase the depth and rate of breathing, with a corresponding increase in the output of blood from the heart. The muscles also have to respond efficiently. Most children tend to be naturally active and are fit. As they get older many become rather sedentary in their habits, having to sit for lessons at school, and spending prolonged periods watching television or reading.

Sporting activities provide a way of maintaining physical fitness, and being a member of a team which works together as a group develops social skills as well as agility. Little is to be gained by making children who are unenthusiastic participate frequently in sport, but an active lifestyle in childhood is important. Walking, swimming and cycling all contribute, and many habits established in childhood persist throughout life. Adults who regularly take moderate exercise remain healthier than those who have sedentary habits.

Fitness also implies the absence of disease. There is strong evidence that the children of parents who smoke in the home have many more coughs and attacks of chestiness than children from non-smoking households. Parents should remember that smoking adversely affects their children's health as well as their own.

UPPER RESPIRATORY TRACT INFECTIONS

An upper respiratory tract infection, or URTI, can affect the nose, throat or air sinuses. In adults and older children most such infections are mainly of nuisance value, rather than the cause of significant illness. They may predispose to secondary bacterial infection, which can cause tonsillitis or otitis media (see pages 304 and 290).

The common cold or coryza is familiar to everybody. There are many different cold viruses that provoke the symptoms — initially, a flow of secretions from the nose, often associated with a headache and slight fever. After one or two days the symptoms change to a thick nasal discharge of mucus and pus. The whole illness lasts about a week. Treatment is directed at the symptoms, with paracetamol to relieve fever and a decongestant to inhale.

Babies cannot suck effectively if their nose is blocked, so that feeding is a problem, and the malaise (general feeling of being unwell) associated with the cold may also be more pronounced. Sometimes the virus that causes the cold symptoms also infects the lower respiratory tract. This can lead to croup or to bronchiolitis (see pages 253 and 244).

ASTHMA AND WHEEZY BRONCHITIS

Between 5 and 10 per cent of children have some degree of asthma. In many it is mild and attacks are infrequent, but in some children it causes a marked disruption of normal life. Severe asthma attacks may be life-threatening.

Some individuals have an inborn predisposition known as atopy: atopic people are prone to develop asthma, and also eczema, allergic rhinitis and hay fever (see pages 239, 231 and 272 for details). These diseases often run in families. Very often children who have infantile eczema will subsequently develop asthma. Atopic individuals are liable to develop allergies, and some attacks of asthma are precipitated by exposure to allergens in the air or in food. Other precipitants for asthma attacks include upper respiratory tract infections (URTIs), exercise and emotion.

Asthma consists of episodes in which the small airways in the lungs become narrowed, due to a combination of contraction of the bronchial wall muscles, swelling of the mucous membrane lining the respiratory tract, and blockage of the airways by thick secretions. This makes breathing more difficult, and the air moving in and out through narrowed tubes makes a wheezing sound. There may also be a cough and there may be abdominal pain. Asthma attacks often start in the middle of the night.

It is uncommon for asthma to start much before the age of 1 year, and in the majority of affected children the first attack is between the ages of 1 and 2. The development of asthma is often not recognized immediately. Typically the child has a cold, which after a day or two becomes chesty, and he begins to cough and wheeze. At this stage a diagnosis of chest infection or wheezy bronchitis is often made, as it is considered that the infection that caused the cold has spread to the lungs. However, in a majority of cases of wheezy bronchitis and chest infection of small children the URTI causes the airways to narrow, but there is no actual infection in the lungs. The diagnosis of asthma is often made only when it is realized that the child becomes chesty every time he has a cold.

The severity of asthma attacks is very variable. Sometimes the child just has a slight wheeze or cough, or he may be extremely breathless due to a marked narrowing of the airways. The frequency of the attacks is also very variable, some children only ever getting a few, and others being wheezy for much of the time.

Children who do have asthma usually outgrow their attacks some time during childhood. For some this is in the pre-school period, in others not until puberty. Only about 10 per cent of children who develop asthma in early childhood persist with symptoms as adults.

Caring for the asthmatic child

Asthma attacks If a child is having an attack of asthma, treatment can be given to relieve the narrowing of the airways. Bronchodilator drugs are the first choice (see below), and in severe attacks these may be supplemented with steroid treatment. Antibiotics are seldom useful. Furthermore, if it is known that something usually brings on an attack, such as URTI or exercise, treatment can be used before the onset of wheezing to try to ward off the attack.

Parents of asthmatic children should always keep a supply of bronchodilators at home, so that any attack of asthma can be treated promptly. Most attacks can be handled satisfactorily at home, either by the parent, or by parent and family doctor together. More severe attacks may require hospitalization, and children with severe asthma may have repeated admissions in early childhood.

Bronchodilator drugs relax the muscle in the wall of the bronchial airways, and also have some effect in shrinking the swollen

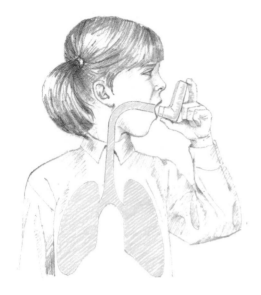

respiratory mucous membrane. A wide selection of different bronchodilator drugs is available. Salbutamol and terbutyline are most widely used as first-choice drugs, and may be given in liquid, tablet or aerosol form. In a severe attack they are most effective when given through a nebulizer, which breaks down a solution of a bronchodilator into very fine particles which are breathed into the lungs.

Sometimes the doctor will feel that the use of a second bronchodilator is necessary because of an incomplete response to the first. One with a different mode of action is chosen, usually aminophylline or one of its derivatives.

In a severe attack where there is inadequate response to bronchodilators steroid treatment may be helpful. Although steroid drugs have disadvantages, including obesity and poor growth, when used for long-term treatment there are few problems associated with their occasional short-term use, and they usually cut short an attack.

Planning treatment both between and during attacks in a child with moderate or severe asthma can be difficult with so many different drugs to choose from. The doctor will need to review progress from time

to time, and tailor the regime to each individual.

Treatment between attacks

Most children have no wheezing or other symptoms between their attacks, and if attacks are infrequent then no specific action is necessary, apart from avoiding anything known to precipitate asthma.

In the child who has frequent attacks of asthma, or who often wheezes or has a persistent night cough, it may well be worth considering whether the attacks can be prevented. There are two approaches to

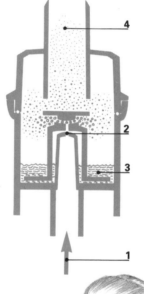

Above left: Using an aerosol inhaler. As the inhaler is pressed a fine mist containing a bronchodilator drug is released. The child must coordinate breathing in with each squirt of bronchodilator.

Below and left: Using a nebulizer. In this method the drug is drawn into the lungs as the child breathes in through a mouthpiece. Compressed air (**1**) is forced through a small inlet (**2**), emerging as a jet to draw up the liquid medicine (**3**). The mixture of air and liquid breaks up into minute droplets (**4**) as it is forced through the outlet.

prevention: avoiding exposure to allergens and other precipitating factors, and the use of medication.

Allergen avoidance In many asthmatics attacks can be triggered by exposure to dust, fur, feathers, pollen, smoke or something to which the child is allergic. House dust often contains a minute insect, the house dust mite, and this has been shown to be a potent cause of attacks in many asthmatic individuals. For any child who has frequent attacks it is worth making sure that pillows and bedding do not contain feathers, and trying to cut down on dust, particularly in bedrooms. Cotton blankets that can be washed frequently are helpful. Covering the mattress with a plastic cover that can be wiped over ensures that it stays clean. Having a vinyl floor covering or a short-pile carpet that can be kept dust free is also wise.

Making beds and house-cleaning stir a lot of dust into the air, and this takes between one and two hours to settle completely. The child should not be in the room while beds are being made or housework is in progress, and should not return to the room for an hour if possible.

Furry pets may be a cause of asthma attacks in some children. Families with an asthmatic child should carefully consider the position before acquiring a new pet. A more difficult decision is what to do about a well-established pet if a child develops asthma. Unless the child is obviously made worse by contact with the animal, or has been shown by skin testing (see below) to be allergic to fur, there is no certainty that the asthma will improve if the pet is given away. However, if the child's attacks are frequent or severe the removal of the pet from the home should be considered.

Skin testing As well as the common air-borne allergens that may precipitate attacks of asthma, some children are allergic to less common substances, and sometimes to food constituents such as cow's milk and eggs. In the child who has frequent asthma attacks skin testing may be helpful in identifying other potential allergies. The test consists of placing minute amounts of various substances on the skin and making a small prick through them into the skin, or covering them with a patch to keep them in skin contact. After thirty minutes there may be reddening where the test was done, and the extent of the reaction gives an indication of the severity of the allergy. (See also the section on allergy on page 231.)

Medication Bronchodilator drugs can be used to prevent attacks, as well as for treating an established one. If the child develops a cold it is often better to give him the bronchodilator drug before chestiness starts rather than waiting until he is wheezy. If a child becomes wheezy with exercise the use of a bronchodilator aerosol at the beginning of a sports session may be helpful. The child who has frequent attacks may be helped by being given a regular dose of a long-acting bronchodilator.

As well as bronchodilators there are other drugs that can be helpful between attacks. Sodium cromoglycate is a prophylactic or preventative drug which is inhaled as a powder or aerosol, or given via a nebulizer two or three times daily, and reduces the frequency of attacks in many children. It has no beneficial effect during an asthma attack, so there is no immediate feeling that it is doing good, but continued use in most children will lessen the severity of asthma. Aerosol steroid preparations are also used in some children with moderate and severe asthma to reduce the frequency and severity of attacks.

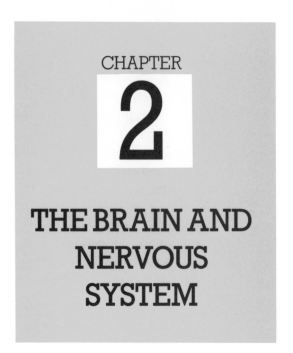

CHAPTER 2

THE BRAIN AND NERVOUS SYSTEM

HOW THE NERVOUS SYSTEM WORKS

The brain, the spinal cord and the nerves together make up the nervous system. The brain has many different functions, including co-ordinating all the actions of the body, storing memories, learning and thinking. The spinal cord consists of bundles of nerve fibres and carries nervous impulses up and down the body. The nerves (called motor nerves) run between the brain or spinal cord and all parts of the body, including the internal organs, muscles, blood vessels, joints and skin, and transmit messages both to and from the brain and spinal cord.

The brain receives information from all parts of the body, transmitted by sensory nerves either directly to the brain or via the spinal cord. Information from the special sense organs, the eyes, ears, nose and tongue, goes directly to the brain. The various sensations of touch, hot and cold, vibration, awareness of body position, and pain from all over the body travel by the sensory nerves to the spinal cord and then to the brain. The brain processes and co-ordinates this information and sends out messages via the nerves to control movement, posture and most of the body's functions.

Much of this nervous activity is unconscious and reflex. Some messages do reach consciousness and people are aware of making decisions about their actions. Only a small proportion of information which reaches consciousness is stored as long-term memory. What is retained forms the basis of experience and knowledge for the future.

Every day we all receive an enormous amount of information about our surroundings, interact with people, and are continuously making decisions big and small. The sensation of tiredness and the necessity for sleep seem to be due to the need to cut off the information input to the brain. During sleep the brain sorts out the day's experiences, and files or discards memories of the various events.

With young children many of their activities or experiences are new and therefore more puzzling than familiar happenings. Talking through the events of each day with an attentive and interested adult provides them with an opportunity to understand and learn from all experiences, whether new or familiar. Parents or grandparents should try to ensure that every child has the opportunity to be 'centre stage' on return home from nursery or school, or at some other opportune moment each day.

INVESTIGATING THE NERVOUS SYSTEM

A doctor seeing a child as a new patient will first want to find out what has caused the parents to seek medical help. Details will be needed of the symptoms themselves and how long they have been present, and of the pattern of the illness.

Because the brain and nervous system are so complex, a wide variety of symptoms may signify neurological disease; some of these symptoms may also be due to a disorder of other systems, and the doctor taking the history will try to work out whether or not the features are related to nervous system disorder. In childhood the most common features of neurological disease are impairment of vision or hearing, weakness or incoordination of movement, including cerebral palsy (see page 246), mental handicap and convulsions. Headaches may also sometimes be due to disease of the nervous system, but are more commonly related to tension or stress.

Having taken the history, the doctor will examine the child. A lot of information about the functioning of the nervous system can be obtained by watching the child at play and moving around the room. A movement disorder because of weakness or incoordination may be apparent, and is often easier to assess when the child is engaged in spontaneous activity than by persuading him to undertake various tests.

The doctor will also want to weigh and measure the child, and do a full general examination including measuring the circumference of the head and testing the nerves and reflexes.

At the end of the examination the doctor may be in a position to make a diagnosis, or may want specialized tests performed. Where a child is known to have some brain damage the doctor is likely to arrange tests of vision and hearing and a developmental assessment, in addition to the general investigation. Other tests, including blood tests, may be ordered. The following are commonly performed on children being investigated for neurological disease:

Lumbar puncture

In some diseases of the nervous system it is necessary to obtain cerebrospinal fluid (CSF), which surrounds the brain and spinal cord, for laboratory investigation, particularly in meningitis and encephalitis (see pages 285 and 261). The sample of fluid is obtained by inserting a needle between two of the lumbar (lower back) vertebrae into the fluid-filled space just below the end of the spinal cord.

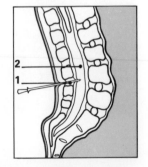

Right: In a lumbar puncture a needle is inserted between two vertebrae of the lumbar spine (**1**) to obtain cerebrospinal fluid from the space below the spinal cord (**2**).

Below: An X-ray of the skull.

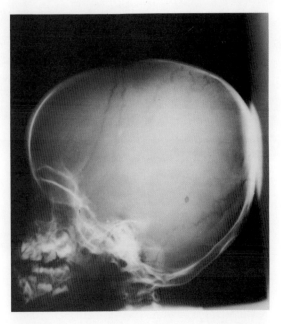

Skull X-ray

An X-ray of the skull from the front and from the side provides useful information about the bones of the skull, and may give some information on the brain and whether the pressure of fluid inside it is raised. The brain itself is not well shown on ordinary X-rays.

Ultrasound

In infants up to the age of 1 year or 18 months it may be possible to visualize the brain and the fluid-filled spaces within by using ultrasound. Ultrasound cannot produce pictures through bone, as the bone absorbs the sound waves. In young children, however, the anterior fontanelle or soft spot – the depression on the top of the head where the three bones of the skull meet – may be open and permit ultrasound examination. This is of particular use in suspected hydrocephalus and for haemorrhage in the newborn period (see pages 277 and 271).

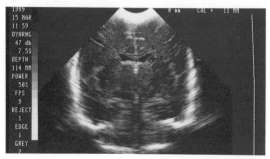

In babies some of the structure of the brain can be seen by means of ultrasound. During a scan the probe is placed over the fontanelle to obtain cross-sections: **left**, from side to side (coronal); and **below**, from front to back (sagittal). Both of these results are normal. **Bottom:** The infant shown here undergoing a scan was suffering from hydrocephalus. He has been treated with a shunt tube which drains the excess of cerebrospinal fluid (CSF) associated with hydrocephalus from within the brain to the abdomen.

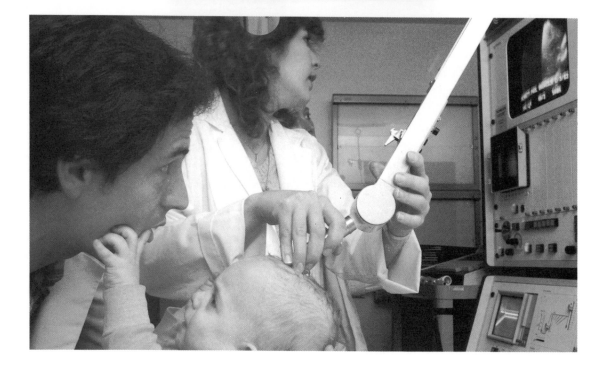

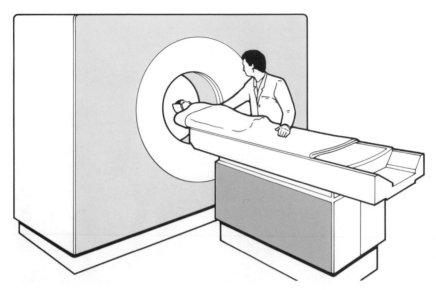

A CT scanner in operation. Computerized tomography (CT), which is also known as computerized axial tomography (CAT), is a highly sophisticated method of forming images from X-rays. The anatomical detail possible with CT is a significant improvement on that obtained from conventional X-ray examinations. Images are displayed on a television screen and can be copied on to film. The technique is invaluable for imaging the brain and is also extremely useful in imaging the chest and abdomen.

Computerized tomography (CT) scan

Computerized tomography can be used to produce scans of the brain which show the soft structures in great detail. The technique produces computed images built up from multiple X-ray pictures taken from many positions as an X-ray tube is moved around the head. After computation the scanner produces images that look like a series of slices through the brain from top to bottom. The internal structure of the brain is shown in great detail.

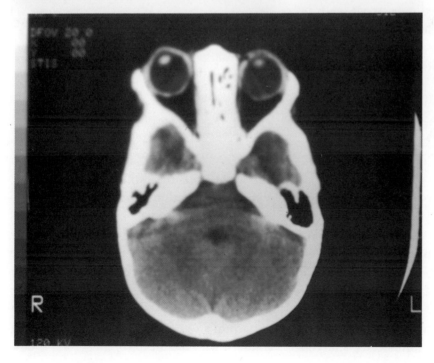

The result of a CT scan, showing a section through the eyes, cerebral cortex and inner ears. The scanner builds up a cross-sectional image or 'slice' by evaluating the X-rays passing through the body. The image it produces can distinguish minute differences in density of structures beneath the surface.

Magnetic resonance (MR) scan

A newer technique than CT scanning is now available in a few special centres. This is magnetic resonance scanning. The patient is placed in a very strong magnetic field, and a special technique is used to produce images which are very detailed, even more so than CT scans. MR can be used to produce pictures which look like slices taken in many different planes through the brain and spinal cord.

Electroencephalogram (EEG)

The electroencephalogram is a record of the electrical activity of the brain. Wires are attached to the scalp to pick up electrical discharges, and a record is taken over a prolonged period. The EEG is principally used in the investigation of suspected epilepsy (see page 262).

Electromyography (EMG)

Electromyography is a recording of the electrical activity of the muscles, both at rest and during a contraction. The recording electrodes may be placed on the skin over the muscle, or a fine needle electrode may be inserted into the muscle. EMG can diagnose damage of the nerve going to the muscle, or disease of the muscle itself.

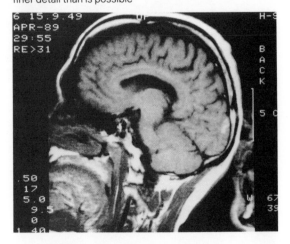

The result of a Magnetic Resonance scan. This technique provides even finer detail than is possible with Computerized Tomography.

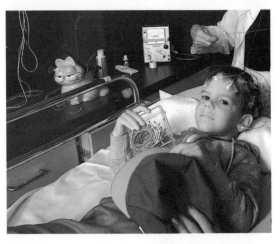

An EEG records the electrical activity of the brain by means of wires attached to the scalp. In the read-out, each wavy line shows the fluctuation in the very small electric current, as detected at different places over the scalp.

MENTAL HANDICAP

The normal range of intelligence for children is very wide; some children may function at school as much as two years above average, and others will be a year or two below the mean. An individual's level of intelligence is not fixed, but is influenced by environment, stimulation, the quality of teaching the child receives, and general health. Intelligence is only one facet of personality; friendliness and the capacity to give and receive love, the ability to communicate, and consideration for others are other equally important qualities which have little or nothing to do with intelligence.

Children are said to be mentally handicapped when their level of intelligence is below the normal range; the handicap can be mild, moderate or severe. This terminology has replaced 'mental retardation' and earlier designations, but does little to convey what the child's problems are. In assessing children with handicaps of all sorts it is now considered more helpful to identify them as children with special needs, and to establish what those needs are, rather than giving them a label which can be stigmatizing.

By identifying and meeting the special needs of mentally handicapped children, and by providing them with a secure, stimulating and loving home and an appropriate education, their intellectual potential can be maximized. Experience has shown that such positive regimes make a significant difference to the ultimate level of ability and independence of the individual.

Causes of mental handicap

It is not possible to find a cause for mental handicap in all affected individuals. Furthermore, for many mildly handicapped children the causes are multiple. For example, children of parents with below average intellect are themselves likely to be below average as regards their intellectual potential. Because their parents are likely to be working class they are more likely to be born prematurely and to be of low birth weight, to be brought up with some degree of deprivation, and to be developmentally understimulated. This cycle of deprivation can mean that children who have the potential to develop within the normal range of intelligence, given an optimal environment, do not achieve it.

Children with severe mental handicap probably all have abnormalities of structure or function of the brain, although these cannot always be recognized. There may be abnormalities of brain development, such as occurs in Down's syndrome (see pages 104 and 259) and in many other syndromes, or the developing brain may be damaged by infection, alcohol or other toxins, oxygen lack or many other factors, some known and many still unknown. There are several rare diseases caused by inherited biochemical defects which can give rise to brain damage,

and these are sometimes progressive. Both road accidents and meningitis (see page 285) can render a previously normal child mentally handicapped.

Identifying the causes of mental handicap so that it can be treated or prevented is of great importance. In the newborn period the introduction of the routine Guthrie blood test for phenylketonuria and for congenital hypothyroidism (see pages 291 and 278) has led to the prevention of mental handicap by the early detection and treatment of affected individuals.

Some handicapping conditions are genetic, and if parents have had one child with a handicap they may be at risk of having another. Genetic counselling should be available to the parents of every handicapped child if they wish it (see page 111).

Recognizing mental handicap in children

It is sometimes possible to know at birth or in the newborn period that a child is going to be mentally handicapped. Down's syndrome is usually recognizable by the appearance of the child shortly after birth (if not identified earlier by amniocentesis or chorionic villus sampling); all children with Down's syndrome are likely to be handicapped, although the degree of handicap is very variable. Other syndromes may also be recognizable early and may be known to cause mental handicap. For many children mental handicap is not suspected until later infancy when their developmental milestones are delayed (see Part One, Chapter 4), and sometimes is not recognized until they start school.

Early recognition enables the child to have special help to encourage development. It is therefore very important that all children have regular developmental screening.

Childhood disability is considered in Part One, Chapter 11.

CHAPTER 3

THE ABDOMINAL ORGANS

The abdomen is a hollow cavity containing the stomach and intestines, which together make up the alimentary tract; the liver and pancreas, organs which play an important part in the digestion and utilization of food, but also have other functions; and the kidneys and urinary system. The various systems have their separate functions but they are in close proximity to each other.

When trying to find the cause of a symptom such as abdominal pain it may be necessary to consider the possibility of dysfunction of any of these organs; injury or some disease processes may affect more than one system.

THE ALIMENTARY SYSTEM AND LIVER

The alimentary system, also known as the gastro-intestinal tract, is primarily concerned with the digestion and absorption of food and fluids, and with the elimination of waste products. These functions are very complex. The liver is closely related to the alimentary tract, and will be considered with it. One of the major functions of the liver is to produce bile to help in the digestion of fat, and there is a special system of blood vessels, the portal system, that carries blood from the intestine to the liver. Absorbed food is also transported by the portal system to the liver, where it is processed before being carried around the body to be used for energy, growth and repair, or to be stored.

A disturbance in the function of the gastro-intestinal tract may be the result of disease affecting the tract itself or another part of the body, or may be a disorder caused by emotional factors.

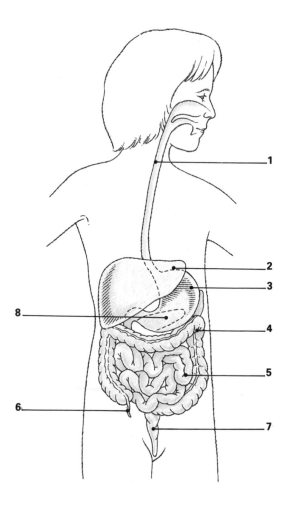

The alimentary system:
1, oesophagus; **2**, liver;
3, stomach; **4**, large
intestine; **5**, small
intestine; **6**, appendix;
7, rectum; **8**, pancreas
(behind stomach).

DIGESTION AND ABSORPTION

After food is bitten and chewed to break it into small pieces and to mix it with saliva, it is swallowed and passes down the oesophagus (gullet) into the stomach. The food remains in the stomach for some time, and there digestion starts.

Digestion is the process by which ingested food is broken down into its constituents: carbohydrate, fat and protein. These are further broken down into smaller molecules in order that they can be absorbed through the intestinal wall and enter the circulation.

In the stomach the food is mixed with the gastric juices, which contain both digestive enzymes and acid; it is broken down into smaller particles by the action of the acid. At the same time the digestive enzymes work on any milk present to coagulate it and form a curd, and the digestion of proteins starts, to reduce them to their constituent peptides and amino acids.

The stomach contents are gradually released into the duodenum, the first part of the small intestine. There they mix with bile from the liver and digestive juice from the pancreas, and digestion of the starches, proteins and fats continues. The small intestine itself contains digestive enzymes to complete the digestive processes, and it is here that the peptides, amino acids, sugars and fats produced as a result of digestion are absorbed. The small intestine has a very large surface area so that absorption can take place efficiently; under normal conditions only minimal amounts of these foods are not absorbed.

Not all constituents of foodstuffs can be digested; the unabsorbed residue is referred to as dietary fibre. Whereas most fibre consists of cellulose from plants, other non-absorbable parts of the diet also contribute to total fibre intake. The non-absorbed residue passes into the large intestine, or colon. In the colon there are large numbers of bacteria and these further degrade some of the food residues.

As what is left of the food passes down the colon much of the contained water is absorbed, leaving a faecal residue. The faeces accumulate in the lower part of the large intestine until defecation, when a bowel contraction moves them into the lowest part of the alimentary tract, the rectum, and then out through the anus.

ALIMENTARY TRACT DISORDER: DIAGNOSIS

Vomiting, loss of appetite (see page 100), abdominal pain, diarrhoea and constipation are all common features of disorders of the alimentary tract, but they all may also be due to other conditions. In making a diagnosis the doctor has to consider the symptoms and look at these together with other features of the patient's history and the results of the examination.

In many cases the doctor will need to carry out further tests to find out more about the gastro-intestinal tract. X-rays can be used to visualize the whole tract. A special contrast medium (barium) that will show up clearly on the X-ray has to be used to outline the various organs. When the contrast medium is swallowed, it can be visualized going down the oesophagus and into the stomach. Any abnormality can be seen. The barium then leaves the stomach via the duodenum and can be followed all the way through the small intestine. The lower bowel can be similarly investigated by a barium enema, with the contrast introduced into the rectum.

Endoscopy consists of passing a flexible fibre-optic instrument through a hollow organ so that the inside can be seen directly.

Endoscopy of both the upper and lower bowel has now become routine, and will often enable diagnosis, biopsy (taking a small sample) and sometimes treatment in the gastro-intestinal tract. Children require a general anaesthetic for endoscopy but in adults this is often not necessary.

VOMITING

Infancy

Babies may regurgitate small amounts of milk after feeds. This is known as posseting and is normal. If a baby vomits in the first day or two of life there is a small possibility of congenital blockage of the intestine, either because part of the intestine has not formed properly or because it has become obstructed. If the vomit is yellow in colour due to staining with bile the chance of intestinal obstruction is even higher, and the doctor will want to do an X-ray as soon as possible to confirm or rule out a blockage. There are other causes of vomiting in the first two days of life, including being upset by a difficult delivery,

having an infection, or having gastric irritation due to blood and mucus swallowed during the delivery.

Vomiting may also occur in slightly older infants. In the condition known as hiatus hernia, part of the stomach pokes through the diaphragm, and the top end of the stomach (the cardia) does not close properly; the baby tends to vomit if laid down. The vomiting is not forceful, but may occur repeatedly until the stomach is empty. Regurgitation from a hiatus hernia can start in the first week and without treatment may persist until the baby is several months old. Treatment consists of thickening the feeds, and propping the baby into a semi-upright position. In some babies regurgitation occurs even though there is no hiatus hernia.

About 1 baby in every 600 develops a condition called pyloric stenosis in the first few weeks of life, which gives rise to severe vomiting. The condition is more common in boys than girls, and often runs in families. There is an overgrowth of the muscle in the wall of the pylorus, the lower end of the stomach where it joins the duodenum, and this causes a constriction which prevents milk from leaving the stomach.

The symptoms of pyloric stenosis start between 2 and 6 weeks of age and consist of vomiting immediately after feeds. Over the space of a few days the vomiting becomes more pronounced and forceful, and almost no milk is retained by the baby. The child loses weight and becomes hungry, fretful and anxious. Hospital admission is necessary. The doctor can often feel the thickened muscle while the baby is feeding, and the diagnosis may be confirmed by ultrasound or X-ray. Once the diagnosis has been made, the baby is given replacement fluids to correct any deficiency caused by vomiting. A small operation is then performed, cutting through the pyloric muscle to relieve the obstruction.

CAUSES OF VOMITING IN INFANCY

POSSETTING is the regurgitation of small amounts of milk after feeding. It is normal and of no significance.

INFECTIONS of all kinds in infancy may be accompanied by vomiting.

INTESTINAL OBSTRUCTION due to congenital abnormality is rare, but may cause vomiting in the newborn period.

HIATUS HERNIA occurs when the top end of the stomach does not close properly. Feeds are regurgitated when the stomach is full and when the baby is laid down.

PYLORIC STENOSIS is a narrowing of the outlet of the stomach which can develop when the baby is a few weeks old. It causes forceful vomiting.

As soon as the baby has recovered from the anaesthetic, feeding can be resumed, and recovery is usually straightforward. The baby can return home in a few days.

Hiatus hernia and pyloric stenosis are structural abnormalities that can cause vomiting in infancy, but vomiting can also be due to infections. Together with diarrhoea it is characteristic of gastro-enteritis (page 266) but may also be a symptom of other infections in infancy, including urinary tract infec-

CAUSES OF VOMITING IN OLDER CHILDREN

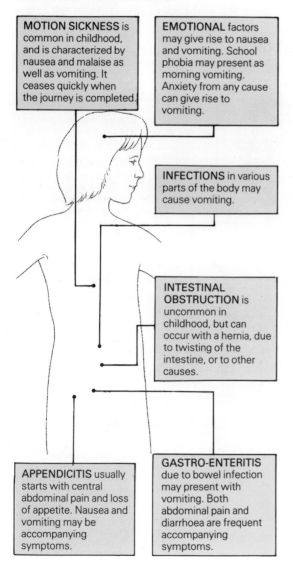

MOTION SICKNESS is common in childhood, and is characterized by nausea and malaise as well as vomiting. It ceases quickly when the journey is completed.

EMOTIONAL factors may give rise to nausea and vomiting. School phobia may present as morning vomiting. Anxiety from any cause can give rise to vomiting.

INFECTIONS in various parts of the body may cause vomiting.

INTESTINAL OBSTRUCTION is uncommon in childhood, but can occur with a hernia, due to twisting of the intestine, or to other causes.

APPENDICITIS usually starts with central abdominal pain and loss of appetite. Nausea and vomiting may be accompanying symptoms.

GASTRO-ENTERITIS due to bowel infection may present with vomiting. Both abdominal pain and diarrhoea are frequent accompanying symptoms.

tions, otitis media and tonsillitis (see pages 171, 290 and 304).

Older children

Nausea and vomiting are frequent symptoms in childhood. Over-indulgence at a party or excitement may cause vomiting, and vomiting as part of travel sickness is very common in young children. Gastro-enteritis is not unusual in childhood and vomiting may be very marked. In small children the combination of vomiting and diarrhoea can give rise to dehydration which may be serious, so prompt treatment of gastro-enteritis is important (see page 266). Other common childhood infections, like those of the ear, throat or urinary tract, and the infectious fevers, may be accompanied by vomiting, and sometimes also by slight diarrhoea.

Migraine may occur in childhood, and often starts with nausea and vomiting before the onset of the headache. Meningitis (see page 285) is rare, but the initial symptoms include headache, fever and vomiting.

Appendicitis (see page 237) may start with vomiting; vomiting and abdominal pain also occur in other causes of intestinal obstruction, due to twisting of the bowel or to a strangulated hernia.

Vomiting does not always have a physical cause: it may be related to emotional stress. Children in households where there is considerable tension as a result of poor housing, marital disharmony, or sickness of another family member may not feel able to express their feelings of fear and insecurity; instead they may manifest as headache, abdominal pain or vomiting. The stress may not be stemming from the home, but from school: perhaps the child is being bullied, or is afraid of a teacher who is unsympathetic or bad-tempered. The apprehension felt by the child before school may cause vomiting.

ABDOMINAL PAIN

Abdominal pain can be due to disease of the alimentary tract, or of other organs in the abdomen such as the liver or urinary tract. It may also be due to pain referred when there is disease in other parts of the body such as the thorax or the pelvis. In children abdominal pain may not be associated with disease at all, but related to emotional factors.

When pain is due to alimentary tract dysfunction it is often colicky, increasing in severity for a minute or two, and then dying away for a few minutes until it recurs. This colic reflects the intermittent contractions of the intestinal muscles. When pain is continuous it is more likely to be associated with localized inflammation. The sudden onset of severe abdominal pain should always be taken seriously, and the doctor consulted if the cause is not apparent.

Sometimes the pain may be known to be associated with food. Some fruits, particularly green apples, and red kidney beans may cause colic. Distension of the stomach or intestines by wind can cause abdominal pain. Inflammation of the upper gastro-intestinal tract can cause pain felt centrally around or above the umbilicus (navel). Pain felt lower

THE CAUSES OF ABDOMINAL PAIN

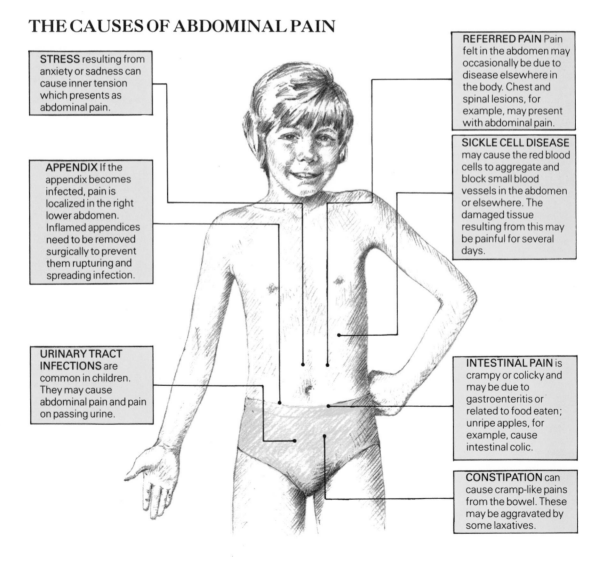

STRESS resulting from anxiety or sadness can cause inner tension which presents as abdominal pain.

APPENDIX If the appendix becomes infected, pain is localized in the right lower abdomen. Inflamed appendices need to be removed surgically to prevent them rupturing and spreading infection.

URINARY TRACT INFECTIONS are common in children. They may cause abdominal pain and pain on passing urine.

REFERRED PAIN Pain felt in the abdomen may occasionally be due to disease elsewhere in the body. Chest and spinal lesions, for example, may present with abdominal pain.

SICKLE CELL DISEASE may cause the red blood cells to aggregate and block small blood vessels in the abdomen or elsewhere. The damaged tissue resulting from this may be painful for several days.

INTESTINAL PAIN is crampy or colicky and may be due to gastroenteritis or related to food eaten; unripe apples, for example, cause intestinal colic.

CONSTIPATION can cause cramp-like pains from the bowel. These may be aggravated by some laxatives.

in the abdomen can be from the colon (large intestine), and may be associated with constipation. Localized pain may indicate inflammation of an abdominal organ in that region.

In appendicitis (see page 237) the pain is often central when it starts, but as the inflammation of the appendix becomes more marked the pain shifts to the lower right side of the abdomen. Other organs in the abdomen may give rise to pain. The onset of infectious hepatitis (page 274) is often heralded by an ache in the right upper abdomen, and infections of the kidneys and urinary tract can give abdominal pain.

Disease in other parts of the body may cause abdominal pain. Small children with tonsillitis or otitis media (see pages 304 and 290) often have tummy ache, and pneumonia (page 292) affecting the base of the lung often gives upper abdominal pain. Some abdominal pain during an asthma attack is common (page 152). In black children who have inherited sickle cell disease recurrent attacks of abdominal pain or pains elsewhere can be disabling (page 299).

Not all abdominal pain signifies disease. Many emotions, including apprehension, fear and sadness, may be associated with abdominal symptoms. Anxiety gives rise to body reactions which may include abdominal pain. In a lot of children where abdominal pain is due to emotional stress the cause is readily apparent, and parents will be able to help. In some children who have recurrent episodes of abdominal pain the precipitating factors are obscure.

Recurrent abdominal pain

Some children have repeated attacks of abdominal pain, which may be severe and may start at any age. Parents will obviously be concerned to know the cause, and the doctor should be consulted. The pain may be associated with nausea and vomiting, and sometimes with headache. In most children with recurrent abdominal pain there is no underlying disease.

We are all familiar with individuals whose constitution makes them prone to headaches. In a similar way the make-up of some children means they are prone to recurrent episodes of abdominal pain. The condition is well recognized, and is sometimes called the periodic syndrome because of the periodic recurrence of symptoms. There is often a family history of migraine, and the syndrome may also be called abdominal migraine, as it is thought that the pain bears a resemblance to migraine attacks. Furthermore some children who have recurrent episodes of abdominal pain in early childhood may go on to have migraine later.

Although it is not known precisely what it is in the make-up of some children that makes them prone to recurrent abdominal pain, it is often possible to identify factors that bring on attacks. They may be precipitated by feelings of anxiety or insecurity arising at home or school. Marital disharmony, family worries over health, employment or finances, or moving house are domestic stresses that affect children. Bullying or teasing at school, or dislike of a teacher can also provoke stress. In children prone to abdominal pain this stress may precipitate an attack. Other children will also be affected by such stresses but may manifest it in other ways.

Not all stress is caused by undesirable situations. Some children put a lot of effort into their school work to achieve good results, and others may concentrate hard on sport or a hobby. Making such special efforts is a very positive action, but may generate stress, and may cause abdominal pain or headache in some children.

Once it is realized that the child who has attacks of recurrent abdominal pain does not have an underlying disease, management becomes easier. Analgesics (painkillers) such as paracetamol may help, and going to bed with a hot water bottle to hold against the abdomen brings relief. If attacks are severe or frequent and are causing absence from school or disruption of normal life, the child may benefit from referral to a paediatrician or psychologist for review and advice.

DIARRHOEA

Diarrhoea – that is, the passage of frequent watery stools – arises because the intestinal contents are propelled rapidly through the alimentary tract, or because little or no water is absorbed in the large intestine. When diarrhoea comes on suddenly it is most commonly due to inflammation caused by infection (see Gastro-enteritis, page 266). Diarrhoea can also be due to the malabsorption of sugars or other food substances (see page 284), rapid bowel transit, or inflammatory disease of the bowel.

The consistency of normal stools is very variable. Some normal children always pass stools which are semi-solid and unformed. If these are not particularly frequent they probably have no medical significance.

CONSTIPATION

Constipation is the passage of hard stools, often requiring considerable straining. Bowel actions are often infrequent as well, but this is not always so: bowel actions may be regular, but they are small and do not empty the bowel. Constipation may occur at any age from early infancy onwards. Constipation in infancy has already been described, in Part One, Chapter 4 (page 62).

Bowel actions vary enormously in frequency in the normal individual. Many newborns will pass a stool after every feed, but some babies, particularly if breast fed, only pass a stool on alternate days. With older children there is also much variation, from two or three bowel actions a day to one every two or three days. Provided there is no discomfort and the stools are not hard, infrequent stools are not positive indicators of constipation.

Some children are rather prone to develop constipation. They tend to pass firm stools, and from time to time they have to strain to have their bowels open. Modification of their diet may be very helpful. Diets which contain a lot of fibre increase the bulk and water content of the stools, so these tend to be more frequent and softer. As such diets are preventative they need to be followed all the time and not just spasmodically; the diet has therefore to be practical and fit in with the child's likes and food fancies.

Fibre in the diet is provided by cereal bran, by fruits and by vegetables including baked beans. Some breakfast cereals have quite a high bran content, but these are not always favoured by children, and the use of wholemeal bread and a generous intake of fruit are more practical ways to increase fibre in their diet (see also page 94).

When constipation is established it is unlikely to be helped by a modification of the diet. The colon (large intestine) is already filled by firm stool, and changing the diet cannot modify that. First the colon needs to be emptied, and then steps must be taken to establish the passage of regular soft stools. A laxative may be needed to soften the stools and make bowel actions more regular. While the choice of a mild laxative like lactulose may seem ideal for children it is so mild as to sometimes be ineffective. The use of senna compounds is more reliable. They should be given first thing in the morning, or on return from school. They take around six hours to work, and if the initial dose is ineffective the amount may need to be increased the next day. Laxatives may provoke abdominal pain as they work in part by stimulating contraction of the muscle of the gut wall.

It is seldom of any use to give a laxative on a single occasion, as constipation is likely to recur. It needs to be continued for a week or more to re-establish a regular habit. At the same time it may be beneficial to increase the amount of fibre eaten, if the child has previously been on a diet that is low in fibre.

A few children have chronic (long-term) constipation with the retention of a mass of faeces in the rectum. They tend to have abdominal distension and a poor appetite, and faecal soiling of underclothes may be a problem. The soiling is often liquid, and the children are sometimes diagnosed as having diarrhoea. This spurious diarrhoea is due to the fact that the colon is partially obstructed, and only liquid stool can pass. Children who are persistently or recurrently constipated need referral to a specialist to see if there is an underlying cause, which may be physical or psychological.

THE KIDNEYS AND URINARY SYSTEM

The two kidneys are situated one on either side of the spine at the back of the abdominal cavity. They filter the blood, and eliminate waste from the body as urine. The urine drains from each kidney to the bladder through a tube called the ureter. The bladder collects the urine, which is periodically emptied through the urethra. In the baby the bladder empties as a reflex action when it is full, but as the child matures and develops, bladder control is acquired, initially during the day and then later at night. The urinary system has a close relationship to the reproductive system as developmentally they are formed together.

The kidneys are essential to life. They have three main functions, each of which is of major importance in the regulation of the body and the maintenance of health. They filter the blood to remove wastes and toxins; maintain the fluid and salt balance of the body, and help to control blood pressure.

Because the blood is filtered by the kidneys they have a large blood supply, and in the adult about 200 ml (⅓ pint) of fluid per minute is taken from the circulation, processed by the kidney and either returned to the circulation or excreted as urine. The filtering system is very sophisticated: substances which the body needs, such as glucose and proteins, are not excreted in the urine, but waste products are excreted in high concentrations.

As well as removing nitrogenous wastes and some toxins from the blood, the kidney also regulates the amount of salts excreted, so the body stays in salt balance. The amount of fluid removed from the bloodstream is also closely controlled so that neither fluid overload nor dehydration occurs. Keeping the amount of water and salts constant in the blood helps to maintain blood pressure within normal limits. Kidney damage may cause high blood pressure, and high blood pressure itself can then cause further kidney damage.

Doctors can investigate kidney function by analysing blood and urine in the laboratory, and can detect urinary infection by studying urine. The kidneys can be visualized by abdominal ultrasound; this will indicate their size and position, and will detect scarring or any other structural abnormality. Intravenous urography involves the injection of a dye which is opaque to X-rays into a vein, and taking a series of X-ray pictures so that the excretion of the dye can be followed from the kidneys through the whole urinary tract.

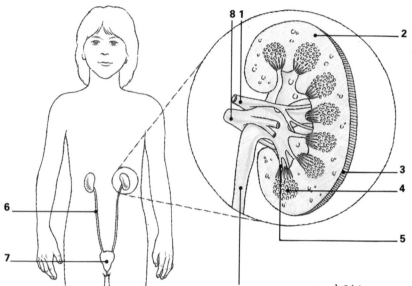

How the kidneys function. Branches of the renal artery (**1**) pass to the cortex of the kidney (**2**). Some of the blood is filtered off by a series of tiny glomeruli (**3**). The filtered liquid passes along tubules through the medulla of the kidney (**4**) where reabsorption of nutrients back into the bloodstream takes place. The remaining fluid is the urine which contains body wastes. It passes via collecting tubules (**5**) into the ureter (**6**), and then down to the bladder (**7**). Blood which has had some of the body wastes and water removed leaves the kidney by the renal vein (**8**).

BLADDER CONTROL AND BED WETTING

The bladder collects urine from the kidney, and periodically empties through the urethra. At first this is a purely reflex action: the bladder wall is muscular and waves of contraction pass over it. When the bladder is full the waves are stronger, and may provoke relaxation of the sphincter, or ring of muscle, that opens the urethra and permits the passage of urine. During the toddler period, the child starts to develop an appreciation of the sensation of having a full bladder, and voluntary control of the sphincter. At this stage many parents will start potty training and leave off nappies. Some mothers and fathers do not have a training routine, but their children also soon develop daytime control as they mature. Apart from the occasional accident it is very uncommon for there to be persistent daytime wetting beyond the age of 2 years; even if there is, introducing structured training usually achieves results.

Remaining dry at night is usually achieved around the age of 3, but there is wide normal variation. Some children acquire the skill at around 2½ years, while about 10 per cent of children are not reliably dry at night at the age of 5. Night-time bladder control is acquired due to developmental progress rather than to training. Inhibiting reflex bladder-emptying while asleep is not something that can be taught in a normal way, as the skill has to be learnt and practised while the child is sleeping! Bed wetting beyond the normal age is referred to as nocturnal enuresis.

There is some evidence that, although the ability to remain dry while asleep is part of normal development, it may be hindered by adverse factors. If there is significant family stress around the time the child should be acquiring the skill – that is, some time between the ages of 2½ and 3½ – there is a greater likelihood of the child becoming enuretic. Such things as the arrival of a new sibling, moving house or marital disharmony may all have an adverse effect, and if several such events occur together there is a greater risk. Boys are more likely to be enuretic than girls, but it is not known why.

Many parents will attempt to help their child acquire bladder control. Restricting evening drinks probably does not make much difference, but going to bed after a period of calm, and emptying the bladder at bedtime do. Some parents will wake the child when they go to bed so that he can pass water. It is important that the child is awake for this, otherwise he is being trained to pass urine while asleep! Most important is encouraging the child and being pleased when there is a dry night. Although finding a wet bed in the morning is depressing for the child as well as the parent, expressing disappointment or being cross does not encourage the child, nor help him improve. It is worth remembering that children do eventually acquire control.

If enuresis is still a problem at around the age of 6 treatment can be tried. Effective treatment is directed at increasing the child's awareness of the enuresis and encouraging him to be involved in trying to prevent it. If the subconscious is primed reflex bladder-emptying during sleep can be inhibited. A combination of support, record keeping and rewards for success can be helpful.

Also very helpful are buzzer alarms. These devices go off if the child passes urine in the night. Provided the buzzer wakes the child each time urine is passed it conditions the subconscious, and within two weeks most children have stopped wetting. It cannot be expected to work if the child does not wake, nor if it is not used consistently. Modern buzzer alarms are miniaturized electronic devices. There is a sensor within an absorbent pad which is put into the child's pants. As the child begins to pass urine an electric circuit is completed, and the battery-powered buzzer goes off. The buzzer can be pinned to the collar of the child's nightwear so it is close to his ear.

Medication with certain antidepressant drugs given in the evening can give temporary control of the bladder at night. The way they work is not understood; they do not assist learning, so there is a relapse when they are discontinued. Their use is therefore very limited.

URINARY TRACT INFECTION

Urinary infections are common. In the newborn period boys and girls are affected equally, but at all other ages infections are much commoner in girls.

The symptoms of urinary infections can be very variable. In infancy there may be fever and malaise (a general feeling of being unwell), poor feeding or slow weight gain, and symptoms may not obviously be related to the urinary tract. In older children there may be abdominal pain, discomfort or a burning sensation on passing urine, and frequent urination. Sometimes the child feels desperate to go to the toilet but cannot then pass water. In some children urinary infection can persist without symptoms.

If the doctor suspects a urinary infection he or she will arrange for urine samples to be examined in the laboratory to determine whether an infection is present and, if so, which germ is causing it. When an infection is found it will be treated with an antibiotic; the doctor may wish to do further tests, such as X-rays or ultrasound, to find out if there is any special reason for the child developing an infection and whether it has had any effect on the kidneys. Kidney damage is most common if infection is acquired in infancy, and if it is not eradicated. If there is any evidence in young children that the infection has affected the kidney or is likely to be recurrent, the doctor may recommend a course of antibiotic treatment for several years to ensure that normal growth of the kidney is not inhibited by the presence of infection.

Even in cases in which there is no evidence of kidney involvement and the child is older, the doctor will want to check that the infection has been completely eradicated by following the child up and re-testing the urine at intervals.

In some children who are prone to urinary infection it is found that the ureter does not function normally: as the bladder empties, some of the urine flows back up the ureter. This abnormality, known as reflux, predisposes to further urinary infections and may be an indication for prolonged antibiotic treatment. If the child can be kept free of infection ureteric function usually becomes normal again and reflux disappears.

In some girls urinary tract infection is a recurrent problem. Sometimes a cause can be found, but not always. Such children are likely to need repeated or prolonged courses of antibiotic treatment. All individuals prone to urinary tract infection find it helpful to drink rather more than most other people. A high urinary flow helps to wash out any bacteria present in the urinary tract and lessens the likelihood of infection.

KIDNEY DAMAGE AND FAILURE

Although it is normal to have two fully functioning kidneys, satisfactory renal function can be maintained with much less. Only when damage has reduced the amount of functioning kidney tissue to about 25 per cent of normal is there any significant impairment of renal function.

This means that scarring affecting a kidney, or even the absence of a whole kidney, is not necessarily of great functional significance to the individual. If a child has any kidney disease, however, it is important to limit any damage, and this is usually possible; sometimes, though, because of either a congenital abnormality or an untreatable disease, it may not be possible to maintain normal kidney function.

If the kidneys gradually stop working properly, the onset of renal failure is slow. At first, blood levels of waste products such as urea (formed from the breakdown of protein) start to rise. There may be a gradual loss of appetite, and growth begins to be affected. As the kidneys gradually grow worse there are problems in getting rid of acid waste from the body, an inability to excrete excess phosphate, an extra loss of calcium, and a failure to activate vitamin D. Renal failure becomes complicated by the development of a bone disease rather like rickets (see page 294) and growth may be markedly affected.

Renal failure is first treated with a low protein diet which lessens the work the kidney has to do, and with medication to counteract many of the harmful effects of kidney failure. If the kidneys get worse this may not be enough, and dialysis may have to be started. This can either involve a machine to filter the blood or the use of fluid inserted into the abdominal cavity in order to remove waste products from the body. Dialysis has to be performed two or three times weekly, so that the patient spends a lot of time having treatment, but it can be continued indefinitely in most patients, and will maintain him or her in reasonable health.

Kidney transplantation is an alternative to dialysis in many patients. A donor kidney is placed in the lower abdomen; its blood vessels are connected to the patient's circulation and its ureter to the patient's bladder. It functions like a normal kidney and the patient recovers rapidly from the operation, but the body's immune system has to be continually suppressed with drugs to prevent it rejecting the donor kidney.

A kidney transplant lessens the time the patient has to spend having treatment, and also improves the general quality of life compared with dialysis. The techniques of renal transplantation are now well established, and most transplanted kidneys work satisfactorily for many years, although rejection is sometimes a problem.

The solid structure of bones seems to imply that they are relatively inert and unchanging, just acting as support and protection and as levers for the muscles. This is not so. In the body bone is a living tissue with a rich blood supply, nerves, and active cells, and bone structure is constantly adapting to meet the stresses placed upon it. Throughout childhood the bones change shape, new bone being added and older bone taken away in response to growth, nutritional status, hormonal influences and the genetically determined blueprint for the skeleton.

The solid matrix of the bones is composed of complexes of calcium and phosphate, but throughout each bone there is also collagen, a fibrous tissue which gives the bone added strength, rather as steel rods strengthen reinforced concrete.

Diseases of the bones and joints do occur in childhood, but are fortunately uncommon. More common are anomalies and deformations, many of them minor but some of major importance. Fractures of bones are also very common in childhood.

GROWTH OF THE BONES

At birth the ends of each bone are composed of a hard gristly tissue called cartilage, while the shaft in the middle is composed of bony tissue. As the bones grow and develop they increase in length and width, and cartilage is gradually replaced by bone, a process known as ossification. Some cartilage persists throughout childhood. At most bone ends another centre of ossification develops as growth proceeds: bone is formed within the cartilage and this is known as an epiphysis. When the epiphysis finally joins with the shaft, growth of that end of the bone is completed.

Doctors can use the appearance and fusion of the epiphyses to estimate the physical maturity of a child. This is usually done by taking an X-ray of the left wrist and hand. There are so many bones in this area that a good estimate of maturity can be made. The degree of maturity is often referred to as the bone age.

In order to grow and ossify, the bones need a plentiful supply of dietary calcium, and also adequate amounts of vitamin D. During

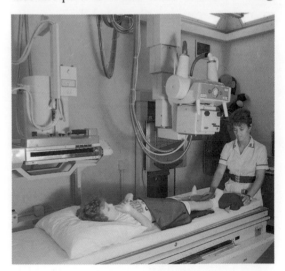

Before an X-ray is taken the patient is positioned precisely so that the beam of the X-ray is restricted to the appropriate area.

Hand and wrist X-ray of a 10-year-old girl. At this age many of the bones are still growing and are not yet in one piece but have a separate growing plate at the end.

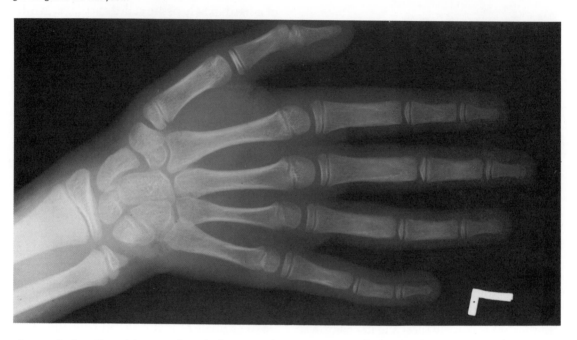

the periods of rapid growth – infancy and adolescence – vitamin D deficiency may be a problem. This gives rise to rickets, in which the bone ends fail to ossify, and become soft and deformed (see page 294). Rickets in infancy can be prevented by vitamin supplementation of the diet (see page 93). In adolescents who eat a mixed diet and are exposed to sunlight, rickets should not occur. It is occasionally seen in Asian girls who eat little meat, butter and milk, and do not go into the sun without being well covered by traditional clothing. At this age rickets may show itself as backache or limb pains rather than deformity.

COMMON SKELETAL ANOMALIES

Some skeletal anomalies are noted at birth or in the newborn period. Others develop as the child grows. Many are not of great significance, but if a parent is worried about the shape of any part of the limbs or spine the doctor should be consulted.

Extra digits

Extra fingers or toes are fairly common, particularly among Africans and Afro-Caribbeans, but as they are usually removed shortly after birth most people are unfamiliar with them. Supernumerary fingers are usually not fully formed and attached to the bones of the hand like other fingers, but are short in length, rudimentary in structure and are attached to the side of the hand on the little finger side. Sometimes they are so rudimentary that they just appear as skin tags. They are easily removed at any stage after birth and only a very small scar is left to indicate that they were once present.

Extra digits that are more fully formed and are an intrinsic part of the hand and foot are not so easily removed. When they are present the doctor will examine the baby carefully, as sometimes when there is a congenital abnormality affecting one part of the body there may be abnormalities in another organ. When the child is a few months old an orthopaedic or plastic surgeon can advise if there is anything that should be done for the hand or foot.

Sometimes digits are joined together at birth, a condition called syndactyly. Partial syndactyly of the third and fourth toes is a common normal variant of no significance. Syndactyly affecting the hand will require surgical correction while the child is a toddler.

Club foot (talipes)

The feet may appear deformed at birth. One cause is so-called club foot, or talipes, in which the foot has been fixed in position in the womb for a prolonged period, so that the bones, ligaments and tendons have grown in a distorted way. Talipes is particularly likely to occur in pregnancies complicated by breech presentations or an inadequate amount of liquor (oligohydramnios). Similar deformities of the feet may occur in children with spina bifida in whom the feet may be deformed as the muscles of the legs are paralysed (see page 301). There are two main types of talipes: the toes may point downwards – talipes equinovarus – or less commonly, the toes may point upwards and outwards – talipes calcaneovalgus.

If the feet can be put into the neutral position then manipulation to stretch the soft tissues and strapping are likely to lead to full correction. If the foot cannot be fully corrected an operation may be needed.

Intoeing (metatarsus varus)

This very common anomaly, often not noted until the child starts to walk, is when the front part of the foot turns inwards. It comes to notice when the toddler starts to walk, as the toes point inwards and the child may stumble because one foot gets caught up with the other. The heel and ankle are normal, which differentiates the condition from club foot. No treatment is needed for intoeing as the foot straightens as the child grows.

Flat feet

The adult foot is arched, particularly on the inner side: while the heel and ball of the foot are in contact with the ground only the outer side of the rest of the foot touches the ground in normal standing and walking. Loss of this metatarsal arch, so that the inside edge of the foot becomes weight-bearing, is the condition of adults known as flat foot. The metatarsal arch does not develop until middle childhood, so that the feet or footprints of small children are naturally 'flat'. The age at which the arch develops is very variable; flat feet are extremely rare in children who have otherwise normal feet, but are sometimes seen in children with a neurological abnormality, and may then require treatment.

Knock knees and bow legs

Both knock knees and bow legs can occur as part of normal development, but may sometimes signify bone disease. Knock knees (genu valgum) can be detected when the child is standing with her knees together, and the ankles are at least 2·5 cm (1 inch) apart. With bow legs (genu varum) the child who is standing with her ankles together has a gap between her knees.

Both bow legs and knock knees may be a normal stage of development between the ages of 1 and 3 years, particularly in children who are either heavy for their age or who started to walk early. These deformities can also signify that the leg bones are not as strong as usual, probably as a result of rickets (see page 294). It is therefore important to seek medical advice if parents are at all concerned.

DISEASES OF THE HIP

The importance of examining the newborn to try to detect congenital dislocation of the hip has been emphasized in Chapter 2. It is not always possible to detect it in early infancy, as some hips are initially in position but slip out later. This is liable to happen when the socket for the hip joint is shallow and poorly formed, the condition of hip dysplasia. Dislocation of the hip and irritable hip are discussed on pages 259 and 280.

FRACTURES

Bones that are strong and in health do not break performing normal activities, but on occasion they may be stressed beyond their limit and a fracture results. The terms 'fracture' and 'break' are used synonymously. Bones may be broken by direct trauma, such as occurs in road accidents, or may break as a result of transmitted force, as for example when the collar bone breaks because of a fall

Below: The main types of fracture. **1**, greenstick fracture, common in children as the flexibility of the bone at this time of life often limits the damage to a partial break on one side only; **2**, simple fracture, in which the broken bone remains in a good position and there may be little damage to the surrounding tissue. **3**, compound fracture, in which the skin has been penetrated by the bone, exposing it and the surrounding tissue to infection. If blood vessels or organs nearby are damaged by bone splinters, the injury is called a complex fracture. **4**, in a comminuted fracture the bone is broken into several small pieces at the site of the injury.

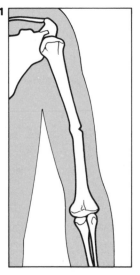
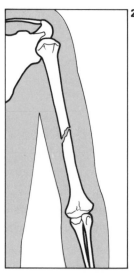
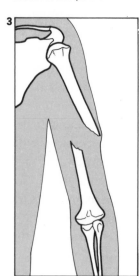
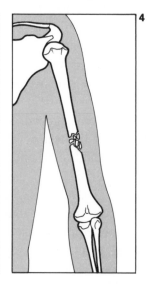

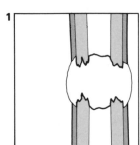
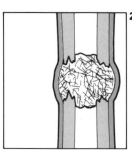
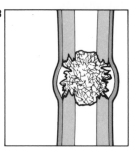
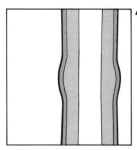

Above: The healing process. Healing begins shortly after fracture as blood collects around the injury site (**1**). During the first week this blood clot becomes fibrous and the periosteum or membrane covering the bone starts to grow around the site (**2**). New bone is then laid down (**3**). The injury has healed when the clot has been absorbed and old and new bone have completely knitted together. The bump indicating the site of the fracture will gradually disappear (**4**).

on the outstretched hand. Most fractures in children affect the limbs.

A fracture should be suspected when there is pain and tenderness over a bone following an injury, and the affected part cannot be used. It may also be swollen and deformed. Medical help will be required and first aid is limited to keeping the part comfortable.

When a bone breaks there is some bleeding from the broken ends, so that blood collects around the fracture site. This soon clots, and the fibrin from the clot forms the framework for repair (see page 149). Over the next few days fibroblast cells, which produce collagen, and osteoblast cells, which make new bone, move into the area, and the bone ends are gradually joined together.

Fractures do not have to be immobilized for the bone to heal, but it is important that healing takes place in the right position, and that long bones are properly aligned. If the fracture has left the bone ends in an unsatisfactory position they will need manipulating under a general anaesthetic into a good position before immobilizing. Encasing the limb in plaster, including the joints above and below the break, is usually satisfactory. For fractures of the femur (thigh-bone), and in cases where there are skin wounds, it may be necessary to immobilize the limb with splints and traction rather than with a plaster cast.

When a plaster is first put on it is important that swelling inside the cast does not cut off the circulation. Broken bones usually heal rapidly in children. Initial union of the bone takes place in 3–6 weeks, and after a period of similar length the repair consolidates so that the bone is almost as strong as before the break.

SPORTS INJURIES

Many sports are potentially dangerous, particularly if they involve speed or body contact. Protective clothing should always be worn when it is appropriate, and team games need to be properly supervised. Although injuries may sometimes be inevitable if sport is played competitively, parents should ensure that their children are not put into unnecessarily dangerous situations. Safety precautions are particularly important for horse riding, swimming and water sports. Furthermore, facilities for the prompt treatment of injuries need to be available in case children are injured.

With some ball games, particularly cricket and squash, the fast, hard ball can inflict damage. The eye is most at risk, and safety glasses should be worn while batting at cricket or playing squash.

If children do sustain a joint injury playing games they must not resume playing until it has fully healed, and medical advice should be obtained if appropriate. The specialty of sports medicine is in its infancy, and little research has yet been done into children's soft tissue injuries and the best methods of treating them. Your family doctor will know if there are any specialized facilities locally.

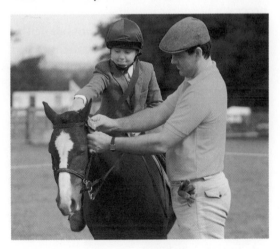

Protective clothing and padding must be worn for any sport that carries a significant risk of injury, such as horse-riding.

CHAPTER

CHAPTER

5

THE SPECIAL SENSE ORGANS

Vision and hearing are the major special sense organs, and any impairment of their function leads to major disability. Both eyes and ears are very closely related to the brain. The interconnection between eye and brain and between ear and brain is fundamental, as the interpretation of the signals received from the sense organs is a very complex brain process.

At birth both senses are present but neither is fully developed; the development of full function is dependent on the maturing of the brain as well as of the eyes and ears.

EYES AND VISION

The newborn infant has some vision: babies will blink in bright light, and follow for a few seconds a face or bright light held about 30 cm (1 foot) in front of their eyes. This visual following is irregular and uncoordinated, but most babies born at term can do it. At this stage the eyes move together most of the time, but intermittent squinting is common (see page 182). By 2 weeks of age the infant shows more interest in large objects, and will watch the face of the person who is feeding her.

Vision depends both on the eyes and on those parts of the brain that interpret the signals received from the retina, the light-sensitive membrane lining the back of the eye. The brain also coordinates and controls eye movements. As the baby grows, visual function gradually develops further. Acuity, the ability to discriminate fine detail, slowly improves and will be fully developed by the age of 2 or 3 years. With improved acuity comes greater visual awareness, which can be recognized when the child begins to follow a moving object or person with her eyes. By 10 weeks the baby can follow a moving object through 180 degrees, and use her eyes to explore her surroundings. The eyes move together in a coordinated (conjugate) fashion, and three-dimensional vision develops with both eyes working together. Colour vision probably does not develop fully until the child is around 18 months old.

The development of visual awareness and ability is partly innate, but also depends on use and practice. The child with defective vision will have difficulty in developing conjugate eye movements, and will be less visually aware than the child with normal vision. Defective vision will therefore affect other aspects of development, and so it is important that vision is tested regularly during early childhood, so that any problems can be detected and treated.

The structure and the function of the eye are often likened to a camera. There is a lens at the front, which focuses images on the retina at the back of the eye. The iris (the coloured part of the eye) dilates and constricts to regulate the amount of light entering the eye, as the variable aperture of the camera does, and the lens can be varied to alter the focus. The retina is light-sensitive like a

How the eye works. An object in front of the eye, such as the tree shown here, sends light rays to the eye. These pass through the transparent cornea (**1**) to the lens (**2**).

The lens focuses an image of the tree onto the retina (**3**), which is sensitive to light and sends messages on the size and shape of the object to the brain via the optic nerve (**4**).

photographic film, and sends messages about what is seen through the optic nerves to the brain, where the images are interpreted.

However, whereas the camera has a relatively simple structure and function, the eye is infinitely more complex. The interconnection between the retina and the brain means that visual images are an intrinsic part of the information received by the brain, and for seeing individuals they have a major influence on development and on a person's perception of the world.

TESTING VISION IN CHILDREN

Testing vision in babies and small children is difficult, as is testing hearing. While a complete absence of a special sense is normally noticed very early, it is much harder to be sure that vision is perfect until a child is around 2 years of age. However, as early detection of problems is important, vision

needs to be tested at every developmental check.

Squints should be looked for in the developmental check. If babies and small children find difficulty in co-operating with visual tests, checking that the reflection of distant light source is seen on the same part of each eye is useful. When relaxed, the axes of the eyes should be parallel; if they are not, a reflected light source will show differently on each eye.

The infant's near vision is first tested by ensuring that he can follow a face or moving object held close; by the time he is 5 or 6 months of age tests will establish whether he can see and pick up a brick. As the child grows older, smaller objects are used. The toddler who can pick up individual 'hundreds and thousands', the tiny beads of coloured sugar used to decorate cakes, has no problem with acuity of near vision.

Testing distant vision in early infancy is done by observing the child, to see whether an interest is taken in distant objects or people. From about 1 year or 15 months more formal testing is possible: for example, watching whether the child can fix and follow rolling balls of different sizes, or fixed balls moved slowly through different parts of the visual field. By the age of 3 years, charts can be used, with the child matching letters or shapes held up with those in a book or on a card.

Children do not realize that their vision is defective, as their only standard of normality is their own experience. Even intelligent schoolchildren will not be aware that they have more difficulty than others in seeing the blackboard, or in doing close work. Parents and teachers have to be alert to the possibility that a child can develop a visual defect at any age, and that the tests done as part of early developmental screening do not ensure that a child's vision will remain normal. Vision should also be formally tested at 5, 8, 11 and 14 years, and at any other time if a defect is suspected.

All children should have routine periodic vision checks during childhood, and a special test should be arranged if there is any specific concern. Formal tests should be carried out at the ages of 5, 8, 11 and 14.

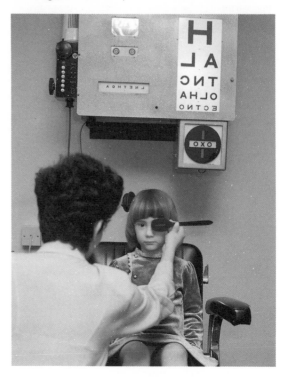

VISUAL IMPAIRMENT

Serious visual impairment is fortunately rare. Vision may be impaired either because the eyes or the visual pathways in the brain have not developed as well as they should, or because of eye disease, or because a refractive error (see below) prevents the eyes focusing properly. Some intra-uterine infections can affect the eye: rubella (German measles) can cause cataracts (lens opacities – see page 245) and also damage the retina, and infection with the toxoplasma micro-organism can cause retinal injury.

Injury of the eye in childhood can cause damage to the cornea (the transparent circular 'window' at the front of the eye) or more severe eye disruption, but most injuries affect one eye only, so do not lead to severe visual handicap. More common is visual impairment as a result of brain damage. The part of the brain specifically concerned with the interpretation of vision is the occipital cortex at the back of the brain. If this fails to develop properly, or is damaged as a result of such things as shortage of oxygen or lack of nutrients while the baby was in the womb, vision will be impaired. If brain damage is more generalized the child may suffer visual inattention and impairment: this is because limited intellect does not permit the full interpretation of the visual messages received from the eye.

If the eye is not in focus vision will be blurred. This may occur because the eye is longer or shorter than usual, and so the lens is unable to make a clear image on the retina at all distances. This is known as a refractive error. Refractive errors are common, and are further described opposite.

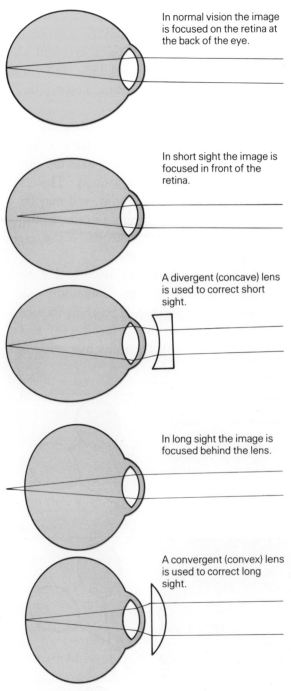

In normal vision the image is focused on the retina at the back of the eye.

In short sight the image is focused in front of the retina.

A divergent (concave) lens is used to correct short sight.

In long sight the image is focused behind the lens.

A convergent (convex) lens is used to correct long sight.

Refractive errors

With the normal eye distant objects are in focus when the muscles in the eye are at rest; focusing on close objects requires contraction of the eye muscles to alter the shape and focal length of the lens. Prolonged reading or other close work can make the eyes feel strained because of the continuous contraction of the muscles in the eye.

In long sight, which is also called hyperopia or hypermetropia, the eyeball is shorter than it should be, and the focal point of the lens at rest is behind the retina. The muscles in the eye have to contract to bring distant objects into focus, and the eye may not be able to bring close objects into focus at all, or only with difficulty and strain. Hyperopia may be noticed in early childhood if a child appears to have difficulty in seeing for close work.

In short sight, or myopia, the eyeball is longer than it should be, so that the focal point of the lens is in front of the retina. Close objects can be seen without difficulty, but distant objects cannot be seen. Myopia does not usually become apparent until midchildhood or later.

Both long and short sight are basically due to an imbalance between the strength of the lens of the eye and the length of the eyeball, and they are known as refractive errors. Another refractive error is astigmatism, where the lens of the eye is somewhat distorted so that at any distance part of the image is not in focus. Astigmatism may occur together with myopia or hyperopia.

The cause of refractive errors is often unknown, but is sometimes familial. Such errors can be corrected by wearing spectacles.

With long sight the use of the appropriate convergent (convex) spectacle lens ensures that with the eye muscles at rest, distant objects are focused on the retina. The eye's own ability to focus means that close work can be carried out without excessive strain. With short sight a divergent (concave) lens is used to ensure that with the eye muscles at rest distant objects are in focus. Astigmatism can be corrected by having a lens with an asymmetry that corrects the asymmetry of the eye's own lens.

Wearing glasses

Parents occasionally think that a child is handicapped by having to wear glasses. The opposite is in fact the case: the child with a refractive error is handicapped without glasses. Children's spectacles can be made tough enough to withstand most normal childhood activities, and the various styles available mean that a design can be chosen to suit anyone's features. If children are found to need spectacles it does not follow that they will have to continue to wear them indefinitely. Children with hyperopia or astigmatism discovered in early childhood may well find that the defect lessens as they grow; children with myopia usually remain short-sighted for life.

Teenagers, like adults, can usually be fitted with contact lenses as an alternative to spectacles.

Squints and lazy eyes

A squint, or strabismus, is a condition in which the eyes do not move together when they look at an object. This is common in childhood. Intermittent squinting in small babies is normal, but by the time the child is 3 months old the eyes should be co-ordinated and always move together. An expert opinion is needed for persistent squints, and for intermittent squints persisting beyond the first few months of life.

The commonest sort of strabismus in childhood is where both eyes have a full range of movement, but their axes are not parallel when they move around. This is known as a concomitant squint, and may be present all the time, or only intermittently. Usually the eyes are convergent – that is, looking in towards each other.

Many concomitant squints are due to defective vision in one eye. Commonly one eye will be long-sighted. The child focuses on close objects with his good eye, and because the eye with the refractive error is

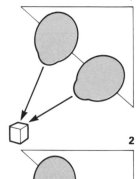

Right: Squints. While in normal sight both eyes focus on the same object (**1**), in a squint only one eye focuses on the object. The squint may be convergent, in which case the defective eye turns inwards (**2**), or divergent, in which case the defective eye turns outwards (**3**).

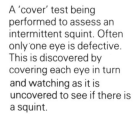

A 'cover' test being performed to assess an intermittent squint. Often only one eye is defective. This is discovered by covering each eye in turn and watching as it is uncovered to see if there is a squint.

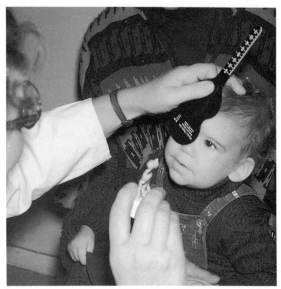

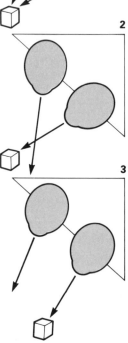

not in focus, binocular vision (with both eyes working together) does not develop properly. Furthermore, if the refractive error is not corrected, the image coming from that eye is ignored by the brain, and will in due course be suppressed, so that the function of the eye deteriorates further. This is known as a lazy eye; if it is not corrected, the eye becomes non-functional even though structurally intact, a condition known as amblyopia.

When a child with a concomitant squint is assessed by an ophthalmologist (eye specialist), vision in each eye will be tested separately. If a refractive error is found spectacles will be prescribed. Often with the use of spectacles the squint corrects completely, as when both eyes focus together on the same object the movements of the eyes become co-ordinated.

Sometimes this does not happen because the defective eye has become lazy. In that case, at the same time as the defective eye is fitted with a corrective lens the good eye is occluded (covered up) with an opaque glass; this treatment needs to be continued for some months. With this so-called selective occlusion the vision in the lazy eye will hopefully improve, but if the eye has been amblyopic for too long vision may be permanently depressed. Even if vision returns in the weak eye a corrective operation for the squint may be necessary, but this is only likely to lead to the development of binocular vision if a lazy eye has been corrected first.

Not all concomitant squints are due to one eye being weaker than the other. The eyes may have developed so that their axes are not parallel. Small degrees of convergence or divergence of the axes are corrected once binocular vision develops, but larger degrees lead to persistent or intermittent concomitant squints. Many of these need corrective surgery. The operation is skilled, but simple in concept. The globe of the eye is moved by small muscles outside the back of the eye. To correct the non-alignment and bring the eye straight and in-line the muscle on one side of the eye is shortened and that on the other side lengthened.

If one or more of the muscles that move the eye is paralysed, a different sort of squint, known as a paralytic squint, develops. When the eyes are turned the lack of action of the muscle or group of muscles becomes obvious: in some directions the eyes seem to be looking together, and in other directions they diverge widely. Surgery cannot restore the movement of paralysed muscles, but can ensure improved appearance by minimizing the deviation of the affected eye.

Colour blindness

Some degree of colour blindness is present in about 12 per cent of boys; it is less common in girls, of whom only about 0·5 per cent, or 1 in every 200 is affected. The defect is hereditary (see Chapter 8), and persists throughout life. In many affected people colour blindness is not severe enough to cause problems, apart from making matching shades of the same colour difficult or impossible. It may pass unnoticed unless specifically tested for. If colour blindness is more severe the child does not do well at learning those activities that make use of colour matching. The child does not know that he has a problem with colours, and teachers need to be aware of the possibility. Unexpected poor performance at tasks involving colour matching warrants a formal test for colour blindness, as does fidgeting or inattentiveness while the child is supposed to be doing such tasks. If the child is old enough, colour vision is tested with special charts with coloured numbers or letters against a background that is only contrasting if colour vision is normal.

There is no treatment for colour blindness, nor is it usually the cause of any significant disability, although in adult life colour blindness may preclude employment in some specialized occupations.

THE EARS, NOSE AND THROAT

The cavities of the middle ear and of the nose both connect with the throat, or pharynx, so that they are anatomically related. Infections in one part will often spread to another, and many of the medical problems of each area inter-relate. Therefore medically the ears, nose and throat are often considered together, and there are many surgeons (ENT surgeons) who specialize in the problems of this part of the body. The nose and throat obviously also relate to the respiratory system, and the throat to the mouth and alimentary tract (see Part Two, Chapters 1 and 3).

The ear consists of three parts: the external ear, the middle ear and the inner ear (see the illustration below). The part that can be seen on the outside is the external ear, and consists of the pinna and the external ear canal. The canal ends at the eardrum, which vibrates in response to sound. The middle ear is situated between the eardrum and the inner ear; it is an air-filled cavity bridged by three small bones or ossicles – the hammer, anvil and stirrup – which conduct the sound waves from the eardrum to the inner ear. The Eustachian tube connects the middle ear cavity with the pharynx at the back of the nose and ensures that the pressure inside the middle ear can be equalized with the atmospheric pressure when the person swallows. The inner ear is embedded in bone and consists of the cochlea, which is the organ of hearing, and the semi-circular canals, which are organs of balance.

During breathing the nose carries air from the nostrils at the front to the nasopharynx at the back. The air then passes

Structure of the ear: **1**, external ear; **2**, bony ossicles; **3**, semi-circular canals; **4**, inner ear; **5**, cochlea; **6**, Eustachian tube; **7**, middle ear; **8**, drum; **9**, ear canal.

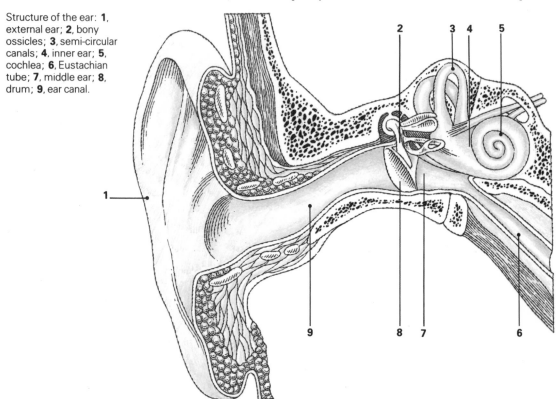

down through the pharynx into the voice-box (larynx), and then into the lungs. During its passage through the nose the air is warmed and humidified. The inside of the nose acts as a heat exchanger so it has a large surface area with lots of bony plates acting like baffles to mix the air, and a good blood supply, and is kept moist all the time. While this structure is ideal for humidifying the inspired air so that it does not have a cooling or drying effect in the lungs, it also explains why the secretions from the nose can be so prolific when a person has a cold, and why nosebleeds may be profuse.

At the back the nose opens into the naso-pharynx. The adenoids, a pad of lymphoid tissue which is part of the body's immune system, are in the roof of the nasopharynx, and the openings of the Eustachian tubes going to the middle ears are on each side. The tonsils, situated on either side at the back of the mouth where it joins the pharynx, are also pads of lymphoid tissue.

Examining children

Examining the ears, nose and throat can be difficult in small children as they may be frightened of the instruments needed. Part of the secret of success is for one of the parents to hold the child firmly but gently, so that the examination can be done speedily and in the least frightening manner possible. The way to hold a baby or child who needs to have his ears examined is shown in the illustration (right). To look into the ears the doctor uses an otoscope which contains a light source and a magnifying lens. To see into the back of the throat requires a good light source, and some-times a tongue depressor to push the tongue out of the way. This is intensely disliked by children, but as the tonsils are a frequent site of disease in childhood a proper examination is necessary. The nose is examined by shining a light into the nostrils.

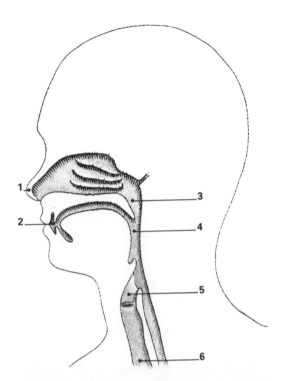

Above: The upper airways: **1**, nose; **2**, mouth; **3**, naso-pharynx; **4**, pharynx; **5**, larynx; **6**, trachea.

Below: Small children dislike having their ears or mouth examined. Provided the child is held firmly such an examination can be performed quickly and with minimal discomfort.

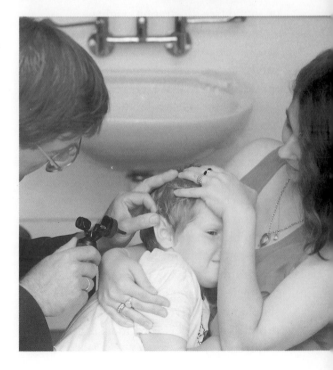

HEARING

Hearing is obviously fundamental to the development of communication and the acquisition of language (see pages 58–9). Disease of the ear, or of its connection with the brain, may affect hearing, and so can interfere profoundly with normal development. It is thus important to ascertain whether babies are developing normal hearing, and to be aware that infants and children may develop hearing impairment at any time due to infections of the ear.

TESTING HEARING IN CHILDREN

Hearing tests are designed to ascertain whether children have normal hearing. They therefore depend on the use of soft sounds. Only if the child does not respond to quiet sounds should louder ones be used. Knowing that a child reacts to very loud noise is nowhere near as informative as the fact that the child stops crying or turns on hearing a soft voice or sound (see illustration, right).

If a child is completely deaf, parents are usually aware of this very quickly. Fortunately this is rare. Parents may not be so quick to realize that their child has a partial hearing loss. Delay in the diagnosis of a hearing loss means that a child might miss out on many of the important early stages of language development, and speech is likely to be delayed. If there is a hearing problem it is important to detect it early.

Parents should check at intervals whether their child's hearing is attaining the normal stages at the appropriate time as set out in the box feature (above). If parents are worried that their child might have a hearing loss they should always have his hearing checked by a professional who is used to assessing young children.

The development of hearing in the first year

By 1 month Loud noises cause the baby to start or blink. A hand clap can be used to test this.

4–6 weeks The baby will pause and listen to sounds when they first start, such as the radio, TV or vacuum cleaner.

16–20 weeks The baby will recognize his parents' spoken voices and will respond by smiling and turning, or by quietening if crying or vocalizing.

26–30 weeks The baby will turn immediately to his parent's voice if it comes from the side or behind, unless he is engrossed in some other activity.

9 months The baby will listen and try to identify the source of all sounds, even if soft.

1 year The baby responds to his own name and to the command 'no'. He shows pleasure in 'talking' – taking turns, babbling and making repetitive sounds like 'dad-dad', or 'mum-mum'.

Formal tests of hearing

In some maternity units many newborn infants are screened to check hearing, using soft sounds and a machine that records responses to sound, such as a change in breathing rate, a slight turn of the head or a slight movement of the body. If the baby makes a definite response hearing is present, but lack of an observable response may be due to the baby being sleepy or cross. If repeat testing does not elicit a response the baby needs more sophisticated tests, and should be assessed by an audiologist or a skilled paediatrician.

Formal hearing tests are carried out as a routine part of developmental assessments, usually at around 6 weeks, 6 months and 10 months, by the health visitor or the doctor.

CHILDREN WITH HEARING DIFFICULTIES

Hearing deficits may be due to a defect in the ear, or in the nerve that carries impulses from the ear to the brain where they are interpreted. If the problem in the ear is in the conduction of sound through the ear canal, eardrum or the interconnecting bones, it is referred to as a conductive hearing loss; if the inner ear or nerve is damaged, it is referred to as nerve deafness.

Nerve deafness may be due to inherited disease, or can follow from intra-uterine infections such as rubella (German measles), or from meningitis in the newborn period or later (see page 285). Some antibiotics used for serious infections can also cause nerve damage as an occasional side-effect. In many cases the cause of a nerve hearing loss is not

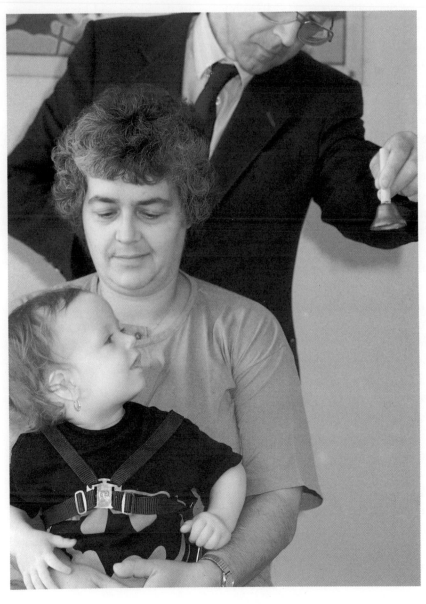

To test hearing in babies and small children, a soft noise is made behind the child, using a rattle or bell. If the child responds by turning to the sound, hearing is satisfactory. If the response is poor the test should be performed again on another day to rule out other causes before more detailed analysis is undertaken.

found. Conductive hearing loss is usually the result of infection or fluid in the middle ear (see otitis media and glue ear, pages 290 and 270).

Children who can hear but have moderate loss of hearing are referred to as 'partially hearing'. The word 'deafness' is reserved for those who are unable or virtually unable to hear. The use of the term 'partially hearing' emphasizes that such children need special help to develop their listening and communicating with others. For them hearing and speech are still going to be the major ways of communicating with other people.

Younger partially hearing children will require special assistance in developing communication skills. They will need to wear hearing aids, and parents and child will all have to learn to use and look after these. Because understanding speech is more difficult for partially hearing children they need to learn ways of augmenting their understanding, including looking at the person speaking, concentrating on what is being said and also watching the lips and mouth. A special teacher needs to be involved as soon as the diagnosis is made, and the child may need primary education in a special unit. Provided the child can communicate satisfactorily he should be able to continue secondary education in a mainstream school.

If hearing loss is profound or the child is completely deaf, alternative forms of communication need to be developed. The child with profound hearing loss will experience great difficulty in learning language, and may well become behaviourally disturbed if unable to communicate. As soon as deafness is recognized the child will need specialist educational teaching and will need to learn alternative forms of communication, including writing and using sign language. Education has to be tailored to his special needs and requirements.

ADENOIDS AND TONSILS

The tonsils and adenoids together form a ring of lymphoid tissue around the walls and roof of the pharynx, at the back of the mouth and nose. In structure both adenoids and the tonsils consist of large numbers of lymphocyte cells together with supportive tissue. These lymphocytes play an important role in preventing and fighting infection, by having a direct toxic effect on micro-organisms, by boosting the number of lymphocytes in the blood and by producing antibodies. The mouth and nose are potential portals for the entry of bacteria and viruses into the body. The location of the adenoids and tonsils in the pharynx therefore provides an important defence against infection, and they have an important role in health maintenance.

The tonsils and adenoids are not very big at birth, but grow rapidly during the first few years of childhood. In many 5- to 10-year-old children the tonsils appear very large, but this is not abnormal. From about the age of 10 or 12 the tonsils and adenoids

Section through the nose and mouth: **1**, mouth cavity; **2**, tongue; **3**, pharynx; **4**, soft palate; **5**, naso-pharynx; **6**, adenoids.

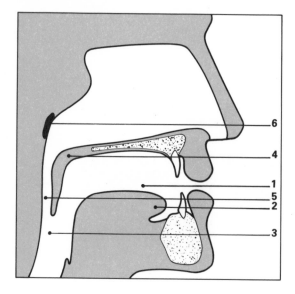

actually shrink in size, so that they are smaller in the adult than in mid-childhood.

Enlarged adenoids in early childhood may cause problems, particularly if they become swollen with infection. They may partially or completely obstruct the nasal airway. The child starts to breathe through his mouth, and may snore at night. The nose tends to run a lot of the time as secretions do not drain away into the pharynx. The opening of the Eustachian tube at the back of the pharynx may be affected. Both otitis media and glue ear (see pages 290 and 270) are more common in children with enlarged adenoids. If adenoidal enlargement is causing significant problems, removal of the adenoids may be necessary.

The tonsils are naturally large in mid-childhood, and can become even bigger when they are the site of infection. Following a bout of infection they usually shrink back to their previous size. This is a sign that the tonsils are functioning as they should in helping to combat infection. Sometimes, however, frequent or persistent infection means that they remain enlarged and infected, and become a source of continuing ill health. Poor appetite, frequent sore throats and intermittent fevers may occur. The lymph nodes in the neck (see page 283) are likely to be permanently enlarged and intermittently tender.

If the enlargement and chronic (long-term) infection of the adenoids or of the tonsils is causing persistent or recurrent symptoms, their removal surgically may be necessary. These operations are called adenoidectomy and tonsillectomy. Tonsillitis is described on page 304.

Adenoidectomy

The adenoids cannot be directly seen from the outside as they are on the roof of the naso-pharynx. They can be seen if the doctor gives the patient a general anaesthetic, and then

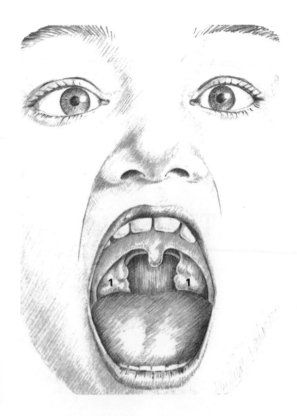

The tonsils (**1**) can be seen on the side of the pharynx, above the back of the tongue. They are often large in children but only require treatment if infected.

opens the mouth wide and uses a mirror to see above the back of the soft palate. The adenoids are removed using a specially shaped instrument, and pressure is applied until the bleeding stops. Recovery from the operation is rapid. Tonsillectomy may be performed at the same time. Hospitalization is only necessary for 2–3 days.

Tonsillectomy

It is rare for tonsillectomy to be performed in children under the age of 5. The operation is carried out with the patient anaesthetized and asleep. Each tonsil is dissected away from the wall of the pharynx and removed, and any bleeding is stopped. Recovery from the operation is usually rapid, but a sore throat persists for some days. Eating ice cream is the traditional treatment for this.

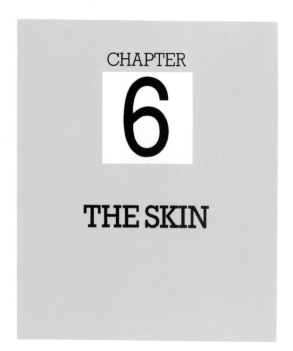

CHAPTER

6

THE SKIN

THE STRUCTURE OF THE SKIN

The skin is made up of three layers: the outer epidermis, the underlying dermis and the subcutaneous tissue. The epidermis consists of cells which are constantly being worn away at the skin surface and constantly being renewed at the base of the epidermis. As the cells move towards the surface they become tougher because of a substance called keratin, which helps to make the skin impermeable and strong. The deeper layers of the epidermis contain pigment cells that give the skin its colour.

Beneath the epidermis is the dermis, which is composed of fibrous tissue and forms a tough but flexible sheet between the epider-

Structure of the skin: **1**, hair; **2**, epidermis; **3**, dermis; **4**, sweat duct; **5**, sweat gland; **6**, sebaceous gland; **7**, hair follicle.

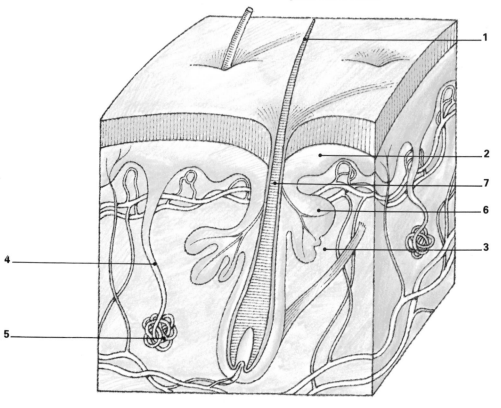

mis and the deeper tissues. The dermis contains nerve endings for the reception of various forms of sensation, including heat and cold, touch and pain. Hair follicles and sweat glands are located within the dermis, although they are derived from epidermal cells. Beneath the dermis is the subcutaneous layer comprising fat cells and some fibrous tissue. The subcutaneous tissue is the major site for fat storage in the body, and this fat provides heat insulation as well as cushioning against injury. The dermis and the sub-cutaneous tissue are both well supplied with blood vessels and nerves.

Hairs and hair follicles, sebaceous and sweat glands, and nails are all appendages that develop as part of the skin.

DEVELOPMENTAL ABNORMALITIES

As the skin develops there may be abnormalities. Birth marks are either abnormalities of pigmentation or of the blood vessels that occur during development. The common types are considered on page 27.

Other developmental abnormalities do occur and are usually of no medical significance. The skin may be dry and flaky, a condition known as icthyosis which is inherited and persists throughout life. Small pits in the skin may be found in front of the ear, at the base of the spine, in the neck and sometimes in other places. Small appendages of skin and cartilage may occur in front of or below the ear. Cysts are occasionally present in the neck (see 'Branchial cysts', page 243). Accessory nipples are not infrequent, above or below the normal pair of nipples. They may be single or multiple, and are usually not well developed. They may be considered to be birth marks rather than being recognized for what they are.

Developmental abnormalities of pigmentation are also possible. Patches of over-pigmentation are familiar as skin moles. Most striking is albinism, where there is a total absence of skin and hair pigmentation. It is inherited as a recessive disorder (see page 108), both parents being carriers, and is more common in pigmented races. It is normally recognized at birth or soon after. The eyes usually also lack pigment and are pale blue in colour. The absence of skin pigmentation in albinism means that affected individuals are very prone to skin injury by the sun, as exposure to the sun does not provoke any protective pigmentation. They need to wear protective clothing or sun cream whenever they are exposed to bright sunlight.

Congenital abnormalities of the nails are sometimes seen, and may be associated with other skin problems such as an absence of sweat glands, or sparse hair.

Developmentally the hair is part of the skin. Developmental abnormalities of the hair are very rare.

EXPOSURE TO SUN-LIGHT AND SUNBURN

The warmth of the sun, if excessive, can give rise to heat exhaustion and heat stroke (see page 223). The sunlight may also be directly harmful to the skin. Both visible and ultraviolet light affect the skin, and exposure should be regulated. Individuals vary widely as to how much sun they can tolerate. Fair-skinned people are particularly prone to sunburn, while those with pigmented skins are relatively protected.

Children should only be allowed out in strong sunlight for short periods until they become adapted, and a high-factor sun cream should be used on exposed skin. As always, prevention of harm is important, and can be easily achieved by gradually increasing sun exposure within the limits of tolerance.

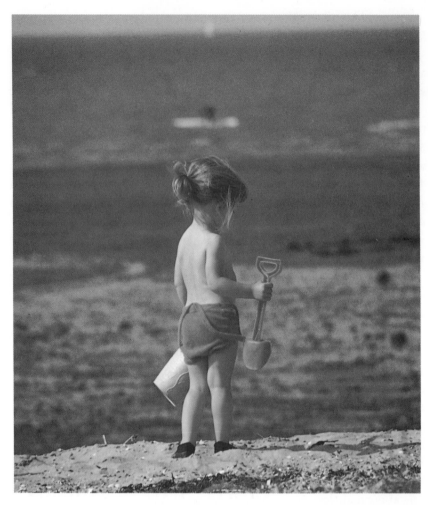

Most children enjoy playing in the open air and especially by the sea. When doing so it is important that they are not exposed to strong sunlight for long periods until they have become adapted. A high factor sun cream will help to protect them from sunburn.

The effects of exposure to the sun are cumulative over a period. The skin may redden soon after exposure starts. This is a heat effect and will settle if the skin is cooled. More insidious is the effect of the light. The reaction takes 6–12 hours to develop and so it is easy to be exposed to a harmful amount of sun before any reaction occurs. First the skin reddens. As the redness develops the skin becomes itchy, swollen and tender, and there may be localized blistering. If a large area of skin is affected the child will be unwell and in great discomfort. This inflamed state of the skin may persist for around twenty-four hours and then gradually settle. Following this, the outer layer of the epidermis may be shed (peeling), but there will also be an increase in the pigment in the deeper layers, so that a suntan develops.

Fair-skinned people who are exposed to strong sunlight over many years sustain damage to the skin and have a higher incidence of skin tumours than those not exposed. This is a rising problem in countries with a temperate climate whose peoples are now taking regular trips to very much warmer parts of the world. Although no evident long-term skin damage is seen in childhood, repeated exposure may have some lasting effects, and is another reason for moderating exposure to sunshine, and wearing protective clothing and sunhats, or applying effective barrier sun creams. The treatment of sunburn is described in the chapter on first aid, on page 225.

CHAPTER

7

CARE OF THE TEETH

People with healthy teeth which last throughout life are very fortunate. Regrettably dental disease is widespread, and much of it starts in childhood. Most childhood dental disease can be prevented by simple measures carried out regularly, but this requires parental will and effort. Parents should encourage their children to care for their teeth, and make sure that they have regular check-ups at the dentist. The reward – children with healthy teeth and no fillings – should persuade all parents to take prevention seriously.

HOW THE TEETH DEVELOP

The first set of teeth, often referred to as milk or deciduous teeth, are the primary dentition. There are twenty in all: each side of the lower and upper jaw has two incisor teeth, a canine and two molars when the primary dentition is fully erupted. The teeth are all formed within the bone of the jaw; they gradually migrate to the surface, and then erupt through the gum. The timing of tooth eruption is very variable, but the first teeth usually appear between 5 and 8 months. The central upper incisors usually appear first, and the other teeth follow gradually. The primary dentition is complete by around 2½ years of age.

There are thirty-two teeth in the permanent secondary dentition. They form in the jaw deep to the milk teeth, and begin to erupt through the gum at around the age of 6; the dentition is not complete, however, until the appearance of the third molars, or wisdom

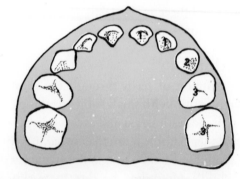

Top: Primary dentition takes place over a long period, beginning when the child is a few months old and ending at around the age of 2½. There are twenty of these so-called milk teeth, which comprise incisors (**1**), canines (**2**) and molars (**3**).

Bottom: Permanent dentition starts at around the age of 6 and is completed when the back molars or wisdom teeth appear, in about the late teens. Full permanent dentition comprises a total of 32 teeth: incisors (**4**), canines (**5**), premolars (**6**) and molars (**7**).

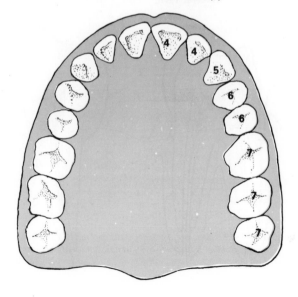

teeth, at around the age of 17–19. As the secondary teeth develop and grow, the roots of the adjacent primary dentition are absorbed. The secondary teeth then move towards the surface, pushing on the milk teeth, which gradually become loose and then fall out. The first of the permanent teeth to erupt is usually the first permanent molar, which appears behind the second milk molar; therefore its arrival is not heralded by a tooth falling out. The full permanent dentition consists of two incisors, a canine, two premolars and three molar teeth on each side in both the upper and lower jaw.

Teething

The eruption of teeth through the gum is often painful. With small babies teething can give rise to restlessness and excess salivation, so that they dribble more than usual. Only if the tooth can be felt close to the surface will the child's symptoms be due to teething. Much of the excess saliva is swallowed and may cause slight looseness of the bowels, but teething does not cause other diseases.

A child who is teething may take comfort from chewing on a teething ring or other hard object. There are also various proprietary preparations available which may help: they

The first teeth usually appear when the child is aged between 5 and 8 months. The eruption of the milk teeth can be a painful experience and toddlers like chewing on a hard object to alleviate the discomfort.

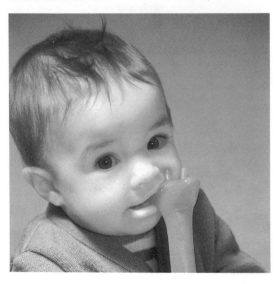

Dental caries is caused by the acid produced by bacteria eroding the layers of the tooth. The illustrations below show the structure of a normal tooth, and teeth with various degrees of decay. **Far left**, a normal tooth, showing the hard outer coating of enamel (**1**), the bony dentine (**2**) and the inner core or pulp (**3**) containing nerves and blood vessels. **Mid-left**, caries has eroded the enamel, but a small filling prevents its progression. **Mid-right**, erosion of both the enamel and dentine requires more extensive filling. Left untreated, caries will eventually extend to the pulp and cause toothache. **Far right**, a dental abscess requires extensive treatment including, if the tooth can be saved, root filling.

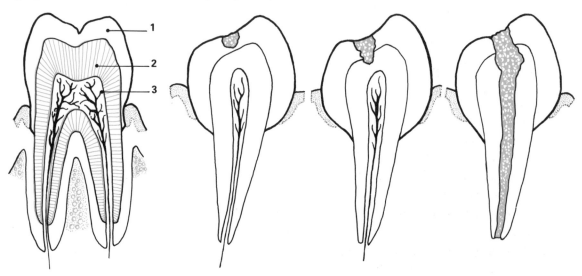

can be applied locally, and contain a local anaesthetic. If the child is restless and uncomfortable a cuddle may be more soothing than other measures.

DENTAL CARIES AND ITS PREVENTION

The teeth are very strong, consisting of hard bone called dentine, which is covered with even harder enamel. They are adapted to withstand the very high pressures generated in biting and chewing, and seldom chip or break. However, this strength can be eroded by the action of minute bacteria, which give rise to tooth decay, or dental caries.

Other than in communities in which there is fluoridation of the water supply, it is regrettably rare to find a child over the age of 10 who does not have at least one tooth cavity or filling, and caries can develop in the incisor milk teeth even before the primary dentition is complete. Erosion of the enamel, and then of the underlying dentine, is due to the acid produced by bacteria, and is preventable.

With the consumption of sugar and sugar-containing foods, and with poor dental hygiene, a hard scale called plaque, consisting of bacteria, food residues and saliva, builds up between the teeth and around the base of each tooth. The plaque bacteria live on the food particles, and produce acidic secretions which gradually dissolve the enamel.

Eating a lot of sugar and sugar-containing foods is one of the major factors causing dental caries. In a Western diet sugar is ubiquitous. It is present in fruit juices and sweet drinks, cakes, biscuits and puddings, and breakfast cereals. Jam, honey and syrup have a very high sugar content, and sweets and confectionery are almost entirely composed of sugar. Pure sugar is put into tea and coffee, and sprinkled on to breakfast cereals. Regular cleaning and a low consumption of sugar are the fundamentals of preventing plaque. They should be supplemented in two other ways: with fluoride and regular dental check-ups.

Eating less sugar

As so many foods contain large amounts of sugar there are practical difficulties in giving a child a low-sugar diet, but with thought it can be done. As well as these practical problems there is a need to overcome cultural patterns. All children like sweets and sweet things and so these are used as treats, presents and rewards. While an occasional sweet may do little harm, regular consumption is hazardous for teeth. Grandparents in particular often like to bring children presents of confectionery, and need to be gently but persistently discouraged.

It is not only a high consumption of confectionery that causes plaque to form, however. Babies given bottles of fruit juice as a comforter or to help them go to sleep often develop severe caries of the front teeth within a few months of their eruption, and other sugar-containing foods also encourage the build-up of dental plaque.

Regular teeth cleaning

Regular cleaning, preferably after every meal and certainly twice daily, can help to prevent the build-up of plaque by removing food particles and sugar from around the teeth. Cleaning the teeth after eating sweets is also useful, as it helps to remove the sugar and reinforces the connection in children's minds between sugar and decay. Small children need to be shown how to clean their teeth, and all children enjoy using plaque discloser, a harmless dye that shows where plaque has built up on the teeth, and where cleaning needs to be more effective. The coloration only persists for a few minutes. An electric toothbrush can be a useful incentive for the small child who is a reluctant tooth cleaner.

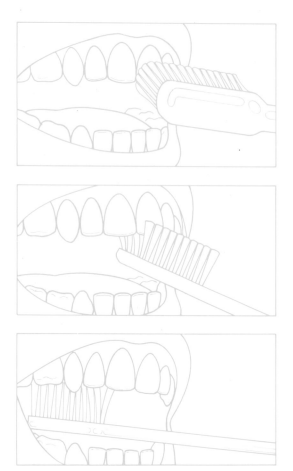

The outer and inner surfaces of the teeth should be brushed well in several directions for at least one minute. This should be done at least twice daily.

Fluoride

Fluoride salts occur in nature, and in the past it was noted that in areas with naturally high concentrations of fluoride in the water the incidence of dental caries was lower than usual. The addition of fluoride to the water in some areas confirmed the usefulness of a high fluoride intake in making the teeth more resistant to decay. In the concentrations being considered fluoride has been shown not to have harmful effects, and in areas where communities have fluoridated water suppply

there has been a dramatic drop in the number of dental caries.

Children can be given fluoride to protect their teeth, in the form of tablets or drops once daily, from infancy until the permanent teeth are fully formed at around the age of 14. Fluoride in water or taken as medication is absorbed into the body and becomes part of the tooth, and this gives the best protection. Protection can be extended by cleaning the teeth with fluoride toothpaste, as some of this fluoride is slightly absorbed into the surface of the teeth. Having the dentist coat and seal the teeth with a fluoride sealant also gives good protection. This is a straight-forward procedure. The fluoride is mixed in a plastic which is applied to the surface of the teeth, and then hardened by an ultra-violet light source. As the permanent dentition starts to erupt around the age of 6, the teeth can be protected by sealing at around the age of 7.

Dental check-ups

From an early age children should have regular dental inspections. These should emphasize the importance of preventative measures, and the dentist can discuss these with the family as a whole. The inspection will also detect any early signs of caries or other tooth or gum disease, enabling immediate steps to be taken. When the secondary dentition starts there may be problems with overcrowding or malalignment of the teeth; the dentist may be able to help with this, or may suggest referral to an orthodontist.

Toothache

Toothache is most commonly due to dental caries (tooth decay). The enamel is eroded and the dentine exposed underneath contains nerve endings and may be sensitive. These nerve endings may give rise to pain if they

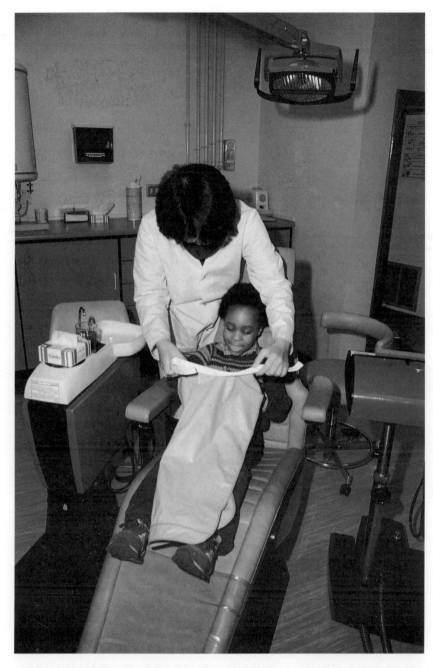

Routine dental inspections should start in early childhood and continue regularly throughout life. Prevention of dental disease is important, as is the early detection of orthodontic problems.

are exposed to heat or cold, or excessive sweetness. Less commonly in childhood toothache may be due to an infection around a tooth.

If a child is suffering from toothache he should be taken to the dentist without delay; all dentists will see children with pain as emergencies. Paracetamol in the correct dose for the child's age may help in the interim.

Treatment of dental caries (tooth decay)

Dental caries can be lessened and almost completely prevented by the measures indicated above. However, when decay has occurred and there is a tooth cavity, the dentist should be consulted and will advise about treatment.

If the cavity is small, not giving rise to any

symptoms, and is in a milk tooth that is likely to be shed over the next few months, treatment may not be necessary. With caries in other milk teeth the alternatives for treatment are either filling or extraction, and the choice will again depend on which tooth is affected, whether it is giving rise to symptoms, and whether it is likely to be shed naturally in the near future. Very small children need general anaesthesia for dental work.

When caries occurs in the permanent teeth it must be treated promptly to prevent it worsening. A cavity acts as a trap for food residues so that plaque bacteria flourish there and do more damage. The dentist will fill the tooth to protect it from further harm. This may be done under general or local anaesthetic, depending on the age and temperament of the child.

If a child does develop a cavity the preventative measures being taken are inadequate, and sugar avoidance, tooth cleaning and fluoride treatment should be reviewed and improved.

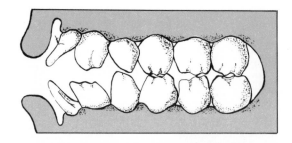

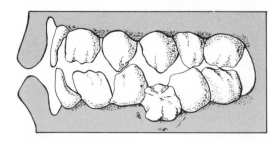

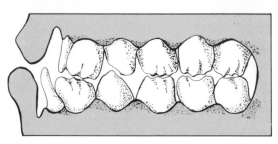

Some common orthodontic problems: **top**, protruding incisors; **middle**, overcrowding; **bottom**, malocclusion or protrusion of the lower jaw.

ORTHODONTICS

The word 'orthodontics' comes from the Greek, meaning 'straight teeth'. The teeth in both the upper and lower jaw should together form a smooth curve, and the upper and lower teeth should fit well together. In most people this happens naturally, but there may be problems with badly aligned teeth, incisors that protrude or recede, loss of the regular curve of the upper or lower jaw, or malocclusion of the teeth where the upper and lower jaws do not fit well together. These are all situations which the orthodontist may be able to help.

The orthodontist is primarily trying to achieve teeth that are regular and functional, so that long-term problems with the teeth and jaw will be unlikely. During the course of the

treatment the appearance of the teeth is usually also enhanced. A course of orthodontic treatment is usually carried out just before and during the puberty growth spurt (see page 82), but if there are special problems it may start much earlier. Children with cleft palates (see page 251) need to be referred to the orthodontist in infancy, and attend regularly throughout childhood.

Orthodontics uses various techniques to improve the shape of the jaws and the position of the teeth. Initially the orthodontist will make a plaster cast of the teeth and jaws and take photographs and an X-ray, so that there

Orthodontic treatment is often lengthy and children who undergo it understandably experience feelings of resentment and frustration. Parents need to be especially supportive and encouraging at these times.

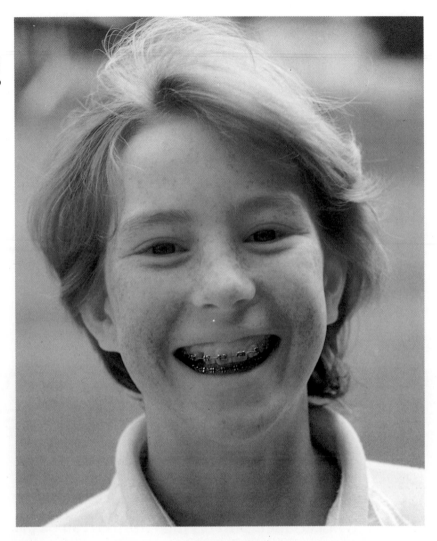

is a record of the state of the child's mouth, and to enable treatment to be planned. The period of treatment may well be as long as two or three years. If the teeth are seriously overcrowded and malaligned it may be necessary to extract some primary teeth, and occasionally some of the permanent teeth.

Braces, wires and rubber bands are used together to apply steady pressure to the teeth and jaws. As the jaws and teeth grow their relative positions will be altered, and the shape of the jaws and the alignment of the teeth favourably influenced. Even when a good position has been obtained it is necessary to continue the treatment for some extra months to consolidate that position and to ensure that there is no regression.

Children undergoing orthodontic treatment often feel discouraged and cross. They are concerned about their appearance and resent the bother and discomfort of braces and wires. They are likely to dread their consultations with the orthodontist, and express their frustrations and anger to their parents. These are all understandable feelings and the child needs encouragement and support throughout the long course of treatment. Parents and orthodontist should point out that this present discomfort will lead to a long-term improvement.

PART THREE

SAFETY

Making the Child's Environment Safe, and Essential First Aid

Most accidents involving children can be prevented. Nevertheless, accidents constitute the major cause of death in children over the age of 1 year. This section begins with advice to parents and other carers on approaches to accident prevention and stresses the need for constant vigilance if 'Thinking Safety' is to become automatic. Parents must possess this awareness before they can educate their children into avoiding dangerous situations. The section goes on to highlight potential danger areas in the home and elsewhere and provides first-aid procedures for many common childhood accidents and emergencies.

1

ACCIDENT PREVENTION

Accidents are a more frequent cause of death or permanent disability in children over the age of 1 year than any single disease, and account for almost half of all deaths of teenagers. Not all accidents can be avoided, but many of those that occur in and around the house are preventable. Parents have a primary role to play here, and can do much to guard against mishaps by adopting a safety-conscious attitude.

For parents there are three important aspects to protecting children from injury: being aware of potential dangers, teaching children how to recognize hazards and how to cope with them, and protecting children by providing a safe environment.

BEING AWARE

Taking an interest in her surroundings is an important part of a baby's normal development. As soon as the ability to crawl is acquired, exploration begins in earnest, and will continue throughout childhood. The child is exploring the real world, not a carefully controlled play area, and hazards are present almost everywhere, in the family home and garden as much as in the world outside.

Parents need to be alert to potentially dangerous situations in which their children could suffer injury. In the home the most common forms of accident are suffocation, burns, falls, cuts, poisoning and drowning. Parents need to be aware of how these could happen, and should think of the child's safety at all times. This is not onerous: initially parents need to make a special effort to survey their surroundings, looking particularly for possible hazards, but soon this becomes reflex behaviour. Every day children acquire new skills, so parents need to think ahead and not just consider what children could get up to at their present developmental stage.

For babies the common serious accidents are choking, suffocation and falls in the home, and car travel is also potentially hazardous if they are not adequately secured.

Babies should not be given a soft pillow in the cot. They will sleep perfectly satisfactorily and safely without, whereas a soft pillow may obstruct the baby's mouth and nose. A pillow is even more of a hazard if the baby is sick. The vomit could collect in a pool on the pillow and obstruct the airway.

It is a normal stage of development for all babies to put things in their mouths during the second half of their first year. Parents cannot stop this, but need to ensure that small objects are not left lying around for babies to choke on. Leaving a baby propped up in a cot with a bottle of milk is also potentially hazardous: some babies have choked and suffocated in this way.

Often when bathing, feeding or changing a baby not everything needed is to hand. Never leave the infant on a raised flat surface such as a bed or shelf while moving away to fetch anything. Even very young babies can

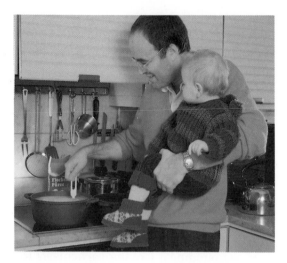

The kitchen can be a dangerous place, especially for young children. It should be made as safe as possible and infants should be supervised when they are there.

wriggle, twist or roll over the edge, and sustain serious injury. Similarly, when carrying a baby, particularly up- and downstairs, parents should hold her securely, and protect her head from knocking against the wall or protruding objects in narrow passageways. While this is obviously common sense, there may be times when safety is forgotten because the parent is busy or fraught.

When the child starts to crawl or becomes a toddler the dangers increase. She may fall against hard or sharp objects. If the home has glass doors she can fall through them and sustain serious lacerations. Stairs and windows are other places where serious falls occur. Windows need to be fitted with safety locks, and stairs with gates at top and bottom until the child is able to walk up- and downstairs safely. Living in rented accommodation is no reason for not modifying your home to make it safe for your child.

The kitchen is especially dangerous for children, containing as it does sharp knives, electric gadgets and a stove. If electric flexes hang over the edge of a shelf the small toddler is bound to hold on to them in trying to reach upwards to see what is going on.

Pulling an electric kettle or hot iron over is a very real risk. Similarly, saucepans on the stove are interesting to a toddler. The handles must always be turned inwards, and not left sticking out. For extra safety a raised rim attached to the top of the stove can prevent pans falling or being pulled off. Remember, too, that low-level oven doors may get hot on the outside when the oven is switched on.

When they are toddlers, children learn the skill of putting things over their heads. Parents must ensure that plastic bags and sheeting are kept well away from small children to prevent the risk of suffocation. Playing with string, cord or rope is also dangerous, as children can put it round their necks and injure themselves.

Accidental poisoning is very common in children aged 1 to 3 years. The house and garage are filled with things that are poisonous to children, such as bottles of alcoholic drinks, bleach, disinfectant, white spirit, weedkillers, medications, and many more common substances. Keep no more than is necessary. Lock all medicines away in a high cupboard and store other packets and bottles that might be harmful on a high shelf. Do not leave pills in a handbag.

Small children should never be left unattended in the bath. If a child slips, her head may go under the water and she may not be able to regain her balance or lift her head out. Garden ponds and domestic swimming pools are intrinsically dangerous for small children and should be drained or well protected with child-resistant fencing and gates fitted with safety latches.

Until a baby arrives the home is probably a reasonably safe place because adults are aware of hazardous activities and dangerous situations and so are usually able to avoid injury. When a baby arrives a complete check needs to be made of the house, to make sure that it is a suitable and safe environment for a child to grow up in and to explore without risk. Examples of the sort of thing to look for are given in the checklists overleaf. These lists cannot be comprehensive, but can be used as a starting point: check whether there are other areas in your own home that could be made safer.

Holidays are a time when accidents are particularly likely to happen. In strange surroundings there may be hazards that have not been appreciated, and new activities such as fishing or boating; the holiday atmosphere may make parents less safety-conscious than usual. If thinking about safety has become a way of life then this will go a long way towards providing protection in unfamiliar surroundings.

TEACHING CHILDREN ABOUT HAZARDS

The word 'no' is the first command most children learn. Used judiciously it can be the beginning of an education about safety. Toddlers need to know not to touch knives,

matches, flames and hot objects, and not to climb into dangerous places. When out in the street they must realize that they have to walk holding hands with an adult, and not try to run away. Even when parents think these lessons have been learnt they still have to remain watchful, as children can forget the rules in a moment of excitement or wilfulness.

As the child gains greater understanding it is important to explain the reasons for the prohibitions and rules of conduct that have been introduced for safety reasons, so that they begin to be aware of the need for self-protection.

Part of growing up is gaining greater independence: although at the toddler stage children will normally be under direct adult supervision, older children will do things outside the home and without close surveillance. By that stage their own understanding of danger has to be good enough to protect them. Children walking along a street on their own must understand traffic hazards and know the code for crossing the road.

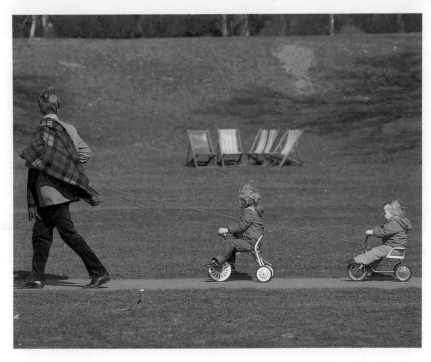

Children need to be made aware of the importance of safety at all times by parents so that they do not expose themselves to danger unnecessarily.

SAFETY POINTERS

In the home

- Ensure all electric plugs and sockets are in good condition
- Do not let children play with sockets or switches
- Put safety plugs into floor-level sockets
- Do not have overhanging flexes that a child can reach up and hold
- Do not have unguarded fires, heaters, hot pipes or radiators
- Always turn saucepan handles inwards
- Keep teapots and cups away from the edge of a table where they could be reached by toddlers, and remember that overhanging tablecloths may be grasped by toddlers
- Do not leave a hot iron unattended where a child might touch it or pull it over
- Do not leave matches lying around.
- Always extinguish cigarette ends thoroughly
- Make sure children's night clothes and dressing gowns are flame-retardant
- Fit smoke alarms, and make sure there are alternative ways out in case there is a fire
- If buying new soft furniture make sure the foam is non-toxic
- Keep all medicines in a high, locked cupboard. Do not keep any more than is necessary. Discard unused medicines
- Keep household liquids on a high shelf or in a garage
- Do not let children play with knives, scissors or sharp implements

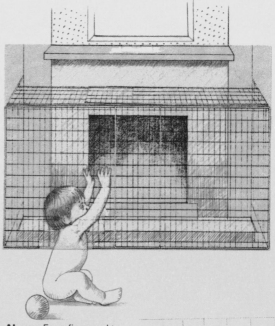

Above: For a fireguard to be effective it must completely surround the fire and be firmly fixed in position.
Below right: A hotplate guard fitted to a cooker is a worthwhile safety device for the kitchen.
Opposite page
Near right: A stairgate is a wise precaution in the home where children are too young to safely walk up or down stairs by themselves.
Far right, top: A custom-built car seat for toddlers or babies.
Far right, below: When being transported by car a carry cot should be firmly fixed in position.

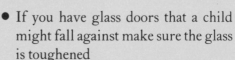

- If you have glass doors that a child might fall against make sure the glass is toughened
- Do not let small children carry glass bottles that they may fall against or drop
- Animals can bite or scratch. Keep them away from small children unless an adult is present
- Install a stair gate if children are at the toddler stage, and do not let·them walk up and down the stairs alone until they are old enough to do so safely

- Check that children cannot climb up the guard rails on the landing, stairs or balcony. If the guard rails are horizontal they may be used as a ladder by a child
- Fit safety catches to all windows, and have stops on them so that they cannot be opened too wide
- Keep plastic bags safely away from children. Remember to put them away every time you come back from shopping
- Never leave small children alone in a bath or near water
- Discourage children from playing with doors. Little fingers can easily be trapped.

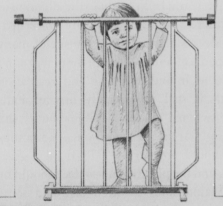

In the car
- Never allow a small child to travel in the front seat
- Have proper car seats fitted for babies and toddlers
- Fit rear seat belts, and always insist they are used
- Have the rear doors fitted with child-proof locks so that they can only be opened from the outside
- Make sure children's hands are out of the way before slamming doors
- Always drive carefully, and avoid sudden stops.

In the garden
- Drain or fence off ponds, swimming pools or other water a child could fall into
- Put all tools away after use
- Make sure fences are secure and child-resistant so that children cannot escape and wander off
- Have safety latches fitted to gates
- Check that all gates are securely fastened before allowing a child into the garden
- Make sure play equipment is safe and in good order
- Do not leave weedkiller or other garden chemicals where they can be found by children
- Keep children away from bonfires or fireworks.

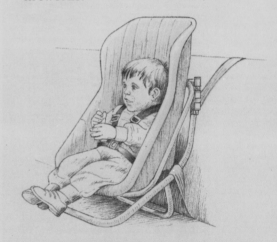

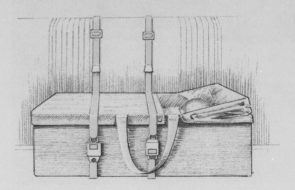

They should not be allowed to cycle on the road until it is safe for them to do so, and parents need to impose restrictions on cycling along busy roads.

As always, children learn more from example than they do from explanation and im-

Many childhood accidents occur in public play areas. Play equipment should be designed to minimize hazards and should also be regularly maintained. Parents can help ensure a high standard of safety by reporting instances of defective equipment to the relevant authority.

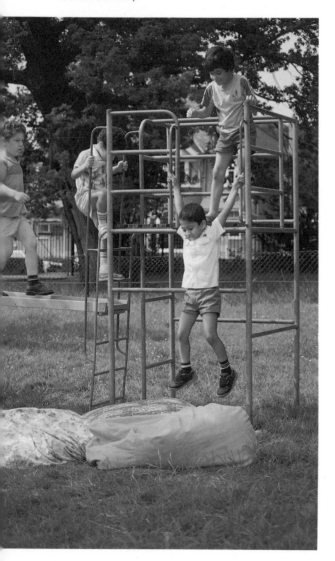

posed rules. Parents who are always safety-conscious are educating their children correctly by their way of life.

MAKING THE ENVIRONMENT SAFE

Parents have direct control over the home and should carry out regular safety audits. Outside the home they have less direct control, but if they make their views known they can sometimes exert pressure to get improvements carried out. Blocks of flats often have dangerous staircases where a child could climb up the protective rail and fall over. Windows in communal areas may not be securely fastened. Slippery or defective stairs or floors may be hazardous. Such shortcomings should be brought to the attention of the landlord or housing authority concerned.

Children's play areas are the site of many childhood accidents. Much of the playground equipment in public parks and recreation grounds is still intrinsically unsafe. Falls from swings, slides, roundabouts and climbing frames are common. The equipment should not permit falls from a great height, and the playground surface should be soft. Maintenance is often lax, and some equipment may be broken. An individual parent can write to or ring up the local authority to point out the hazards, or inform the local councillor. Groups of parents or residents' associations can be effective in bringing about change. Similarly, pressure for road crossings and action against accident black spots can achieve results. If there is widespread public concern over creating a safe environment it becomes a political priority. If unsatisfactory situations are accepted without the authorities being informed, matters are unlikely to improve. In a caring society the safety and health of children should be amongst the highest priorities.

CHAPTER

2

FIRST AID

Although with foresight many childhood accidents can be prevented, parents should know how to cope with those that do occur, and also with common medical emergencies that may affect their children. Usually such contingencies happen without warning, and it goes without saying that parents who have been trained and are practised in first aid are better prepared to deal with them. The Red Cross, St John's Ambulance and other organizations arrange training courses in first aid and you should consider whether such a course would be useful for you. No book can be a substitute for personal instruction and practical learning.

This chapter is designed both to help parents understand the common, as well as the serious, emergencies that may occur in childhood and to provide clear and practical guidance on how to deal with them.

Only a few situations present an immediate threat to life, or involve an injury which is likely to become worse if not immediately treated. The conditions which require emergency treatment techniques include choking, unconsciousness, respiratory and cardiac arrest, burns and severe bleeding. Emergency techniques for these situations are given.

Many other emergencies, although not immediately life-threatening, will require urgent medical help. If the patient is going to be taken to a doctor or to an accident and emergency department, first aid should be limited to any treatment necessary to prevent the situation worsening, preparing the patient for the journey and keeping him comfortable. Only the minimum should be done. If an ambulance is being called, the crew will be skilled in making the patient comfortable, so limiting the first aider's role still further. In cases where the injury is not serious, complete the appropriate treatment, as described on pages 219-226.

Action in emergencies
- Keep calm and do not panic
- Assess the situation to decide what needs to be done
- Summon assistance, if required, before starting emergency treatment
- If the patient is choking, unconscious, burnt or bleeding severely give appropriate treatment immediately
- If the patient does not need immediate emergency treatment, does he need medical help? If so, give only essential treatment and arrange for his transfer to hospital or to a doctor.

EMERGENCY TECHNIQUES

When using this section in an emergency, follow the instructions given in the tinted areas.

Choking
A child may choke because a piece of food or a foreign body (such as a toy or small coin) obstructs the airway. Another cause is the inhalation of vomit into the airway.

Choking is usually easy to diagnose. The child initially coughs forcibly, and this usually displaces the object from the airway. If the foreign body remains in the airway the child continues to cough and splutter, and rapidly becomes severely distressed and unable to breathe in or out. The child makes tremendous efforts to breathe and his face turns red or purple and may appear swollen.

If the obstruction is not relieved within a few minutes the child becomes unconscious from lack of oxygen and the struggle lessens. The aim of emergency treatment is to dislodge the foreign body and then to give artificial respiration, if necessary.

STEP-BY-STEP TREATMENT
Choking

1. First put your finger into the child's mouth. Clear any mucus or vomit and remove any dental plates. If you feel a foreign body in the mouth remove it if you can, but be careful not to push it further in.

2. To dislodge the foreign body use the following methods, depending on the age of the child.

3. Smaller children and babies. Hold the infant face downwards and support his chest and abdomen while you sharply slap him over the upper spine.

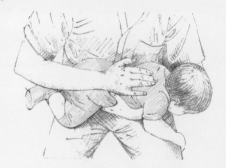

4. If Step 3 fails, try the following. Sit the infant on your lap with his back towards you. Place together the tips of two fingers of each hand and jerk them into the upper abdomen just below the ribs.

5. Older children. Place the child face downwards over your knees and give a sharp slap between the shoulder blades with your hand. At the same time, support the chest with your other hand. If this is unsuccessful at first, repeat it several times. The slap needs to be quite forceful.

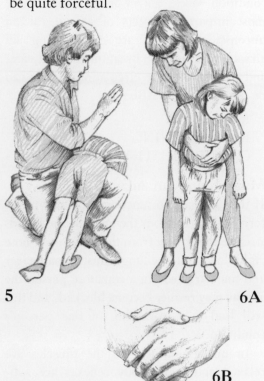

5
6A
6B

6. If Step 5 fails, try the following. Standing behind the child, put your arms around him (**A**). Join your hands together as shown (**B**), then jerk them inwards and upwards to force air out of the lungs.

7. Give artificial respiration, if it is required (see page 212 for procedure).

8. After a serious choking episode, arrange for the child to be seen by a doctor to check that there are no complications requiring treatment.

The unconscious child

Unconsciousness, or coma, may be due to such varied causes as head injury or poisoning, or may follow convulsions. It is a serious emergency and medical help should be obtained as quickly as possible. Whatever the cause, all unconscious patients need to be looked after carefully to make sure their condition does not worsen. The three most important aspects of caring for an unconscious person are maintaining an airway, making sure breathing is adequate, and maintaining the circulation. These can be remembered as ABC:

> A = AIRWAY
> B = BREATHING
> C = CIRCULATION

Maintaining an airway

If the lungs are to function properly, transferring oxygen from the air into the bloodstream, the airway from the mouth and nose right down into the lungs must remain clear and unobstructed. In a comatose person the airway may readily become blocked, and this will lead to a worsening of that person's condition.

In unconsciousness all the muscles are relaxed and many body reflexes are suppressed. When a comatose patient is lying on his back, his relaxed muscles allow his jaw and tongue to sag backwards, and the tongue may completely obstruct the airway. A further hazard of the 'face-upwards' position is that any secretions or vomit in the mouth can run back into the throat. The reflexes that normally prevent aspiration of food and fluid into the lungs and that provoke coughing are suppressed in unconsciousness, so the windpipe can become blocked.

Blockage of the airway can be prevented by placing the unconscious patient semi-prone in what is known as the recovery position. (This position is also used for patients recovering from the effects of anaesthesia.) In the recovery position the tongue and jaw fall forwards rather than backwards, and any blood or vomit will drain out of the mouth and not collect in the throat. It is therefore a

STEP-BY-STEP TREATMENT
Unconsciousness

1. Seek skilled assistance urgently. If you are alone place the child in the recovery position, face downwards and with the elbow and knee on one side bent.

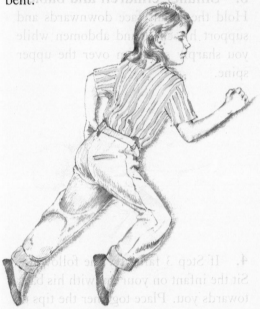

2. Go for help or 'phone for an ambulance, then return to the child as soon as possible.

3. Remember the ABC:

A = AIRWAY
B = BREATHING
C = CIRCULATION.

4. Check whether the child is breathing adequately. If you can see the chest moving and the lips and tongue are pink, breathing is satisfactory. If the chest is not moving or is only moving slightly, and the lips are blue or pale, good position for the patient, provided that breathing and circulation are also adequate: the recovery position *cannot* be used if mouth-to-mouth respiration or heart massage is to be performed.

breathing is not adequate and mouth-to-mouth respiration is required (see page 212 for procedure).

5. If the child is not breathing adequately, check the circulation. If you can feel a pulse at the wrist (**A**) or in the neck (**B**), the circulation is adequate. If the child is not breathing and you cannot feel a pulse, heart massage may be needed as well as mouth-to-mouth respiration (see pages 214 and 212 for procedures).

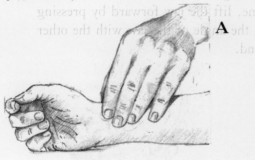

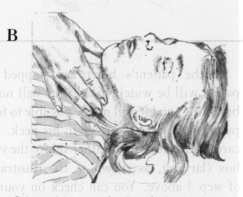

6. If breathing and circulation are adequate, keep the child in the recovery position. Continue to observe the child until help arrives, and check breathing and circulation regularly.

Absence of breathing

If a person is fully conscious the amount of oxygen in his blood is adequate. The first aider only has to consider the use of artificial respiration (also called artificial ventilation) in the unconscious patient. In choking or suffocation a lack of oxygen causes unconsciousness, but coma from any other cause can be complicated by inadequate amounts of oxygen entering the body. Coma may depress respiratory effort, and may also be complicated by airway obstruction, as described above.

Respiratory effort is inadequate if breathing is absent or slow and shallow and the lips and tongue have a bluish tinge. Check the airway first. Make sure the tongue has not fallen back, and there are no secretions blocking the passage of air. If the airway is clear, but the respirations are shallow or absent, artificial respiration will be needed to provide the patient with enough oxygen.

The most effective method of artificial respiration is mouth-to-mouth respiration, which has also been called the kiss of life. The principle of mouth-to-mouth artificial respiration is that the first aider breathes in normally and then out into the patient's mouth. As only a small amount of the oxygen breathed in is absorbed, exhaled air still contains a lot of oxygen. If there is no air leak the patient's lungs can be inflated and oxygen will then be absorbed into his bloodstream. When the first aider removes his mouth to take another breath, the air escapes from the patient's lungs, and the sequence can be repeated. The patient will gradually become adequately oxygenated, and his condition will improve.

As no equipment is needed for mouth-to-mouth respiration it can be done in almost all circumstances; it is a relatively simple technique and many people have done it successfully without prior training.

STEP-BY-STEP TREATMENT
Mouth-to-mouth respiration

1. Summon assistance.

2. When examining an unconscious child, first check for signs of breathing. If the respirations are shallow, or absent altogether, and the lips and tongue are blue or pale, breathing is inadequate and treatment is required.

3. Before beginning treatment, first ascertain whether the heart has also stopped by checking the circulation. (If the heart has stopped, heart massage is required — see pages 214-5 for treatment.) Look at the child's pupils to see whether they are widely dilated or small.

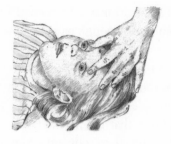

Then feel for a pulse in the neck. If the pupils are small and/or you can feel a pulse, the heart has not stopped.

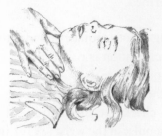

4. Prepare the child for treatment by laying him face upwards on a flat surface. Kneel beside the child's head.

5. Make sure the airway is clear by bending the head slightly backwards, holding on to the nose. At the same time, lift the jaw forward by pressing on the angle of the jaw with the other hand.

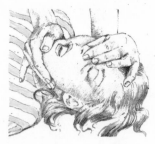

Absence of heartbeat

In some patients whose breathing is inadequate the heart will also have stopped or will be beating inadequately. The heart may also stop as a result of severe electric shock. If the heart has stopped blood will not be circulating around the body. In this situation mouth-to-mouth respiration alone is unlikely to be of benefit, as oxygen will still not reach the body tissues. It is occasionally possible to maintain circulation and restart the heart by performing heart massage at the same time as artificial respiration.

If the patient's heart has stopped his pupils will be widely dilated, he will not be breathing, and it will not be possible to feel a pulse in the carotid artery in his neck. The carotid arteries run on either side of the voice box (larynx), as shown in the illustration of step 3 above. You can check on yourself where they are.

Performing cardiac massage if the heart has not stopped is potentially dangerous, as the force needed to compress the chest may lead to rib fractures and internal injuries.

6. Smaller children and babies.
Breathe in, then place your mouth over
the infant's nose and mouth. Breathe
out, but blow only part of each breath
into the infant.

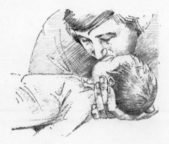

7. Older children. Breathe in, then
place your mouth over the child's
mouth; breathe out while squeezing the
nose to prevent an air leak.

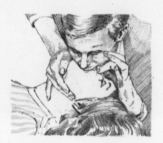

8. Look towards the child's chest to
make sure it is expanding. If it is not,
check that the head is tilting backwards,
the nose is blocked, the jaw is forward
and that the tongue is not bent back.

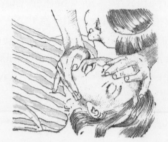

9. After you have breathed into the
child, remove your mouth and take a
normal breath. Do not try to breathe
more deeply or faster than normal.
Repeat the sequence.
10. If your efforts are successful the
child's lips and tongue should become
pink. Stop occasionally to see whether
the child can breathe adequately unaided. If he cannot, continue with treatment until a doctor or ambulance
arrives.

The technique of heart massage is carried
out by pushing rhythmically on the breastbone (or sternum) with the heel of the hand.
This action effectively compresses the heart
between the breastbone and the spine and
squeezes the blood out. When the pressure is
relaxed, more blood then flows into the
heart. Once this cycle is complete, com-
pression can then be repeated. Because the
heart contains valves the blood flows the
correct way round the circulatory system.
Heart massage is performed at a rate of
around fifty to seventy times per minute.

Heart massage restores some circulation
of the blood. If at the same time the amount
of oxygen in the blood is increased by
artificial respiration, this oxygenated blood
will be carried by the circulation to the brain,
to the heart muscle, and to the other organs.
The heart may start beating again, but even if
it does not, maintaining some circulation of
oxygenated blood prolongs the time during
which resuscitation efforts by a medical team
may be successful. It is therefore essential to
call an ambulance before beginning artificial
respiration and heart massage.

STEP-BY-STEP TREATMENT
Heart massage

1. Summon assistance.

2. Check the circulation before proceeding with the treatment. First, look at the pupils to see whether they are widely dilated or small (**A**). Second, feel for the pulse in the carotid artery in the neck (**B**). If the pupils are small or you can feel a pulse, the heart has not stopped.

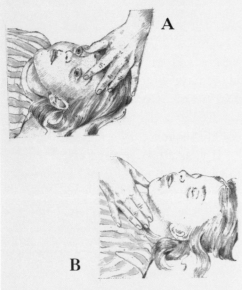

A

B

3. Do not start heart massage unless you are certain that the heart has stopped — otherwise, the patient may be harmed.

4. If you are sure the heart has stopped, you will need to perform mouth-to-mouth artificial respiration as well as heart massage. This is most easily done by two people: one to perform artificial respiration while the other performs heart massage.

5. Place the patient on a firm, flat surface, face upwards. The floor or the ground is usually the best place readily available. Kneel beside the patient.

6. Make sure the airway is clear by tilting the head slightly back, holding on to the nose. At the same time lift the jaw forward by pressing on the angle of the jaw with the other hand.

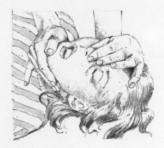

7. Smaller children and babies. Breathe in, then place your mouth over the infant's nose and mouth. Breathe out, but blow only part of each breath into the infant.

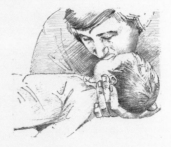

8. Older children. Breathe in, then place your mouth over the child's mouth; breathe out while squeezing the nose to prevent an air leak.

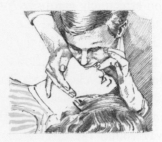

9. Then locate the massage point by running your hands up the lower margin of the rib cage until you find the breastbone. The massage point is situated just above the bottom of the breastbone — marked with an 'x' in this illustration.

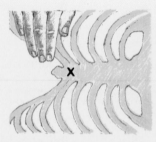

Begin heart massage —

10. Smaller children and babies. Use two fingers only to compress the chest at the massage point. Relax and repeat at a rate of about eighty beats a minute.

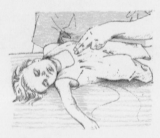

11. Older children. Place the heel of your hand on the massage point and, keeping your arm straight, push down firmly so that the breastbone moves about 2.5 cm (1 inch). Relax and repeat the action about once a second.

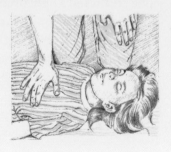

12. Cardiac massage should not be performed while the chest is being inflated. If two people are attempting resuscitation the heart massager should pause after every five compressions to permit one breath of respiration. If only one person is attempting resuscitation, the sequence should be about fifteen compressions of the heart followed by two breaths of respiration, and so on.

13. Every few minutes you should pause for a few seconds to see whether the heart has restarted and breathing has resumed. If the heart starts to contract spontaneously it will be possible to feel a pulse in the neck. Heart massage can then be discontinued. Otherwise continue with treatment until the ambulance arrives.

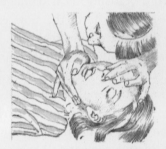

14. If heart and breathing resume place the child in the recovery position (see Step 1, page 210), but observe him closely to ensure that breathing remains adequate and that you can still feel the neck pulse.

Burns and scalds

The kitchen is a dangerous place for children as they may touch hot plates or oven doors, pull boiling pans over or touch naked flames. In the toddler age group accidents involving hot drinks are very common.

The heat involved in burns and scalds leads to damage or death of tissue; whether the heat injury is caused by dry heat giving a burn or moist heat giving a scald, the problems are similar. Burns are usually extremely painful, because of damage affecting the pain receptors in the skin. Shortly after the burn takes place fluid leaks out of the circulation into the burnt area, and blistering may occur. Raw areas gradually scab over. If the full thickness of the skin is destroyed healing will inevitably leave a scar, but fortunately in many heat injuries the damage is superficial. If burns are extensive healing is slow, and scarring may be marked.

As well as causing local damage, burns may have general effects; the more extensive the burn the more serious these are. Fluid is lost from the circulation into the burnt area, and the burn itself may lose fluid both by evaporation and from a weeping discharge. In severe burns this fluid loss is marked; the circulation may become impaired and intravenous fluid replacement will be needed.

Burns also provide a ready portal for the entry of infection into the body. The combination of a breach in the skin and damaged tissue permits bacteria to invade.

Prompt treatment at the time of the burn can lessen some of the problems. When someone is burnt he instinctively moves away from the source of heat if possible, but even away from the heat further damage takes place while the tissue itself remains hot. It is important therefore to cool the whole of the burnt area thoroughly and rapidly to limit the extent of the damage. Cooling is also the best immediate way of lessening the pain.

STEP-BY-STEP TREATMENT
Burns and scalds

1. Immediately remove the child from the source of heat.

2. If hot or boiling fluid remains on the child's clothes, remove them immediately. Cutting or tearing them may be quicker than trying to remove them in the usual way.

3. Plunge the part affected by the burn into cold water, or pour cold water over it, or hold the affected part under cold running water. The colder the water, the better. Continue this treatment for at least five minutes, to allow the cold to penetrate deeply and to cool the tissues thoroughly.

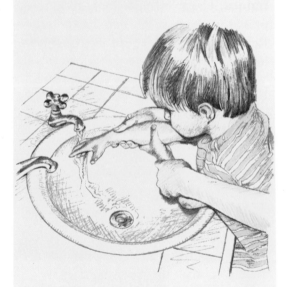

4. If the burn is minor, cover it with an antiseptic cream and a light dressing. If it is severe enough to require medical attention, cover it with a clean wet cloth and seek help immediately.

Bleeding

Bleeding from cuts and other injuries usually stops within a short time. The body has two complementary mechanisms that stop the flow of blood: constriction of the blood vessels and clotting of the blood (see page 149). When tissue is damaged various substances are released which cause the muscle in the wall of the local blood vessels to contract, so that the flow of blood to the wound area is diminished. At the same time these tissue substances trigger an accumulation of platelet cells from the blood in the injured area; these platelets obstruct blood flow and also help to start the blood-clotting process. Clotting then proceeds over the space of a few minutes so that the liquid blood becomes converted into a solid clot. Over the next few hours the clot consolidates, and the process of repair commences.

Treatment of bleeding aims to help the natural process. This is achieved by slowing or stopping the blood flow so that a clot can form and not be washed away by continuing haemorrhage; at the same time care should be taken not to introduce infection into the wound. If the wound is extensive or the blood flow profuse and continuous, medical help will be required.

The main way of slowing the rate of blood flow is by applying direct pressure to the wound. A dressing consisting of cotton wool, gauze or any other clean piece of cloth such as a towel, flannel or handkerchief, or a wad of paper tissues is pressed on to the wound. This dressing can be kept in place by a firm bandage, but if one is not available just pressing it firmly is enough. If the wound is small only gentle pressure is required; if bleeding is marked firm pressure should be applied and kept up for at least five minutes, and then only released when it is apparent that the blood flow has ceased. If bleeding continues through the dressing do not remove it, but place another dressing over it to apply more pressure.

Elevating the bleeding part also slows the rate of haemorrhage: children with head wounds, for example, should be placed in a sitting position unless they are feeling faint or are unconscious; similarly, bleeding from a hand wound will slow if the arm is lifted above the level of the head.

For wounds to the arms or legs where bleeding does not stop in spite of continuing firm direct pressure, compressing the main artery in the limb may help. There are pressure points in the groin and upper arm which can be used, as shown in the illustrations overleaf. Pressing on these points with either one thumb or both simultaneously will reduce the flow of blood to the limb or stop it altogether.

When blood loss from a wound is considerable – for example, with extensive injuries or where a large blood vessel such as an artery or a varicose vein has been damaged – there may be consequent circulatory problems. The body can compensate for some loss of blood by constricting the blood vessels and quickening the heart rate. The patient looks pale, may feel faint or nauseated, and the pulse rate is rapid and may be difficult to feel. The first aider should lay the patient down, keep him calm and make sure that the bleeding has stopped. If the patient still seems faint, his legs can be elevated. An ambulance should be called as soon as possible; in cases where there has been great loss of blood, a blood transfusion will be required.

There is no treatment the first aider can give to stop bleeding from inside the mouth, or help when blood is vomited up or passed in the motions. In such cases medical advice is urgently required and should be sought at the earliest opportunity.

STEP-BY-STEP TREATMENT
Bleeding

1. If facilities and time allow, wash your hands thoroughly before giving treatment.

2. If bleeding is marked or severe, promptly apply direct pressure to the wound, pressing a dressing, towel, clean material or even a bundle of paper tissues firmly on to it. If possible, use a bandage to keep the dressing in place. If not, just maintain the pressure manually. Slight wounds only require gentle pressure. Maintain pressure for at least five minutes.

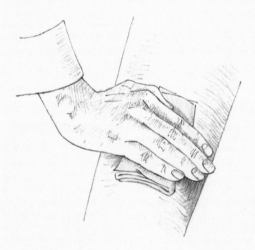

3. If bleeding continues through the dressing, do not replace the dressing but place a further dressing over the top to apply yet more pressure.

4. If appropriate, elevate the bleeding part (for example, head or hand), as this will slow the flow of blood.

5. If bleeding continues from an arm or leg wound in spite of direct pressure, apply indirect pressure over the main artery to the limb. The two main pressure points are in the brachial and femoral arteries:

● The brachial pressure point is found on the inner side of the upper arm (**A**).

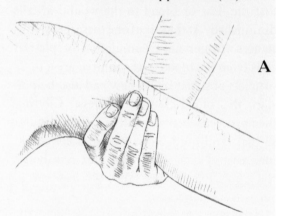

A

● The femoral artery can be felt pulsating in the middle of the groin crease at the top of the leg (**B**).

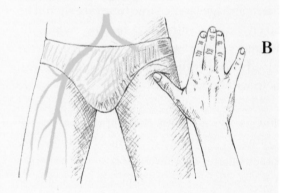

B

6. If the wound is extensive or likely to require stitches, or if blood loss has been considerable, seek medical advice promptly.

AN A-Z OF ACCIDENTS AND EMERGENCIES

Animal bites

The commonest bites sustained by children are from dogs or other pets such as gerbils or rats. Usually such bites cause a puncture wound which is small but deep. Bleeding is not normally a serious problem, but because the wound is deep it is not easy to clean. It should be washed thoroughly, using an antiseptic solution, and covered by a dry dressing. If children are bitten by an animal and are not up to date with their tetanus immunizations they should start a course or have a booster injection, whichever is appropriate. Rabies is not a risk with bites from domestic animals in developed countries.

Blisters

Blisters arise when friction causes damage to the skin, perhaps by rubbing footwear or from scalds. Tissue fluid accumulates within the skin, and the overlying skin layer is likely to burst. All the while the skin cover is intact there is little risk of infection. Small blisters should be protected against bursting and infection by a dry dressing, and healing will take place naturally. It may be necessary to burst larger blisters with a sterile needle before applying the initial non-stick protective dressing.

Bruising

Bruising results from bleeding in the skin or deeper tissues due to injury with a blunt object, but does not involve a break in the skin. Small bruises need no treatment but large bruises in deep tissues can be very painful. The area should be protected with a sling or bandage, and strenuous activity should be discouraged. The blood in the bruise may work its way up to the skin over

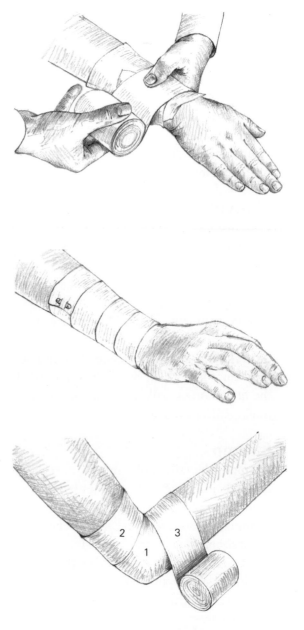

Applying a roller bandage. **Top and middle:** The bandage should be kept flat and the first turn applied at an angle to fix the bandage firmly in position. Each successive spiral turn should cover two thirds of the preceding one. The bandage should give support and protect but should not be so tight that the circulation is impeded.

Bottom: When applied around a joint, the bandage is initially taken over the joint itself and then passed alternately above and below this first, central turn. Each of the successive turns should cover just over two thirds of the preceding turn. Bandaging should finish above the joint.

the first day or two after the injury; the colour of the bruise changes to yellow during healing. Bruises normally disappear within about five days.

Concussion

Concussion is a temporary unconsciousness due to a blow to the head, but does not involve brain damage. See Head injuries (page 223) for treatment.

Convulsions

Convulsions in small children are most commonly provoked by fever (see Febrile convulsions, page 265), but may also be due to epilepsy (page 262). Most convulsions cease spontaneously without the need for specific treatment. The child should be placed in the recovery position (see page 211) and tight clothing should be loosened; if the child feels hot, the clothing should be removed. If the fit continues, call an ambulance or summon medical aid urgently.

Cramp

Cramp is the failure of a muscle to relax; in children it is likely to occur either during vigorous exercise such as swimming or running, or sometimes at night when they are asleep. Massaging the affected part brings relief, and the spasm in the muscle gradually eases, although the muscle may continue to be painful for an hour or so later.

Cuts and lacerations

The skin may be cut by a sharp object, or may split because of a blunt injury. In either case there will be bleeding, and this should be stopped by direct pressure (see page 218). The wound should be assessed when the bleeding has stopped. First wash your hands. If the wound is small it should be cleaned by washing it with water or mild antiseptic, and then covered by an adhesive dressing.

Cuts that go through the full thickness of the skin will result in some scarring. Wounds that are longer than about 1 cm (½ inch), particularly if they are gaping, will heal better if stitched, and often stitching will lessen the amount of scarring. Cuts on the face may also require stitching to lessen the scarring. If you think a laceration may need stitching it should be covered with a dry dressing, and you should seek a medical opinion.

Drowning

In drowning accidents respiration stops because water enters and blocks the airways. The child should be held head downwards for a few seconds to drain out any water in the upper airways. Then, if breathing is poor, mouth-to-mouth artificial respiration should be started (see page 213).

With prolonged immersion, particularly in very cold water, the patient's body may have cooled down. The first aider should not attempt to warm up a patient who is not breathing, however, as a low body temperature reduces the body's need for oxygen. The priority is to establish mouth-to-mouth respiration, and if necessary also to start heart massage (see pages 213 and 214).

Ear, foreign body

Small children sometimes put beads or other small objects in their ears. Unless the object is protruding from the ear canal, attempts to remove it are likely to push it further in. The foreign body can sometimes be removed if the child lies down on his side, with the affected ear uppermost, and the first aider runs tepid water or slightly warm olive oil into the ear, causing the object to float or be washed out. If this is unsuccessful a doctor should be consulted.

Electric shock

If a child touches faulty electrical apparatus

or a live wire and sustains an electric shock, there are two possible serious consequences: the shock may cause the heart to stop, and the electricity may give rise to serious burns.

- Switch off the current before approaching the child
- If the child has sustained an electric shock and is unconscious and not breathing, it is likely that his heart has stopped. Call an ambulance and start mouth-to-mouth respiration and heart massage, as described on pages 213 and 214.

If a child is conscious after an electric shock the heart will not have been seriously affected but he may still have sustained an electrical burn at the point of contact. Electricity causes severe heating of the tissues and the burns may be quite deep and more serious than they appear at first sight. The affected part should be immersed in cold water for at least five minutes. Except for the most trivial burns medical advice should be sought, as the burns may extend deeply.

Eye, foreign body

Sand, dust, small insects and other small particles may get into the eye and stick to the eyeball or under an eyelid. They are very painful, causing the eye to water and the child to hold his eyelids tightly shut. Often, foreign bodies may be washed out by tears.

The child should be restrained from rubbing his eyes, as this could cause damage to the eye, as could attempts to remove foreign bodies. Do not try to remove a foreign body which is embedded in the surface of the eye, or is lying over the pupil. If the foreign body can be seen on the white part of the eye or the inside of the lower lid and if the child is co-operative, it may be possible to remove it with a moist cotton-wool bud or the corner of a clean handker-

chief. The child should sit facing the light. Foreign bodies lodged under the upper lid are more difficult to remove, and should be left to professionals.

Medical help should be obtained if the foreign body is embedded in the eye, or cannot be removed, or is over the pupil, or if the child is not co-operative. If a foreign body cannot be seen but the eye continues to be watery and painful, a medical opinion should also be sought.

Eye injuries

Soap or splashes of other liquids may get into a child's eye, causing intense pain and irritation. Wash the eye with water to dilute the liquid immediately: gently pour water on to the side of the eye, holding the child horizontally and keeping his eyelids partially open. Fortunately soap and most household liquids are not likely to cause serious damage, but if in any doubt seek medical advice.

The eye may also be injured by a direct blow. Cover the eye with a pad, and seek a medical opinion urgently.

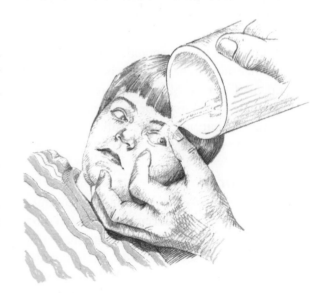

Washing out the eye to remove irritant liquid or a foreign body.

Fainting

Fainting is due to a temporary reduction in the flow of blood to the brain, so that it cannot function properly; as a result unconsciousness ensues. Faints are not common in early childhood but often happen during adolescence. They may be brought on by emotion or by pooling of blood in the lower part of the body, perhaps on prolonged standing or on suddenly getting up after prolonged sitting. Being in a warm room (which promotes dilatation of the blood vessels in the skin) and fasting both predispose to fainting.

Unless someone intervenes, the person who faints falls to the ground, and immediately the blood flow to the brain improves. Treatment for someone who feels faint, or who has fainted, consists of lowering the patient's head to restore the blood flow to the brain. He should not be supported in an upright position. Lowering the head is most easily done by laying the patient down on the floor, and then loosening any tight clothing around his neck. Recovery of consciousness is very rapid, usually occurring within a minute. There may not even be time to put him in the recovery position before he recovers! Once consciousness returns, the patient should lie still for about another minute; he may then be allowed to sit up, and can be offered a drink. He may continue to feel dizzy or nauseated for a few minutes, but after this full recovery is normally very quick.

Fractures

Fractures (broken bones) are very common in childhood, as children are active and often sustain falls and other injuries, subjecting their bones to severe stresses. Falling with a hand protectively outstretched can lead to breaking an arm or collar bone; falling awkwardly while running may lead to a leg fracture.

A fracture should be suspected after a fall if there is pain which persists for more than a few minutes, and if the child is reluctant to use the limb or to walk. The injured part may also be swollen and possibly deformed. The site of the injury will be tender to the touch.

If a fracture is suspected a medical opinion is needed. First aid is limited to preventing movement of the limb to minimize pain, comforting the child, and taking him to the doctor or hospital. For an injured arm a sling will be helpful. It may be possible to prevent leg movement by carefully lifting the child while protecting the injured limb; if moving the leg is painful, you may need to bandage both legs together so the good limb acts as a splint for the injured one.

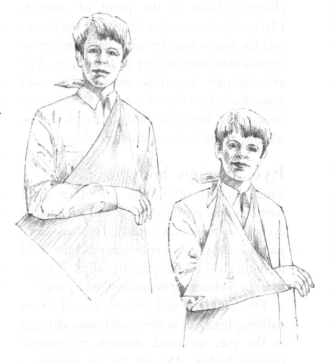

A sling is useful for protecting and supporting a fractured or injured arm, hand or shoulder. To make a basic sling, place an open triangular bandage between the chest and forearm, with the point of the triangle extending beyond the elbow (**left**).

Bring the upper end over the shoulder on the uninjured side and round the back of the neck. Take the lower end to meet the top end and tie the two together (**right**). If a triangular bandage is not available, improvise by using a headscarf or other piece of material.

Grazes (abrasions)

Grazes consist of the loss of the surface of the skin by friction. They usually occur when a child falls over while running, and scrapes his hands, knees or elbows on the ground. Most grazes are fairly superficial, but they are often very painful: this is because a relatively large area of skin surface is affected, and the nerve endings that produce pain are located in the superficial parts of the skin.

Bleeding may initially be profuse, but will stop rapidly with direct pressure. The wound must be properly cleaned. Any bits of sand or gravel not removed may remain in the skin after the wound has healed, and can produce a permanent tattooing effect. Soak the wound in a detergent antiseptic and then clean it gently but thoroughly with cotton wool. Once the wound is clean it can be left exposed. The surface dries and forms a scab, which will come off when the skin below has healed.

Head injuries

Children sustain bangs on the head fairly frequently in play and the majority of such injuries are trivial. However, prompt medical advice should be sought if a head injury results in any of the following:

- Loss of consciousness, however brief
- Confusion or drowsiness persisting after a head injury or coming on afterwards
- Severe or persisting headache
- Vomiting in the twenty-four hours following a head injury.

If a child is unconscious after a head injury an ambulance should be called immediately. While waiting for the ambulance, you should care for the unconscious child as described on page 211, checking airway, breathing and circulation.

The majority of children in whom there is transient loss of consciousness, or in whom the injury is followed by headache, drowsiness or vomiting, will not have sustained serious injury. However, because in a few children head injury gives rise to a build-up of pressure on the brain which can be very serious, all children with any symptoms that might indicate brain irritation need to be seen and assessed by a doctor.

The scalp is well supplied with blood, and if the skin is lacerated as a result of a head injury bleeding is likely to be profuse. Direct pressure over the area which is bleeding should be maintained for five minutes, and is usually enough to stop the flow, even if the exact site of the wound is obscured by blood and hair. If the laceration is long or gaping stitching may be required.

Heat exhaustion and heat stroke

Small babies exposed to severe heat, and children undertaking strenuous exercise in hot weather may suffer from the heat. When the ambient temperature is high the body is only able to prevent itself from becoming too hot by sweating and by reducing energy expenditure. If a baby or child becomes listless in the heat this suggests heat exhaustion. If heat exhaustion goes unchecked and is not corrected by removing the child to a cooler place and giving him plenty of fluid to drink, then dehydration can develop, leading to heat stroke. If sweating ceases, body temperature then rises and the child becomes seriously ill. Urgent medical treatment is required to correct the fluid deficit and to bring down the body temperature.

Babies are at risk from heat exhaustion because they can rapidly become dehydrated. Prevention is important. In hot weather babies should not be over-dressed, although they do need protection from direct sunshine. Give them extra fluid to drink, and do not leave them in hot environments such as inside a parked car.

Older children should not be allowed to undertake strenuous sports or other games when the weather is very hot; give them plenty of fluid to drink. If they become listless you should ask them to rest in a cool place and give them several glasses of water or soft drinks.

Insect bites and stings
A sting from a bee or wasp is very painful; the skin rapidly becomes red and there is local swelling. Holding a piece of ice against the sting, or placing the affected part in icy water is soothing. If pain and swelling persist the doctor may prescribe an antihistamine drug. Stings around or inside the mouth can lead to marked swelling, and urgent medical attention may be needed.

Stings and bites from smaller insects, such as mosquitoes or cat fleas, usually give rise to multiple small, itchy bumps on the skin. Calamine lotion may be soothing. If cat fleas are suspected the animal should be treated with a flea powder.

Joint injuries
An injury to a joint which causes pain and swelling and restricts movement is serious enough to need medical attention. At its most severe, injury to a joint can cause dislocation, where the joint is disrupted so that the articular ends of the bones are no longer in contact. Shoulders and fingers are the joints which most commonly dislocate, although occasionally other joints may be affected. A dislocated joint needs putting back into place by the doctor, and then the joint must be immobilized until the injury has healed. Damage to the ligaments which hold the joint together is also serious, and sometimes needs an operation to repair it.

Minor joint injuries in which there is pain but no significant swelling or loss of function can be treated at home with a supportive bandage, but if symptoms persist for more than a couple of days your family doctor should be consulted.

Nail damage
A bang on the end of a finger or toe may lead to bleeding under the nail. It is very painful and tender, and the nail looks black. With time a new nail grows under the old one, and the old nail separates.

When just the nail has been injured the pain can be relieved if the doctor makes a hole through it to let out the blood that has collected under pressure.

Nose, foreign body
Children sometimes push beads, berries or other objects up their noses. Attempts at removal by the inexperienced usually result in the foreign body being pushed further in. Removal is usually easy for the doctor, who has a special hooked instrument which gets behind the foreign body. Occasionally removal under anaesthetic is required.

Nosebleed
Bleeding from the nose, or epistaxis, may either occur spontaneously or as the result of a blow on the nose. Nosebleeds will usually stop on their own within a few minutes. It helps to keep the patient upright, and to tell him not to breathe through his nose or swallow until the blood has had a chance to clot. Sit the patient down, telling him not to talk, and ask him to breathe in and out through his mouth with the head bent forward. Place a dish or tissues under the nose to catch any blood. Do not attempt to squeeze the nose. If the bleeding does not stop, or if a child is having frequent recurrent nosebleeds, medical help should be sought.

Poisoning

Medicines, white spirit, paraffin and domestic cleaners are all toxic and must be kept away from children. Nevertheless children do sometimes ingest substances that are potentially dangerous.

If tablets or medicines have been swallowed it may be possible to induce vomiting by putting a finger to the back of the child's throat. If this is successful it helps to remove some of the poison. Vomiting should not be induced if oily or corrosive substances have been swallowed; instead the child should be given a glass of milk to drink, which has some protective effect.

Whatever the child has swallowed or might have swallowed, either the doctor should be consulted or an ambulance called. Remember to take along the bottle or carton that contained the ingested substance.

Snake bites

If a child is bitten by a snake that may be venomous medical assistance should be sought immediately. The bitten part (usually limb) should be held still, but the first aider should *not* attempt to incise or suck out the wound, or to apply a tourniquet.

Suffocation or strangulation

Children may suffocate from putting their heads into plastic bags, or they may sustain a strangulation injury if cord or rope gets caught around their necks by accident or in play. Suffocation and strangulation result in the child's oxygen supply being cut off, and unconsciousness rapidly ensues.

- Immediately remove the object causing suffocation or constriction
- If the child is not breathing start mouth-to-mouth respiration (see page 213) and, if necessary, heart massage (see page 214)
- Summon an ambulance urgently.

Sunburn

Over-exposure to the ultra-violet rays in sunlight can give rise to sunburn. Therefore children should not have unrestricted exposure to the sun but should be protected by light clothing or a barrier sun cream until they have developed a protective tan.

There is a delay of about six hours before the symptoms of sunburn begin. The skin becomes red and hot, may be quite painful or very itchy, and is tender to the touch. The child is usually quite distressed, and may have difficulty in sleeping.

Cold sponging, calamine lotion or cold cream may give some relief. When severe, symptoms may persist for a couple of days; during this period further exposure to strong sunlight should be avoided.

Swallowed objects

If a child swallows a coin, toy or other object it will probably pass through the alimentary tract over the next few days, and be expelled in the stools. However, if the object is sharp or gets stuck it may cause problems, so your doctor should be consulted. He or she may order an X-ray to check on progress. Occasionally objects put in the mouth get into the windpipe and provoke coughing. If you think this has happened you should call an ambulance or take the child to hospital immediately. If the child is choking, carry out emergency treatment as on page 209.

Teeth, bleeding sockets

When milk teeth gradually loosen and fall out, there is seldom any bleeding. However, if teeth are extracted by the dentist bleeding may occur from the tooth socket several hours later. The bleeding can be controlled by getting the child to bite on a wedge of tissue placed over the site of the extraction. You should consult your dentist or, if he or she is not available, your doctor about further management if the bleeding continues.

Tooth injury

Teeth may be broken or loosened by a child falling and hitting his mouth, or being hit in the mouth by a hard ball or similar object. The dentist may be able to splint a loose tooth or repair a cracked one and should be consulted as soon as possible.

The family medicine cupboard

Families should have a lockable medicine cupboard or box in which to keep supplies for first aid, common emergencies, and any medicines that have been prescribed for family members. Unwanted and old medicines should be disposed of: they should be flushed down the toilet and not simply discarded in a dustbin. Medicine cupboards or boxes can be bought complete with contents, or parents can put together their own supplies.

The basics that will suffice for most family medical emergencies are the following:

A good supply of assorted adhesive dressings
A reel of adhesive tape
Cotton wool
Two or three small crepe bandages
An eye pad

Safety pins
Scissors
Thermometer

A bottle of mild antiseptic for cleaning wounds
A tube of antiseptic cream
Eye lotion
Calamine lotion
Paracetamol liquid
Antidiarrhoeal medicine

PART FOUR

AN A-Z OF CHILDREN'S MEDICINE

A Glossary of Disorders, Diseases and Medical Terminology

This quick-reference glossary covers a large number of health problems and diseases of childhood and provides clear explanations of symptoms and treatment. Also included is information on different medicines and other therapies.

Words in *italics* indicate that an entry on that particular subject will be found in this section of the book.

ABDOMINAL PAIN

The possible underlying causes of abdominal pain are too numerous to be covered in this section — including as they do disease of the alimentary tract, liver or urinary tract, appendicitis and constipation, as well as emotional factors. They are therefore discussed in full on pages 62 and 166-68.

ABO INCOMPATIBILITY

An occasional cause of *jaundice* in the newborn period is when mother and baby are of different ABO blood groups; antibodies from the mother affect the red blood cells of the fetus. The mother usually has group O blood and the baby group A or B. Although mothers are often of different groups from their babies, ABO incompatibility jaundice is rare.

ABSCESS

A collection of pus surrounded by a wall of inflammatory tissue. It is a reaction of the body tissues to local bacterial infection, and develops to limit the spread of the infection to other parts. Abscesses are painful, swollen, hot and tender, and if near the skin tend to point in one place where, if untreated, they will burst. The abscess is accompanied by fever, malaise (a general feeling of being unwell) and other general symptoms.

Abscesses in the skin are common, and often arise from minor injury which allows infection to be introduced. They may also occur internally with some infections, or following surgery. Before an abscess has fully developed, *antibiotic* treatment may allow it to heal, but if pus has formed, surgical drainage will normally be required.

Sometimes an abscess forms at the root of a tooth; this is called a dental abscess. If treated early with antibiotics it may settle down but drainage of pus requires the tooth to be drilled or extracted.

ACHONDROPLASIA

A skeletal abnormality characterized by extreme short stature associated with disproportionately short arms and legs. It is genetic in origin and present from birth. Achondroplasia is the commonest of several different diseases associated with short limbs. All are rare.

ACNE

A skin disease affecting the face, chest and back. It is most common in adolescence, and is due to hair follicles becoming blocked with sebaceous secretions. These appear as 'blackheads', or comedones. The blocked follicles may become red and swollen due to secondary infection, and then come to a head and discharge a small amount of pus.

In adolescence the sebaceous glands produce more secretions than previously as a result of the rise in the levels of circulating sex hormones; having some spots at this age is almost universal. Exposure to sunlight is beneficial, and not eating

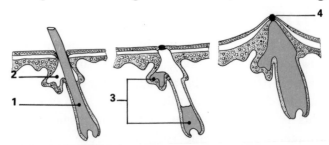

Hair follicles (**1**) contain sebaceous glands (**2**). Acne occurs when fatty secretions called sebum (**3**) build up in a follicle that has lost its hair. The follicle becomes distended and inflamed as the sebum builds up. The sebum dries at the duct opening (**4**) to form a blackhead.

chocolate is often recommended. Frequent washing of the affected areas with soap helps to remove some of the sebaceous plugs and lowers the number of skin *bacteria*. Sometimes mild detergent lotions are used for the same reason. Squeezing blackheads and spots makes secondary infection more likely and should be avoided.

If the acne is severe it may be helped by an acne lotion, which contains an antiseptic. Thick, greasy skin preparations are best avoided. Secondary infection with the development of lots of red, angry spots may be helped by prolonged treatment with an *antibiotic* for some months. If the acne is very severe the doctor may consider referral to a skin specialist.

ADENOIDS, ENLARGED

The adenoids together with the tonsils play an important role in defending the body against infection. They actually reduce in size from around the age of 10 or 12, but can cause problems before then, especially if they become infected. The resulting swelling may block the nasal airway, causing the child to breathe through his mouth. Secretions will not drain into the pharynx but run down the nose instead. The opening of the Eustachian tube at the back of the pharynx may also be affected. Children with enlarged adenoids are more likely to suffer with both otitis media and glue ear (see pages 290 and 270).

Adenoidectomy (surgical removal of the adenoids) may be necessary if a child suffers persistent or recurrent infection.

SEE ALSO pages 188-89

ADRENAL GLAND

The adrenal glands are situated in the abdomen just above each kidney. They produce vital hormones called cortisol and aldosterone, which are concerned with the regulation of glucose and minerals within the body, and also the sex hormones –

oestrogens and androgens. The inner part of the gland produces adrenaline, which regulates blood pressure and heart rate, and is particularly important in preparing the body for sudden action.

SEE ALSO illustration on page 269

AIDS

If a person becomes infected by the human immunodeficiency virus (HIV), the *virus* persists in the body, and the person can be tested and shown to be HIV positive. After a variable period, usually of several years, those infected with HIV may develop symptoms due to a breakdown of the immune systems of the body. This is known as Acquired Immune Deficiency Syndrome, or AIDS. The symptoms are variable and can include enlarged *lymph nodes*, weight loss, persistent infections which tend to be of an unusual type, or sometimes the development of tumours.

HIV is spread by sexual contact, by sharing syringes for intravenous drug abuse, or by the donation of blood or blood products from an infected individual. HIV infection has affected a number of children with *haemophilia* who were given clotting factors contaminated with the HIV virus. Other possible sources of infection for children are *blood transfusions* and spread from the mother while the baby is in the womb or via breast milk. Now that blood and clotting factors are screened and tested for HIV, it is hoped that, in future, cases of AIDS from transfusion will be rare. The major risk to children in future is likely to be HIV acquired from the mother while the baby is in the womb.

Children who do have HIV infection are rarely an infectious risk to others, because the virus can only be passed on by sexual activity, sharing syringes or blood donation.

ALBINISM see page 191

ALBUMINURIA

The finding of albumin, a protein, in the urine; this is abnormal. It may indicate disturbed kidney function and if it is consistently present the doctor may want to do further kidney tests. However, occasionally it is not associated with any disease.

ALCOHOL ABUSE

Many children are introduced to alcohol in their teens by parents on a special family occasion; provided it is done sensibly and they are not permitted too much, this can constitute a useful introduction to the adult world in which social drinking plays a part.

Young people rely on their parents for guidance over drinking and what limits are acceptable. As in so many things, parental example is important, and if parents on occasion drink to excess this can provide a role model suggesting that this is acceptable adult behaviour.

Parents should be aware of the sort of activities their children are involved in, and should set rules for drinking and be prepared to be firm. Although young people may appear to resent restrictions, these nevertheless provide a framework that helps them in controlling their own actions.

Preventing alcohol abuse by children is best, but if a parent discovers that a child is covertly drinking on a regular basis, this needs to be controlled. Parents may not be able to cope on their own and should go to see the family doctor, who may wish to refer them for specialist help.

ALLERGIC RHINITIS

The mucous membrane lining the nose can be affected by an allergic tendency. *Hay fever* is one form of allergic rhinitis, caused by an *allergy* to grass pollen. Hay fever is seasonal, being limited to the early summer when there are a lot of pollen particles in the air, whereas symptoms of allergic rhinitis can persist throughout the year. Symptoms include a blocked and watering nose. Dust, feathers, animal fur, pollen and the spores of fungi can bring on the symptoms, as can smoke and vapours. Treatment is with decongestant medicines, or nasal inhalations of sodium cromoglycate or locally acting steroids.

ALLERGY

Some individuals react adversely to contact with or ingestion of substances which are harmless to other people. The reaction provoked, known as an allergy, is an activation of the body's immune system in response to a hypersensitivity to a particular substance (known as the allergen). Most allergens are proteins, but some drugs may also provoke allergies. The symptoms will generally consist of a skin rash if the allergen is ingested by mouth, or *allergic rhinitis* or wheezing if inhaled.

Individuals with *eczema*, asthma (see page 152) or *hay fever* are known as atopic, and they have a predisposition to develop allergic reactions which aggravate their disease. The exact form their disease takes will be determined by the substances they become allergic to, and the organs affected.

In most eczematous children no apparent allergic element provokes the rash, although exacerbations may be associated with skin contact with various washing powders or ointments, and in some children with allergens in the diet.

Allergy is also a factor in some other diseases such as *dermatitis*, and some forms of intestinal *malabsorption*. In these diseases it is often important to know which substances act as allergens for a particular individual. Dust, pollen, feathers and animal fur provoke an attack in most asthmatics, and should be avoided where possible. However, other allergens may also be involved, and these can be either foods or inhaled particles. Skin testing and dietary manipulations are the main ways of determining what are allergens for a particular individual.

Skin testing is usually done by placing liquid extracts of various common allergens on the skin of the forearm, and making a small needle prick through the liquid so that a minute amount of the substance enters the outer layer of the skin. After about half an hour there will be a red reaction surrounding the prick mark if the substance being tested is an allergen for the patient. Skin testing can also be performed by sticking adhesive patches containing the substance on to the skin. Skin testing measures skin allergy; in asthma or food allergy substances which provoke a reaction in the skin do not always do so in the lungs or intestine, and vice versa. With skin testing some atopic individuals will have a reaction to most of the common allergens.

Food allergy may be part of the atopic syndrome, or may occur without associated problems. It can cause symptoms related to the stomach and intestines, or may give more generalized symptoms. Cow's milk allergy can start in infancy as soon as a baby is started on an artificial formula. The usual manifestations of the allergy are that the baby is slow to gain weight and may have loose stools. The milk protein causes an allergic reaction in the wall of the intestine, so that it becomes inflamed and absorption of nutrients is depressed. In severe allergy the cow's milk protein may cause vomiting shortly after ingestion. Many children who develop an allergy to cow's milk will also develop allergies to other foods. including soya-based infant formulas. As well as possible diarrhoea, vomiting and poor weight gain, food allergy may cause symptoms remote from the alimentary tract; skin rashes and wheezing are the most' common. In individuals who are allergic to cow's milk the sensitivity usually improves as they get older, and many have lost their allergy by the age of 2 years.

In suspected food allergy dietary manipulations are sometimes used to determine the allergens. These are difficult to do, and the results are not always easy to interpret, so they should only be done if an individual has major symptoms and only under the supervision of a qualified dietitian. The individual is first put on a very limited diet for two weeks. If the symptoms improve during this period it may be because the provoking allergens have been removed. Single additional foods are then gradually reintroduced, and if symptoms recur it is presumed that the reintroduced food is an allergen.

Allergic reactions have a very definite immunological basis. The term 'allergy' has been used incorrectly by some practitioners to describe conditions which are believed to be idiosyncratic reactions to common food substances and food additives (see page 95).

SEE ALSO *Drug rash*

ALOPECIA

Hair loss; it may occur secondary to treatment with radiotherapy or certain drugs, particularly those used for the treatment of *leukaemia* and malignant diseases.

Many children accept this as part of the treatment but wigs can be supplied. The hair regrows in a few months. Alopecia may rarely have no obvious cause, affecting either isolated patches or the whole scalp. A dermatologist should be consulted in such cases.

AMENORRHOEA

The absence of menstrual or monthly periods. Amenorrhoea may be either primary or secondary. It is termed primary when a girl has never started her periods and the usual cause is that the onset of puberty is delayed (see page 83). Secondary amenorrhoea is when previously established periods cease. Missing an occasional period is not unusual in adolescence, and can be associated with examinations or other stress. If secondary amenorrhoea is persistent, the commonest causes are pregnancy or *anorexia nervosa*.

ANAEMIA see *Iron deficiency anaemia; Sickle cell anaemia; Thalassaemia*

ANAL FISSURE

A split in the skin margin around the anus is known as a fissure. The usual cause is passing a hard stool. Anal fissures are painful on defecation, and may take a long time to heal as they split open whenever a firm, bulky stool is passed. Small children will often refuse to defecate if they have a fissure and can become more constipated (see page 168). Fissures can be treated by giving *laxatives* in sufficient quantities to make the stools soft. A cream containing a local anaesthetic applied to the anal region can also be helpful.

ANALGESIC

Analgesics are drugs that relieve pain. Simple analgesics, such as paracetamol, are used in childhood for discomfort such as *headache* and abdominal pain (see page 166). Aspirin is not now recommended to be taken routinely by young children because its widespread use has been linked to a rare but serious disease called Reye's syndrome. Both paracetamol and aspirin are also effective in lowering the body temperature in fever.

Strong analgesics such as pethidine and morphine have their use controlled because of the possibility of addiction, and are reserved for severe pain such as that following burns, accidents and operations.

ANENCEPHALY

A rare congenital abnormality in which there is severe maldevelopment of the brain, the cerebral hemispheres being missing. The fetus cannot survive outside the womb.

ANGIOMA

A *congenital* malformation of the blood vessels or lymph vessels, which are enlarged and distorted. Skin angiomas may be present from birth or shortly after as birth marks and may be unsightly. Angiomas in other organs may give rise to swelling or tumours.

SEE ALSO Birth marks (page 27)

ANOREXIA NERVOSA

A psychological disturbance, almost exclusively limited to females, which usually develops around the age of 15–17 years, but may start as early as 12. The affected individual perceives herself to be too fat and develops a compulsion to lose weight. Some girls are obese at the onset, but others are of normal weight.

All adolescent girls are interested in their appearance, and going on a reducing diet is common, but it is seldom very strict or kept up for long stretches at a time. In anorexia this interest in food and body weight becomes an obsession, and the diet is continued even when a lot of weight has been lost.

Minor degrees of anorexia are common and not serious. In more serious cases the affected young woman has an altered perception of her body image, and will still feel she is too fat even when others perceive her as thin or wasted. Food intake is progressively reduced and starchy and sugary foods are particularly avoided. *Laxatives* may be used covertly to encourage weight loss, and vomiting may be induced in secret. Weight is gradually lost, the breasts shrink and the ribs become prominent, periods may stop (see *Amenorrhoea*), hands and feet always appear cold, and there may be excess growth of hair on the arms and legs. Loose clothing is often favoured to disguise the extent of the weight loss.

The obsession with body weight and food in anorexia nervosa is a symptom of an underlying psychological disturbance, which is complex and different in each individual. The young woman may feel very insecure and have a poor self-image, and she may be apprehensive about her developing sexuality or reject it. Stresses are likely to be present in family relationships. Often the girl feels that the family has high expectations of her in academic or employment terms, but insufficient respect for her as an individual.

The aim of treatment is to help resolve the stresses and emotional problems of the patient and at the same time to encourage her to gain weight. This is not something that can be done by the girl alone or even with assistance from her family although, of course, treatment can not be successful without co-operation from the patient. In all cases of anorexia nervosa the family doctor should be consulted as soon as possible, so that he or she can refer the patient to a specialist, usually a psychiatrist.

If the patient has suffered severe weight loss, hospitalization may be necessary. A target weight is set and at the same time as food intake is increased and weight is being regained, the psychiatrist will attempt to understand the inner conflicts and relationship difficulties that have led to the development of anorexia in the patient, and help her to overcome them.

ANOXIA

Anoxia (also called hypoxia) is a deficiency of oxygen in the blood and body tissues. It arises from inadequate breathing, obstruction of the airways, heart or lung disease. Minor degrees of anoxia usually provoke greater respiratory efforts in an attempt to compensate for the oxygen lack. If anoxia is more severe, the deficiency of oxygen interferes with the workings of many of the body organs. The brain and heart are both very dependent on an adequate oxygen supply to continue working efficiently. The treatment of anoxia will depend on its cause.

ANTIBIOTIC

The treatment of infectious disease was revolutionized by the introduction of antibiotics in the 1940s, and there are now a wide range of different antibiotics available for the treatment of common bacterial infections. They are drugs which kill *bacteria* and some other micro-organisms, but are not toxic to man. Some antibiotics are naturally occurring substances produced by other micro-organisms, but many of them are synthetic.

Antibiotics can be used for the treatment of common bacterial infections such as *tonsillitis* and *otitis media*. It may not be known which bacteria are causing the infection when the child first falls ill, and therefore a so-called broad-spectrum antibiotic is chosen. In other situations, such as urinary tract infection (see page 171) and *meningitis*, the doctor takes specimens first to try to determine which antibiotic will be best at eradicating the infection.

Antibiotics are ineffective against *viruses*, so there is no point in taking them for colds and other known viral infections. Unless a child is allergic, frequent courses of common antibiotics do little harm. The development of infections caused by bacteria which are resistant to antibiotics is more of a theoretical than a practical risk. Thrush, a fungus infection, may develop in the mouth after an antibiotic course, as the normal bacterial organisms in the mouth are altered by the antibiotic; the fungus becomes an opportunist invader.

ANTICONVULSANT DRUGS

Anticonvulsant drugs are used in the treatment of *epilepsy* to prevent convulsions. They can also be given during a convulsion to bring it to an end. The anticonvulsant used will depend on the type of epilepsy and on the patient's response. For major epilepsy the commonest anticonvulsants used in children are carbemazepine, phenytoin and sodium valproate. During a convulsion diazepam may be given either intravenously or rectally to stop the seizure.

ANTIHISTAMINE DRUGS

Histamine is produced in the body and triggers allergic reactions (see *Allergy*). Some of the reactions to histamine can be suppressed by antihistamine drugs. They are widely used in *hay fever* and *allergic rhinitis*, but may cause sedation in large doses.

ANUS, IMPERFORATE

Occasionally the anus is not properly formed and a newborn baby does not have an anal opening. If there is just a thin membrane across the anal canal it may be ruptured easily by a paediatric surgeon, but more commonly there is a thick block of tissue that needs to be fashioned into a functional anal canal. This cannot be done until the child has grown sufficiently, so a colostomy, in which the bowel is brought out to open on the abdominal wall, is done for the first few months of life.

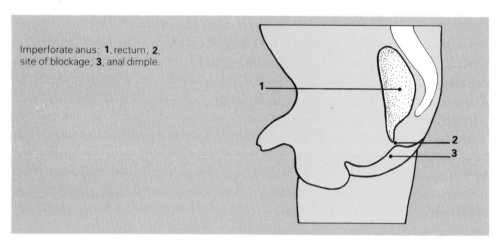

Imperforate anus: **1**, rectum; **2**, site of blockage; **3**, anal dimple.

AORTIC VALVE STENOSIS

A stenosis, or narrowing, of the aortic valve of the heart gives rise to a heart murmur (see page 145). If the narrowing is sufficient to obstruct the flow of blood,

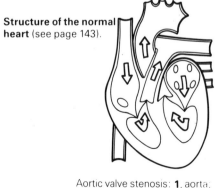

Structure of the normal heart (see page 143).

Aortic valve stenosis: **1**, aorta; **2**, left atrium; **3**, left ventricle; **4** narrowed aortic valve.

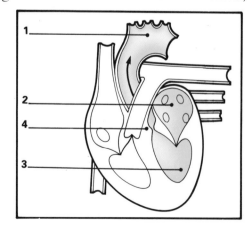

the heart has to work harder than usual. This does not usually cause problems in childhood but may give rise to heart strain in adult life, so an operation is often recommended if the stenosis is severe. Many children with mild aortic stenosis do not require treatment.

APGAR SCORE see pages 20-1

APNOEIC ATTACKS see page 42

APPENDICITIS

The appendix is a short, narrow, blind-ended structure which is hollow; it arises from the bowel where the small and large intestine join, in the lower right side of the abdomen (see page 162). Anatomists call it the vermiform appendix as it resembles an earthworm in size and shape. Occasionally it becomes infected, and appendicitis results. Around 5 per cent of children have appendicitis at some time during childhood. It usually leads to perforation of the appendix wall, and then the intestinal contents can leak out and cause peritonitis, an inflammation of the abdominal lining; an operation to remove the appendix is required as soon as the diagnosis is made.

The onset of appendicitis is marked by malaise (a general feeling of being unwell), loss of appetite and central abdominal pain. At first the pain is not very

The appendix (**1**) is situated at the junction of the large and small intestines. It plays no role in digestion but can become inflamed, and even burst, if a blockage occurs.

In appendicitis the pain usually moves from the centre of the abdomen to the right side, as shown. There is tenderness over the appendix (marked with an 'x').

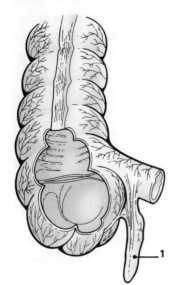

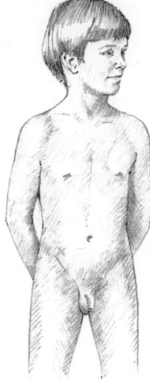

noticeable, but it becomes more so over the space of a few hours. The patient may have nausea and vomiting, but these are not marked. The temperature is usually slightly raised, the tongue is furred, and the breath may smell unpleasant. If the doctor examines the child at this stage and there is tenderness in the right lower abdomen over the site of the appendix the diagnosis is probably appendicitis; the child should be admitted to hospital.

In hospital the child will be seen by a surgeon, and may have a blood test and abdominal X-ray. If appendicitis seems likely an operation to remove the appendix is indicated and should be performed as soon as possible: the longer the wait, the more likely the appendix to perforate, and this worsens the patient's condition. There is much less risk to health in operating and removing a normal appendix than in delay if the appendix is inflamed, so even if the diagnosis is not certain an operation will probably be recommended.

The incision is made through the abdominal wall either over the appendix or in the midline of the abdomen. The appendix is removed, the hole in the bowel wall is stitched together, and the wound is then closed. The child will continue to have a sore tummy and feel unwell for a couple of days, but recovery is usually rapid.

Recurrent abdominal pain is sometimes attributed to a 'grumbling appendix' due to persisting mild infection. This is in fact rare. When the appendix becomes infected it usually perforates within a short space of time and gives rise to peritonitis, so that it is very unlikely that low-grade chronic (long-term) infection will occur.

ARRHYTHMIA

The heart normally beats with a regular rhythm. The term 'arrhythmia' is used when the rhythm is not regular. A variation in heart rate with respiration is very common in children, the rate increasing with inspiration (breathing in) and decreasing with expiration (breathing out); this is normal and is called sinus arrhythmia. Other rhythm disturbances are more serious. In paroxysmal tachycardia the heart may have episodes of going much too fast. With heart block the heart may drop a beat or stop for longer periods. Arrhythmias need investigating, and the more serious ones need treatment with a pacemaker.

ARTHRITIS IN CHILDHOOD

Arthritis is an inflammatory process affecting one or several joints. Fortunately it is not common in childhood. In septic arthritis the inflammation is the result of infection with *bacteria*, and only one joint is likely to be affected. Treatment with *antibiotics*, with or without surgical drainage of the joint, usually leads to complete recovery.

Inflammation of a joint due to infection with *tuberculosis* is now hardly ever seen in industrialized countries, but is still encountered in parts of the Third World where it is a major problem.

Not all arthritis is infective. Some children develop an inflammation of the tissues of the joints without having an infection. Although this inflammatory arthritis has some similarities to the rheumatoid arthritis that can affect adults, it is a different condition. Usually arthritis in childhood causes stiffness of the joints but not much pain, and after a few months or years will disappear entirely. The arthritis responds to treatment with non-steroidal anti-inflammatory drugs (NSAIDs), but sometimes treatment with steroids will also be required. As well as drug treatment, mobility should be encouraged and restriction of joint movement prevented, so a *physiotherapist* needs to be involved. Occasionally special schooling will also be needed.

ASPIRIN

An *analgesic* and anti-inflammatory drug. It is no longer recommended for general use in children under 12 as there is evidence that it may rarely cause a serious disease called Reye's syndrome. For specific purposes such as the treatment of *arthritis* it is still used for children.

ASTHMA see page 152

ASTIGMATISM see page 181

ATAXIA

Ataxia is a problem with the co-ordination of movement which results from disorder of the part of the brain called the cerebellum, or the spinal cord, or may be provoked by toxic doses of certain drugs including *anticonvulsants*, in which case the dose should be reduced.

ATHLETE'S FOOT

A fungal infection of the skin which causes redness and sogginess between the fourth and fifth toes (and rarely between the third and fourth ones as well). It starts because sweat collects in this area when the feet are hot, and this makes the skin vulnerable to the infection. It can be prevented by wearing open-toed sandals and no socks, or treated by the regular application of an anti-fungal dusting powder or cream.

ATOPIC ECZEMA

Atopic eczema usually appears between the ages of 2 months and 2 years. Often there is a family history of eczema, *dermatitis*, asthma (see page 152) or *hay fever*. The first signs of eczema are likely to be red, itchy patches on the trunk, limbs and cheeks. Sometimes other areas can be involved, and if severe the whole body can be affected. At first the rash may show vesicles (small blisters) which weep clear fluid if scratched. As a result of the scratching and chronic (long-term) inflammation, the skin often becomes dry, thickened, pigmented and scaly.

Although the tendency to develop atopic eczema is inborn the skin may be made worse by allergy either to something that comes into contact with the skin, such as soap or certain clothing materials, or to certain types of food. If the eczema is particularly severe and does not respond to treatment it may be worth trying dietary exclusions, particularly of eggs, milk and milk products. Dietary exclusions should be supervised by a dietitian who can advise on which foods to avoid, and can ensure that the diet retains adequate essential nutrients.

After the first year the eczema is usually not so extensive, but some degree of it may persist throughout life, particularly behind the knee, around the wrist and in front of the elbow.

Eczema is best controlled by continuous skin care. The skin always tends to be dry and flaky, and may flare up to become itchy and inflamed. The avoidance of soap, which tends to dry the skin further, and the use of an emulsifying ointment instead, both as a soap and in the bath water, helps to keep the skin smooth and supple. This preventative treatment should become a routine.

If, in spite of this approach, patches of eczema do develop the doctor should be consulted. Eczema can usually be brought back under control with a mild steroid cream, such as hydrocortisone cream, but if there is a secondary infection an *antibiotic* may also be required. Severe eczema may require dressings to keep the medication in continuous contact with the skin, and to prevent scratching. Severe bouts of eczema may require hospital admission.

ATRIAL SEPTAL DEFECT (ASD)

Atrial septal defect is a form of *congenital* heart disease in which there is a hole between the left and right atria, the upper chambers of the heart; some blood passes through this hole. The right ventricle, one of the two lower chambers of the heart, then has to pump this extra blood around the lungs. With time this can put a strain on the heart, and an operation to close the defect during childhood may be recommended.

SEE ALSO page 146

Structure of the normal heart (see page 143).

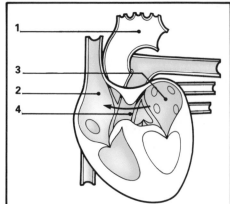

Atrial septal defect: **1**, aorta; **2**, right atrium; **3**, left atrium; **4**, defect or hole between atria, allowing blood to pass through.

AUSTRALIA ANTIGEN

A substance found in the blood of people who have been infected with *hepatitis B*. The antigen was so named because it was first discovered in an aborigine.

AUTISM

A rare psychiatric disturbance of children characterized by a profound inability to relate to people. Features of autism include lack of eye contact and social smiling, an ability to play alone for long periods, and the development of repetitive, compulsive rituals of behaviour. Interruption of these rituals may provoke fierce outbursts of temper. Frequently noted behaviour includes an apparent fascination with water, repeated rocking of the body, or being engrossed in watching movements of the fingers.

The cause of autism is unknown. It is often impossible to test intelligence because the child will not co-operate with the tests, but in some autistic children some abilities are within the normal range. Mental handicap (see page 160) can be associated with autistic features in some children.

BACK PAIN

Back pain is uncommon in children. It may arise as the result of a strain and will quickly settle down. Persistent back pain in teenagers may be the result of *vitamin D deficiency* (see page 93) or of a condition called osteochondritis which affects the growing ends of the vertebrae. A few boys develop back pain in adolescence as a result of *arthritis* of the spine, ankylosing spondylitis.

BACTERIA

Bacteria are micro-organisms that are widespread in nature. Those that are medically important are divided into pathogens and commensals. The pathogens may cause disease, whereas the commensals are normal inhabitants of the skin, intestine or other mucous surfaces of the body. Some bacteria can be commensals in one place and pathogens in another. Urinary tract infections (see page 171) are usually the result of intestinal commensals invading the urinary tract. Bacteria can be killed with the use of appropriate *antibiotics*.

BAD BREATH

Also called halitosis. An unpleasant mouth odour may be the result of having eaten something which smelled strong. If bad breath is persistent it is usually due to dental disease or poor dental hygiene (see Chapter 19). Other causes include *sinusitis* and foreign bodies in the nose.

BALANITIS

Balanitis is an inflammation of the tip of the penis and the foreskin due to bacterial infection. It can usually be treated by an *antibiotic* cream. Repeated attacks of balanitis may mean that *circumcision* is necessary.

BED WETTING see page 170

BILIARY ATRESIA

A *congenital* blockage of the bile ducts, which carry bile from the liver to the intestine. The blockage may be inside or outside the liver. The baby has *jaundice* in the first few days of life, and this persists. Early assessment in a specialized centre is needed as it is sometimes possible to correct the defect with surgery.

BIRTH MARKS see page 27

BLEPHARITIS

Inflammation of the eyelids, which may be caused by infection or *allergy*. It may be associated with *conjunctivitis* or may occur alone. When due to an infection *antibiotic* treatment is needed.

BLOOD TRANSFUSION

Blood transfusions can save the lives of those who are bleeding severely or are unable to make their own blood cells. They have also enabled advances to be made in paediatric surgery by making it possible to perform prolonged or difficult operations which are inevitably associated with bleeding. They are also needed for people with severe *anaemia*.

Blood should be taken from the patient for grouping and cross-matching against the donor blood. In the past, blood transfusions have occasionally led to the transmission of infection. Donors are now screened for health and the blood is tested for *hepatitis* and *AIDS*, so transmission of infection is unlikely.

BOIL

Boils result when hair follicles become infected with pathogenic (disease-causing) *bacteria*. The infection causes pain, swelling, redness, and then the formation of pus in the centre. When the pus has discharged, the boil heals. The bacteria which cause boils are staphylococci, and if they have colonized the patient's skin or nose there may be recurrent crops of boils. Treating each boil with an *antibiotic* does not usually prevent further recurrences. The use of an antiseptic soap and nasal cream to eradicate the pathogenic staphylococci may be more helpful.

BORNHOLM DISEASE

This uncommon infection is due to a *virus*, and is associated with malaise (a general feeling of being unwell), fever and sharp chest or upper abdominal pain coming on suddenly and lasting about two days. Small epidemics sometimes occur. Full recovery occurs in a few days without treatment.

BOW LEGS see page 175

BRAIN DEATH

Traditionally death was defined as the irreversible cessation of the heart beat. However, some people who have sustained catastrophic brain damage can be maintained on a ventilator so that they remain oxygenated and the heart continues beating, even though there is no hope of recovery and the brain is so damaged it cannot sustain any vital functions, including breathing.

In the persistent absence of all fundamental reflexes needed for the maintenance of life, a diagnosis of brain death may be made and ventilator support withdrawn as a consequence.

BRAIN TUMOUR

Children occasionally develop brain tumours that may be benign or malignant. They are signalled either by features of raised intracranial pressure (pressure within the skull), such as *headache* and vomiting (see page 164), or by signs such as the onset of a squint (see page 182), difficulty in swallowing, or weakness of a particular part of the body due to the involvement of or pressure on a particular part of the brain. There is a tumour which may be noted in mid-childhood called a craniopharyngioma; it retards growth as it prevents the production of the growth hormone.

Brain tumours may be treated by surgery, radiotherapy or *cytotoxic drugs*. The success of treatment depends both on the type of tumour, and its location within the brain.

BRANCHIAL CYST

Young children are sometimes found to have cystic (fluid-filled) swellings in the neck. These are remnants of a phase of embryonic development. Branchial cysts are found to the side of the midline. Thyroglossal cysts are found in the midline above the larynx (voice box). Cysts may become infected, so surgical removal is usually recommended.

BREAST ENLARGEMENT: in boys, see page 82; in newborn babies, see page 27.

BREATH-HOLDING ATTACK

When they are hurt, upset or cross, some children have attacks in which they hold their breath. This is most likely to happen between the ages of 1 and 2 years; it is more likely when the toddler is tired or unwell. An incident occurs, such as a fall or another child snatching a toy away, which provokes an immediate upset in the child. Often one cry is given but then the child holds his breath, goes tense, and becomes red or blue in the face; the attack may end when he starts to cry. If the child does not start crying he may become unconscious and will fall down. After a period of less than a minute consciousness is regained, and the attack is over. Breath-holding attacks are a reaction to stress, and are not voluntarily produced.

If a child is observed to be starting a breath-holding attack, it may be possible to halt it by shaking him or blowing in his face to restart breathing. These attacks can appear frightening, but recovery is complete and the tendency soon outgrown.

BRITTLE BONE DISEASE

In brittle bone disease, or osteogenesis imperfecta, all the bones and sometimes the teeth are abnormally brittle and break easily. Osteogenesis imperfecta is an inherited condition and there are several types. In the most severe forms the baby may sustain fractures before birth, while in the milder forms the affected individual will only have occasional fractures. Brittle bone disease is due to defects of collagen, the fibrous tissue that gives strength to the bones (see page 173). Because there is a reduced amount of collagen, the white part of the eye, the sclera, looks blue in many people with brittle bone disease. Treatment is limited to protection from injury and immobilization of fractures.

BRONCHIOLITIS

Infections with the respiratory syncytial virus are common. Usually they only cause upper respiratory tract symptoms of a runny nose and cough, but may cause more serious illness in infants and young children. In them the *virus* may give rise to bronchiolitis, a generalized infection of the airways and lungs.

In bronchiolitis the infection starts as a head cold, followed rapidly by the onset of coughing and wheezing. Initially the baby may not be particularly ill, but the wheeze and cough tend to worsen over the next few days. Feeding may be difficult, and in severe cases the baby becomes quite breathless. The infection persists for about a week or ten days.

If the attack of bronchiolitis is severe the infant may need hospitalization. *Antibiotics* are ineffective, and there is no curative treatment. Nevertheless careful nursing, tube or intravenous feeding if the baby is breathless, and oxygen if necessary are all helpful, and almost always will succeed in keeping the baby in a satisfactory condition until the body's defences overcome the infection. Many infants have a further attack, and some subsequently develop asthma.

BRONCHITIS see page 152

BRONCHOPNEUMONIA

Infection of the lung is called *pneumonia*. When the infection has spread into the lung from the air passages, it tends to be patchy and is known as bronchopneumonia. Infection by the pneumococcus bacterium affects one or more lobes of the lung, and is known as lobar pneumonia. The symptoms include a cough and fever, and treatment with an *antibiotic* is needed.

CAFE AU LAIT SPOT

Light brown patches on the skin with irregular edges are known as *café au lait* spots or patches. Many normal people have one or two and they are not of any special significance. When they are numerous, they may be a sign of the disease neurofibromatosis, in which lumps may grow on the nerves and in the skin.

CANCER

Malignant disease in childhood is fortunately rare, but tumours of various organs may sometimes occur. Tumours of the kidney, brain, bone, lymphatic tissue (a lymphoma) and sympathetic nervous tissue (a neuroblastoma) are the commonest types. The symptoms will vary depending on its site: a swelling, weight loss, or the effects of pressure from the tumour on adjacent tissue. Pain is seldom a feature.

Diagnosis depends on detecting an abnormality by a combination of X-rays or scans, and removing a piece of tissue surgically for microscopic study. Treatment may be surgical; chemotherapy (treatment with drugs) and radiotherapy are also widely employed. The results of the treatment vary with the type of cancer and where it is located, but many children make a full recovery from treatment.

CAPUT SUCCEDANEUM see page 22

CATARACT

Cataracts are opacities in the lens of the eye. In childhood they are uncommon, but they can result from *rubella* (German measles) infection during pregnancy; they also occur in some rare metabolic diseases. Cataracts can be removed by operation.

CELLULITIS

An infection affecting the subcutaneous tissue (that is, just beneath the skin) or other soft connective tissue. Cellulitis is usually caused by *bacteria* and the skin is red, swollen and tender. It responds to treatment with *antibiotics*.

CEPHALHAEMATOMA see page 22

CEREBRAL PALSY

Some parts of the brain co-ordinate body posture and movement by controlling the various muscle groups in different parts of the body. If these parts of the brain are damaged in early life or do not develop properly there will be problems with posture and movement: this is known as cerebral palsy. Cerebral palsy results from brain damage during fetal life, around the time of birth or in the first two years. The extent of the damage and its effects can vary from minimal or slight to very major.

There are many different causes of cerebral palsy, and often no cause can be identified. Sometimes in fetal development a part of the brain becomes damaged or does not develop properly, or the brain may be damaged by intra-uterine infection (infection in the womb), placental insufficiency, oxygen shortage or other factors. At birth or in the newborn period brain damage may occur because of oxygen or glucose shortage, infections, severe jaundice or extreme prematurity. (These problems are all covered in Chapters 1–3.) After the newborn period accidents, dehydration, infection or other causes may lead to cerebral palsy.

Whatever the cause, brain damage that occurs before or while the child is still developing posture and movement control affects that development. There are many similarities between the problems experienced by different children. Although damage of the nervous system in cerebral palsy is non-progressive and does not worsen with time the effects of the damage will vary as the child grows and reaches different developmental stages. The treatment of the child has to be in harmony with the appropriate stage of development.

Cerebral palsy is a movement disorder, but it may be associated with other problems if there are disorders of function of other parts of the brain. Thus cerebral palsy may be associated with mental handicap (see page 160), *epilepsy*, impairment of hearing and/or impairment of vision.

A child with cerebral palsy may not have any obvious postural or movement abnormalities at birth. Sometimes the baby feels floppy or stiff on handling. Parents may gradually realize that their child has difficulty in moving a limb or other part of the body; that head control is slow in developing; that the child tends to adopt a particular posture; or that the child's achievement of milestones in motor development is delayed. If parents are at all concerned about development, movement or posture the child should be taken to the family doctor, who may wish to get a specialist opinion.

Children in whom it is known that there is a possibility of brain damage, such as those who have had *meningitis*, who suffered oxygen shortage or convulsions in the newborn period, or who were of very low birth weight (see Chapters 2 and 3), will be followed up carefully by the paediatrician and will be examined regularly for any postural abnormality or movement disorder.

The examination of the neuromuscular system in infants requires skill, and often examinations need to be repeated before definite conclusions can be drawn. The doctor will be interested in the way the baby lies and the movements that he makes, being particularly concerned to detect any asymmetry between the left and right sides. Children with cerebral palsy often have stiffness (spasticity) of the muscles, and this will be looked for, although it often does not develop until the child is a few months old.

The doctor will want to know whether the baby's basic reflexes, such as starting at a sudden noise or movement and grasping with the palm of the hand, are normal, and will also test his reaction to being turned over and placed in different positions. A general examination of other parts of the body will also be done.

No specialized investigations are necessary in most children with suspected cerebral palsy. The doctor may be able to make a diagnosis that cerebral palsy is present at the first examination, or may need to see the child on several occasions. Even when a diagnosis can be made, the severity of the condition and what effects it will have on the child's development may need time to be established.

The child with cerebral palsy requires treatment to encourage movement and develop head control, balance and posture. Although this treatment may be planned and supervised by a *physiotherapist*, parents will need to be involved in carrying out the regular treatment sessions. A developmental approach is adopted to therapy, so that the child is encouraged to acquire skills in sequence as they develop naturally. A new baby first learns to control and balance the head, so this is one of the priorities in starting treatment. The child then needs to progress through prone and supine lying (face down and up), and to acquire a sense of balance.

If the muscles are stiff and spastic they will tend to hold many of the joints in a fixed position. An important part of the treatment will be to move all the child's joints through a full range of movements every day. Positioning the child when lying or sitting is also important, to ensure that no deformity develops because of an imbalance in the pull of the muscles. Sometimes in cerebral palsy orthopaedic operations are helpful in improving mobility and preventing or correcting deformities, so that very often the paediatrician will want an orthopaedic specialist to be involved in the continuing care of the child.

If the muscles of the mouth and lips are affected by cerebral palsy the child is likely to have problems with sucking and swallowing, and later with the acquisition of speech. *Speech therapists* have special training in ways to encourage movement of the mouth, and should be involved with the child early on if it is apparent that there is an oral problem.

The paediatrician and therapists will want to follow the progress of the child together, and will arrange regular assessments across the whole field of development. These checks identify problems, set goals and plan future treatment.

There are likely to be a large number of people involved in the care of the child who is handicapped. As well as family members there will be the family doctor, health visitor, paediatrician and therapists as a minimum, and workers from the social services and education are also likely to be involved at some stage in early childhood. If the child has other medical problems as well as cerebral palsy the number of people involved may be even greater. Unless the provision of help and treatment is co-ordinated by the team looking after the child, parents are likely to be confused over what is going on, and about the function of every person in the team; the management of the child and his disability will suffer as a consequence. Child development centres, where handicapped children can be assessed and treated, and where all the professionals meet and work together, go a long way towards providing co-ordination. If parents feel that they are not fully aware of what is planned for their child they should ask the therapist or paediatrician to clarify what is happening, and why.

The Peto Institute in Hungary has been treating children with cerebral palsy for many years with an intensive and well-planned regime known as conductive education. Specially trained conductors are responsible for the care, therapy and education of the children who are resident in the institute; this enables the child to develop a very strong relationship with the conductor, and provides a unified approach to management of the disability. Not all children are suitable for the conductive education approach, and the Peto Institute carefully selects those it feels will benefit from the method. With those that are judged suitable the results are good.

There has been a lot of interest expressed in many parts of the world about conductive education, and the approach is now being adopted and adapted in various centres in several different countries. Information on conductive education should be available from the local services for handicapped children.

CHICKENPOX

Chickenpox, or varicella, is a highly contagious viral infection giving rise to a typical skin rash. The illness starts with a slight fever and malaise (a general feeling of being unwell); spots start to appear on the first day, and further crops occur over the next three days or so.

The spots, which are very itchy, start as little pink pimples and soon change to a fluid-filled vesicle (blister). The fluid inside the vesicle becomes cloudy and purulent, and then scabs over. The rash is most marked on the trunk, but can occur all over the body and limbs. Sometimes spots may also be found inside the mouth.

The incubation period from exposure to the onset of the illness is between 11 and 21 days, and the patient is infectious for about twenty-four hours before the appearance of the rash until the spots have scabbed. There is no immunization available for varicella and treatment is directed at the symptoms, mainly calamine lotion to relieve the itching. An attack confers immunity for life.

In children being treated with *cytotoxic drugs* for *leukaemia* or malignant disease chickenpox can be very serious, and the injection of special *gamma globulin* may be necessary.

CHILBLAINS see *Frostbite*

CHILD ABUSE

Babies and small children are dependent on adults for protection and for all their needs. If they are neglected or harmed instead, this constitutes child abuse. Abuse may be deliberate, but is often due to parental inability to cope with the demands of caring for a child. Child abuse takes many forms: physical injury or neglect, emotional neglect, mental cruelty, poisoning and sexual abuse are common types of maltreatment. In some infants poor weight gain may be the only sign of lack of emotional stimulation.

Everybody who looks after babies or children for any length of time knows that it is hard work. Children can be very demanding at times and providing continuous care can be stressful. Child abuse often results from the carer being overstressed and therefore reacting in an impulsive or unthinking way towards the child. The baby who cries continuously and will not settle may be shaken or hit in desperation, or the wilful child may be slapped. If a mother is depressed or under stress she may not be able to respond to the baby's needs for love and stimulation, and emotional deprivation results.

When a child has been physically harmed, the term 'non-accidental injury' is often used to differentiate it from a genuine accident. Doctors and social workers know that in most cases this does not mean that the child was deliberately harmed, but understand that the child's injuries arose as a result of the parent or carer being stressed beyond breaking point.

Many parents will know when they are having difficulty in coping with a child and may be frightened that they could harm him if the problem continues. Sometimes this situation can be helped by talking it over with an experienced friend, or by enlisting the part-time help of a grandparent. If these solutions are not available it may be helpful to talk to the health visitor, family doctor or child health clinic about the difficulties. No experienced professional will be shocked if a parent expresses anxiety about harming the baby, and practical help should be forthcoming.

The management of child abuse is planned both to protect the child from further harm and to provide help for the family so that the child can be better looked after. When a child is known to have been abused or when abuse is suspected, a meeting of health care professionals and social workers will be held. This meeting, known as a case conference, will discuss how the child has been harmed, the family background and how best to prevent further abuse.

SEE ALSO *Sexual abuse*

CHILD GUIDANCE CLINIC

Child guidance clinics are set up to advise and help in the management of children who have behavioural problems or other difficulties at home or school. The staff include an educational psychologist, a child psychiatrist, social workers and others experienced in the emotional problems of children and families.

CHOANAL ATRESIA

A *congenital* abnormality in which a membrane at the back of the nose blocks the nasal airway. As babies normally breathe through the nose this is serious. The baby will have difficulty in sucking, and may become blue at rest because of inadequate breathing. Emergency surgery is required to relieve the blockage.

CHOLERA

A severe diarrhoeal illness, due to the cholera *bacterium*, endemic in many tropical countries. Cholera immunization is necessary before travel to undeveloped countries (see page 118), and travellers should also try to ensure that they avoid water or food that might be contaminated.

CHOLESTEROL

A fatty substance that is present in the blood and is an essential constituent of cell membranes. It can be synthesized in the body when it is needed. High blood levels of cholesterol have been found to predispose to coronary heart disease in adult life, and may be due to an inherited defect or to excess fat consumption (see Chapter 7). **SEE ALSO** *Familial hypercholesterolaemia*

CHRISTMAS DISEASE see *Haemophilia*

CIRCUMCISION

The operation of circumcision consists of removal of the prepuce, or foreskin, in the male. Until around the age of 2 or 3 years no attempt should be made to retract the foreskin as it is often still attached to the glans (head) of the penis. Beyond that age it should be possible to retract the foreskin and older boys should be taught to pull it back and wash under it while bathing.

The situations where circumcisions are medically required are a very small urinary opening which is obstructing the flow of urine, a non-retractable foreskin beyond the age of 3, or repeated attacks of infection (*balanitis*). Alternatives to circumcision can include stretching and separating the foreskin under a general anaesthetic, or making a split in the foreskin so that it is retractable. Most circumcisions are done for religious or cultural reasons.

The operation of circumcision can be performed surgically and should be done under a general anaesthetic. The penis is sore for several days afterwards and urination may be painful. Although the wound itself appears swollen for several days after the operation, complete healing occurs in about a week. An alternative method is to use a plastic cone that is specially shaped to fit under the foreskin, and then to tie round a piece of thread. The foreskin withers and falls off over the space of a few days.

CLEFT PALATE

During embryonic development the palate forms by tissue growing out from either side to form a roof to the mouth. This tissue meets and fuses in the midline. In cleft palate this fusion fails to take place, and the child is born with a defect in the palate. The severity of the defect is variable. The cleft may just be a small hole in the soft palate, or a large cleft in the hard and soft palates. There may also be an associated cleft in the lip, a *hare lip*.

The presence of a cleft palate causes feeding difficulties in the newborn period as the baby cannot suck properly. This can be overcome with either a small dental bridge to cover the defect, or special teats, or spoon feeding. The cleft may interfere with the development of speech, and orthodontic problems are likely (see page 198). The palatal defect will be surgically repaired towards the end of the infant's first year. Affected children need orthodontic follow-up, and will also need to be supervised by a *speech therapist*.

CLUB FOOT (TALIPES) see page 175

COARCTATION OF THE AORTA

A narrowing of the aorta, the main artery taking blood from the heart around the body. The narrowing occurs at the point where the ductus arteriosus joined the aorta in fetal life (see page 44). If the coarctation is causing severe obstruction, the baby may show signs of heart failure in infancy, and the defect will require surgical correction at that time.

Coarctation is often picked up incidentally because of the presence of a murmur (see page 145). If it is untreated, it leads to high blood pressure in the upper part of the body, and this can be harmful in the long term, so surgical correction of the defect is recommended. The surgeon cuts out the narrowed part of the aorta and rejoins the cut ends. The operation is usually very successful.

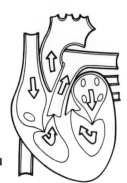

Structure of the normal heart (see page 143).

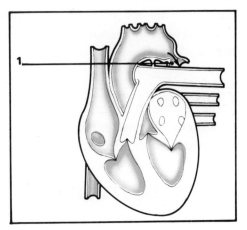

Coarctation of the aorta: **1**, narrowed segment of the aorta, obstructing the flow of blood.

COELIAC DISEASE

Coeliac disease, or gluten enteropathy, is a disease characterized by intestinal *malabsorption* as a result of damage to the lining of the small intestine by gluten, the protein present in wheat and rye, in certain individuals with an inherited tendency. The symptoms of coeliac disease are very variable. It may be noticed as soon as the infant starts to be weaned on to cereals, with weight loss, poor appetite, abdominal distension, malaise (a general feeling of being unwell), and sometimes diarrhoea (see page 168) being the usual indicators. Often the onset of symptoms is more insidious, and some patients show poor weight gain or growth failure, but have very few abdominal features.

The diagnosis of coeliac disease requires a small sample to be taken of the intestinal lining; this can be done either with a special capsule that is swallowed, or through an endoscope (see page 163). The sample is then looked at under the microscope. Once the diagnosis is established the child should start and remain on a gluten-free diet.

COLD see page 152

COLIC see page 62

COLOSTRUM see page 24

COLOUR BLINDNESS see page 183

COMA

A state of unconsciousness from which a patient cannot be roused. In light coma many of the reflexes are preserved, so that painful stimuli provoke a response and the pupils react to light. In deeper coma these reflexes are lost.

Coma is due to a cessation of many of the normal activities of the brain and may be caused by head injury, poisoning or low blood sugar. As well as treatment of the cause, patients in coma need close observation to make sure the airway remains clear and breathing is adequate.
SEE ALSO Recovery position (page 211)

CONGENITAL

An adjective that means present from birth. It is often applied to deformities but is also used for fetal infections and birth injuries.

CONJUNCTIVITIS

Infection of the conjunctiva, the membrane that covers the outside of the eye and the inside of the eyelid, gives rise to redness, a gritty painful feeling, watering of the eye, and the formation of pus. Small children often hold their eye tightly closed so that pussy secretions build up inside the conjunctival sac.

Conjunctivitis is usually easily treated with *antibiotic* cream or drops. Severe conjunctivitis in the newborn period, usually coming on in the second week of life, may be due to infection with the chlamydia bacterium from the mother's genital tract. Prolonged treatment with eyedrops or oral antibiotics is needed.

Recurrent episodes of conjunctivitis in infancy may be due to blockage of the tear duct. It may be possible to clear this by gentle massage just below the inner corner of the eye, but if it is persistent an eye surgeon can clear the duct by passing a thin probe through it.

CONSTIPATION see pages 62 and 168

CONVULSION see *Epilepsy; Febrile convulsion*

COT DEATH see page 137

CRADLE CAP see *Seborrhoeic eczema*

CROHN'S DISEASE

Crohn's disease is rare in childhood. It is a chronic inflammation of the small intestine, and sometimes other parts of the intestinal tract. The cause is unknown. Abdominal pain, poor appetite, anaemia and loss of weight are the main features. The condition is usually controlled with steroids and other drugs. Surgery is occasionally needed.

CROUP (LARYNGEAL STRIDOR)

If infection affects the larynx (voice-box) it may be more or less confined to the vocal cords and may just affect the voice, a condition known as *laryngitis*. Infection may, however, be more widespread so that the larynx, trachea and the airways of the lung are both affected, a condition known as laryngo-tracheo-bronchitis. This can lead to narrowing of the laryngeal airway, so that the child becomes breathless and distressed. Breathing in through a narrowed larynx produces a characteristic noise, known as croup or laryngeal stridor. Breathing out is usually quieter. There is an associated cough with a barking quality. Croup usually occurs at night after a child has had a cold for a couple of days, but it can occur at any time.

If there is only mild narrowing of the airway, noisy breathing is the most noticeable feature, but the narrowing can worsen as the illness progresses. The child will first compensate for the laryngeal narrowing by putting more effort into breathing, and the respiratory rate rises so that enough air can be breathed in. This extra work is tiring. If the narrowing gets worse the child may not be able to breathe in enough air. Because the main airway is narrowed in croup, the condition is potentially dangerous, and the doctor should always be consulted. Unless the croup is very mild the doctor is likely to have the child admitted to hospital for observation.

The laryngeal obstruction may be helped by keeping the child in a warm, humid atmosphere. Most cases of croup are due to *viruses* and are not likely to be helped by *antibiotics*. In most cases of viral croup no specific treatment is indicated, and the croupy breathing and the cough settle down after a few days. During the illness the amount of respiratory obstruction varies, often being worse at night than during the day. Only if the obstruction becomes life-threatening is intervention necessary, and the purpose of admission to hospital is so that if this does happen the child can quickly be given emergency treatment.

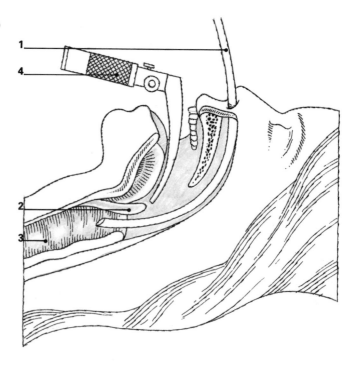

Emergency treatment for croup involves passing an endotracheal tube or ET (**1**) through the nose and past the larynx (**2**) into the trachea (**3**). This is done with the aid of a laryngoscope (**4**), which visualizes the larynx.

Emergency treatment consists of putting a tube into the larynx and pushing it past the obstruction so that air can get in and out easily. This intubation is done under a general anaesthetic, and once the tube is inserted it will need to remain in position for two to six days. This can be both uncomfortable and frightening for the child as it prevents speech. He is likely to need nursing in a high dependency or intensive care unit. Once the swelling in the larynx has settled down the tube can be removed, and the child soon returns to full health.

SEE ALSO *Epiglottitis*

CRYING see page 63

CUSHING'S SYNDROME

The features of Cushing's syndrome are caused by an excess of hormones produced by the *adrenal glands*. Cushing's syndrome occurs rarely as a result of pituitary gland tumours which stimulate the adrenal gland to overproduce cortisol (the hormone concerned with the regulation of glucose and minerals), but the features of Cushing's syndrome are also seen with treatments utilizing steroid hormones such as prednisolone. The features include weight gain with obesity of the face and trunk, a ruddy complexion, poor growth, *acne*, hairiness and muscle wasting.

There are several conditions that require treatment with steroid drugs because these exert a very strong anti-inflammatory action, but the dose must always be kept as low as possible to minimize the Cushing effects.

CYANOSIS

The term used to describe the blue colour of the complexion due to the presence of blue unoxygenated haemoglobin in the red blood cells (see page 147). Cyanosis of the arms and legs (peripheral cyanosis) is seen in normal people in cold weather, and is not of particular significance. Cyanosis affecting the lips and tongue (central cyanosis) suggests a disorder of the heart or lungs which is causing the amount of circulating oxygen to be reduced.

CYST

A fluid-filled cavity, lined with mucous membrane. In children cysts are often remnants of a phase of embryonic development, particularly when found in the neck (see *Branchial cyst*), and may require surgical removal.

CYSTIC FIBROSIS (CF)

A disease inherited in a recessive fashion (see page 108) affecting about 1 in every 2,000 children. The principal features are a *malabsorption* syndrome due to a defect in the workings of the pancreas (see page 163) and a propensity to develop lung infections. It is also sometimes signalled by an intestinal obstruction in the newborn period. In time the recurrent lung infections lead to irreversible damage.

Malabsorption may be suspected in children who have loose stools and are gaining weight slowly. CF is characterized by a raised sodium and chloride content in the child's sweat, so if it is suspected a sweat test is performed: localized sweating is provoked, the sweat is collected and the sodium content is measured. Pancreatic function can be tested by passing a tube into the upper intestine to collect digestive juice, and then testing it for enzyme activity.

Cystic fibrosis may be suspected in children with recurrent or severe chest infections; again, a sweat test is done to confirm or exclude the condition.

The treatment of CF consists of giving replacement pancreatic enzymes by mouth before meals, maintaining nutrition, and preventing or vigorously treating any chest infections. Most children have daily chest physiotherapy at home, and many are on long-term *antibiotics*. While CF remains a serious disease, the outlook with vigorous treatment is improving, and about half of affected individuals now survive until adulthood. The introduction of heart/lung *transplantation* is likely to extend the lifespan of affected children still further.

Where a child is found to have CF, any others in the family should be tested, as there is a 1 in 4 risk that they may also have the condition. Parents should have genetic counselling (see page 111), and it is now often possible to do antenatal screening for CF in early pregnancy, provided genetic studies have been done on other family members.

CYTOMEGALOVIRUS

The cytomegalovirus (CMV) causes trivial or no symptoms of infection in children or adults, unless they have poor immunity. It may, however, affect the fetus if the mother becomes infected during pregnancy. Fortunately this is uncommon. Even in congenitally acquired CMV, many infants are unaffected, but in around 10 per cent the disease may be serious and can cause *jaundice*, an enlarged liver and spleen, and skin rashes. In some severely affected infants, brain growth is affected and they develop *microcephaly*. The eyes may also be damaged by severe *congenital* CMV infection.

CYTOTOXIC DRUGS

The treatment of leukaemia and other malignant diseases utilizes drugs which kill cancer cells, but are also harmful to normal cells. They are known as cytotoxic (cell-killing) drugs and have to be used with care so that the malignant cells are reduced in number and hopefully eradicated completely without dangerous repercussions for normal tissues. Frequent blood tests are needed to monitor their effects. Cytotoxic drugs can also be used to suppress immune reactions as they interfere with the working of some of the cells of the immune system. They are therefore useful in some inflammatory diseases, and are often used in transplantation to prevent rejection.

DEHYDRATION see page 223

DEPRESSION

Depression is uncommon in childhood but can occur as a reaction to separation from other family members, family crises or lack of emotional support. Recognizing that the child's lack of interest and periods of apathy are due to depression may not be easy. The factor that triggered the depression may be readily apparent, and could be parental separation, moving house and losing friends and security, or the death of a grandparent. Treating depression may require specialist help from a child psychiatrist or psychologist.

DERMATITIS

An inflammation of the skin as a result of contact with an irritant or allergic substance. It occurs mainly in atopic individuals (see *Allergy*) and may be associated with *eczema*. The substance which provoked the initial reaction should be avoided there-after.

DIABETES INSIPIDUS

A rare condition in which there is an inability to concentrate urine; the child passes large quantities of dilute urine to excrete waste from the body. Diabetes insipidus may be the result of damage to the pituitary gland at the base of the brain so that the production of anti-diuretic hormone (which reduces water loss from the kidney) is halted. It can also be due to a problem with the kidney tubules not concentrating the urine properly (see page 169).

Patients with diabetes insipidus drink a lot to maintain fluid balance, and children with the condition must be differentiated from those who have a habit of drinking large quantities of fluid; this is more common, particularly in children aged 1 to 3 years.

DIABETES MELLITUS

The common form of diabetes; in childhood it is always due to inadequate amounts of insulin being produced by the body. Insulin is a hormone produced by the pancreas gland which enables glucose to enter the body cells and be utilized for energy. It also controls the level of glucose in the blood.

If glucose cannot enter the cells the child is weak and easily tired; if the level of glucose in the blood is too high, the excess is excreted in the urine together with water, so large quantities of urine are produced and the child is excessively thirsty. If the situation is allowed to progress there will be loss of weight and the onset of more severe metabolic disturbances, along with nausea and dehydration.

Diabetes may run in families, but the cause is unknown. In some children the onset can be associated with viral infections, but in most cases it gradually develops without obvious antecedents. Once diabetes has developed it is present for life. About 1 schoolchild in every 1,000 has diabetes.

The treatment of diabetes consists of giving injections of insulin once or twice daily, regulating the amount of carbohydrate in the diet so that the levels of glucose in the blood remain as near as possible to the normal range, and regularly checking the levels of glucose in the blood or urine to ensure that control is good. Diabetic children should attend a specialist diabetic clinic for regular review, treatment and information.

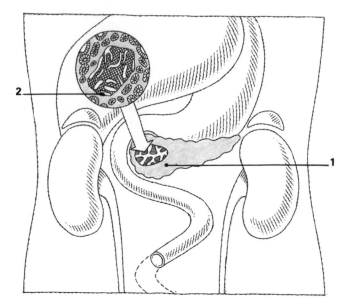

Insulin is produced in a part of the pancreas (**1**) called the islets of Langerhans (**2**). The rest of the pancreas produces digestive enzymes that are secreted into the duodenum.

Diabetes imposes restrictions on the lifestyle of the diabetic child and the family, and emotional problems are common, particularly during adolescence when the constraints seem particularly irksome. Meeting other diabetics may be helpful, and holidays where children go away together may be arranged.

DIALYSIS see page 172

DIAPHRAGMATIC HERNIA

Failure of the diaphragm to develop on one side is an uncommon *congenital* abnormality. As a consequence of this abnormality, the abdominal contents are pushed upwards into the chest, and the lung on that side does not develop properly. Diaphragmatic hernia is signalled at birth by difficulty in breathing, or may be detected on fetal ultrasound in late pregnancy. Emergency treatment is required immediately after birth. Referral to a paediatric surgeon who can repair the defect in the diaphragm is necessary, but the baby's survival also depends on whether lung function is adequate.

DIARRHOEA see page 168

DIPHTHERIA

A serious infection affecting the throat and upper airway, which may cause airway obstruction. The infection also causes the release of a toxin into the circulation which can affect the heart and the nerves. Immunization has eradicated diphtheria from developed countries, but it could return if immunization rates dropped. It is still prevalent in parts of the Third World.

DIPLEGIA

In *cerebral palsy* the muscles are stiff and weak as a result of brain damage. The parts of the body affected vary. Diplegia is the term used to describe cerebral palsy which affects both legs. In quadriplegia all four limbs are affected.

DISLOCATION OF THE HIP

Any asymmetry or restriction in movement of the hip noted in infancy should be reported to the doctor, and at the well baby clinic the doctor should check the hips from time to time. If there is any limping when a child starts to walk or any other concern at that time medical help should be sought.

Whenever *congenital* dislocation is detected it should be treated. The principles of treatment are to hold the hip joint in its correct position and to allow time for the bony and soft tissues to grow and develop to maintain that position. In early infancy splinting alone may be adequate, but later an operation to correct the defect may be needed.

Children with *cerebral palsy* sometimes develop hip dislocation because some of the muscles around the hip joint are often in spasm and put unusual stresses on the joint. An operation may be needed if the hip starts to become unstable, or if it dislocates.

SEE ALSO page 28

DOMINANT INHERITANCE see page 107

DOWN'S SYNDROME

A disorder in which there is an extra chromosome 21. The chromosomal aspects of Down's syndrome are discussed on page 104.

Down's syndrome is characterized by typical facial features, short stature, stubby fingers and broad hands, and some degree of mental handicap. Facial features include slanting eyes which are rather widely set, a round face with a small mouth and a tongue that often protrudes, small ears and a rather flattened back of the head. The head is usually rather small. About a quarter of all patients with Down's syndrome have *congenital* heart disease, and a smaller proportion have an intestinal obstruction present at birth due to *duodenal atresia*.

Babies with Down's syndrome often feel rather limp due to laxity of the muscles. They may feed poorly initially. Improvement occurs gradually during the first few months, although weight gain is usually less than in other babies.

Although Down's syndrome is characterized by developmental delay and mental handicap, the degree of disability is very variable and is also influenced by early experience. Children with Down's syndrome, like other children with developmental problems, need extra stimulation and encouragement and this improves their developmental progress.

DRUG ABUSE

The abuse of drugs is common among teenagers and other young people. No longer is the problem confined to big cities; it occurs in towns and villages too. This means that all children are at risk. Most prevalent is the use of cannabis, but other and more dangerous drugs are widely available. Prevention is important, and parents play a vital role. Children need to be warned of the dangers of drugs in realistic terms, without these being exaggerated. Many youngsters will know someone who has experimented with cannabis, so will also know that this does not have immediate disastrous effects. More importantly parents have a responsibility to know where their children go, who they socialize with, and the activities that take place. Provided this is just one part of being generally interested, involved and supportive of the child's welfare, it will not be seen as being intrusive. Parents can also set an example. The parent who appears to be dependent on alcohol or medication is not in a strong position to offer guidance on the dangers of drug abuse.

Even with a happy and supportive home, some children will experiment with drugs. Parents should be alert to this possibility, and should try to ascertain the reason if their child does become secretive, has sudden mood swings, or seems withdrawn.

If a child is experimenting with drugs or has become habituated, the sooner this problem is tackled the better. Professionals are available to provide advice and support: the problem can be discussed with a family doctor or a social worker, or a specialist advice group may be contacted.

DRUG RASH

Some medicines are likely to provoke skin rashes as a side-effect in some people. These drug rashes may be red and blotchy, or may be itchy and have little weals; the latter type is known as *urticaria*, and resembles nettle stings. Most drug rashes come on about 7–10 days after the drug has been started, but reactions can occur sooner, particularly if the child has been given that drug before. Most drug rashes settle rapidly when the drug is stopped, but it is important to avoid it in future; any doctor who sees the child should be told of any known drug allergies.

DUODENAL ATRESIA

The duodenum is the first part of the intestine and joins on to the stomach. Sometimes a child is born with a *congenital* blockage, or atresia of the duodenum. The child will start to vomit after the first or second feed after birth, and the vomit is likely to be yellow bile-stained milk. If duodenal atresia is suspected an X-ray is performed. If this confirms the diagnosis an operation will be required. Operating directly on the duodenum is technically difficult, so the surgeon joins a loop of small intestine to the stomach to bypass the blockage.

DYSARTHRIA

A difficulty in articulating words, which may result from incoordination of the muscles of the tongue or lips, or from an abnormality of the mouth, such as a *cleft palate* or tongue disease. Speech therapy may help to improve articulation.

DYSENTERY

An intestinal infection causing severe diarrhoea (see page 168). Often the child also has crampy abdominal pain. It may be due to *bacteria* such as the shigella organisms, or in the tropics to microscopic animals called amoebae. In children the prevention of dehydration is very important. There is no specific treatment for bacterial dysentery because antibiotics are ineffective in either controlling or eradicating the infection. Usually the diarrhoea and other symptoms of the infection clear up naturally in around 3 to 5 days, and patients rarely become carriers of the organism.

DYSLEXIA

A specific difficulty in learning to read and write, in children who are of average intelligence and ability in other fields. Severe dyslexia is more common in boys and often runs in families; affected children may show cross-laterality – that is, being right-handed but left-footed, or vice versa.

Children who are dyslexic still have to learn to read and write, or they will be severely handicapped in all their future activities. They require additional help in learning from parents and teachers. The techniques of teaching reading and writing skills are essentially the same as those used in teaching other children, but dyslexic children take much longer to learn.

EARACHE

Earache may be associated with infection of the middle ear (*otitis media*), the onset of *mumps*, or blockage of the external auditory canal by water or wax. If it persists medical advice should be sought.

ECZEMA see *Atopic eczema*; *Seborrhoeic eczema*

ENCEPHALITIS

An inflammation of the brain. It may be due to infection; sometimes the cause is uncertain but it is thought to be some form of allergic reaction. Rarely it may complicate *mumps* or *measles*. Symptoms vary: a headache is likely and this may be severe. Drowsiness and even unconsciousness can occur. The treatment and outcome will depend on the underlying cause, but usually recovery is complete.

ENCOPRESIS

Defecation into the pants or in inappropriate places is known as encopresis. It is often associated with constipation (see pages 62 and 168); sometimes the stool passed is loose and very smelly, and is thought to be diarrhoeal, but in fact is due to partial bowel obstruction from constipation. In this case, clearing the bowel and using *laxatives* and a training regime to re-establish a normal bowel habit are likely to be successful. If encopresis is not associated with constipation, a psychological cause is likely to be present and psychiatric help may be needed.

EPIGLOTTITIS

Although most cases of *croup* are due to infections with *viruses*, there is a severe form of respiratory stridor (strained, noisy breathing) which affects the voice-box (larynx), known as epiglottitis. This infection, caused by the bacterium Haemophilus influenzae, is characterized by the rapid onset of obstructed breathing and laryngeal stridor, due to inflammatory swelling. Very often there has been no preceding cold or other illness. The infection causes rapidly worsening swelling which affects the back of the throat and the larynx. The child becomes short of breath and may have a fever. Breathing is usually noisy. Swallowing is difficult so that saliva drips from the mouth. The child will want to sit upright and will be making a great effort to breathe.

Urgent treatment is required, and an ambulance or doctor should be called at once. If the swelling continues to worsen the airway can become completely obstructed unless an endotracheal intubation (a tube inserted into the windpipe) can be performed (see *Croup*).

EPILEPSY

The terms 'seizures', 'fits' and 'convulsions' are used synonymously, and describe attacks in which there is intermittent disturbance of the electrical activity of the brain, causing features such as stiffness of all the body muscles, jerking of the limbs and loss of consciousness. The word 'epilepsy' is used to mean a tendency to have seizures. Epilepsy is not a single disease as there are many different causes and types of seizure. Furthermore, not all seizures are due to epilepsy. Convulsions as a result of developing a fever are very common in young children (see *Febrile convulsions*), and convulsions can also occur because of low levels of sugar or calcium in the blood, and infections of the nervous system.

Examination and investigation of the child who has convulsions may sometimes reveal a cause which was not previously recognized. There may be an area of scarring or maldevelopment of the brain, and very occasionally a *brain tumour* may be found. In other children epilepsy may be associated with known brain disease or damage. Children with mental handicap (see page 160) and those with *cerebral palsy*, in whom it is known that there is some damage to the brain, may also be prone to fits. These may start in infancy or arise at any time subsequently.

Many children who have seizures have no other symptoms, and a cause for their epilepsy may not be found even after investigation. This is often known as idiopathic epilepsy, idiopathic being a medical word which signifies that the disease process is unknown. Epilepsy itself does not predispose to mental handicap or behavioural disturbance.

The commonest type of convulsion is called a tonic-clonic seizure, or a grand mal convulsion. Such convulsions usually start with the child going stiff (the tonic phase) and becoming unconscious. The eyelids usually remain open and the eyes often roll upwards. Because of the stiffness the child's breathing is stopped. In less than a minute this tonic stiffness gives way to jerking movements which can affect the body, head and all the limbs (the clonic phase). During this period of jerking, regular breathing ceases, and the child may become red or blue in the face. The clonic phase stops, usually after a minute or two, the child's body relaxes and breathing restarts. Incontinence of urine is common during a fit. The child usually regains consciousness after a few minutes, but may then complain of a severe headache and want to go to sleep. Sometimes a series of convulsions will occur together. Children almost never come to any harm during a short fit, but if a fit is prolonged medical attention should be sought urgently. Injections of *anticonvulsant drugs* usually rapidly terminate a convulsion.

Other types of fit occasionally seen include petit mal, in which there is a momentary 'absence': the child looks blank for a few seconds, but does not fall or make any abnormal movements. There are also drop attacks, in which the child goes limp and falls, but without jerking and without loss of consciousness. If a child has had a short episode of unconsciousness it is sometimes difficult to be certain whether it was a fit or a faint.

In temporal lobe epilepsy, attacks may start either with the patient having the sensation of a strong smell or taste, or with him carrying out co-ordinated but automatic actions, such as undressing, without any subsequent awareness that he has performed them. The attacks may terminate at that stage or go on to a major seizure. In some cases there may be diagnostic uncertainty as to whether attacks are temporal lobe epilepsy or behavioural disturbance. Temporal lobe epilepsy may respond well to anticonvulsant treatment.

Any child who has a convulsion for the first time, or has an episode of unexplained unconsciousness, should be taken to see a doctor. Following an examination the doctor may want to refer the child for further investigation and a specialist opinion. A skull X-ray and EEG may be arranged, and sometimes a CT brain scan will also be performed (see pages 157-160).

Treatment with anticonvulsant drugs is indicated for most children with epilepsy. There are several different anticonvulsants available. Either sodium valproate, carbemazepine or phenytoin are most commonly used as the initial treatment for children prone to fits. The doctor will advise on the most appropriate drug, and will adjust the dose and modify the treatment depending on response.

With treatment fits can be completely controlled in about half of all children with epilepsy, and the frequency and severity of fits can be reduced in most of the others. A few children are very resistant to the effects of anticonvulsant treatment. It is important to achieve the best control possible, as having convulsions can interrupt a child's education and social life, and may result in him being stigmatized by his peers. Side-effects of anticonvulsants do occur, particularly if the dose is too high. They include unsteadiness and drowsiness, and occasionally mood changes, the child becoming withdrawn or aggressive.

If a child is having an epileptic fit, he should be put in the recovery position (see page 211) and no other treatment should be attempted.

The activities of the child with epilepsy do not need to be restricted if the fits are completely controlled. If fits persist, unaccompanied swimming and bike riding in traffic are potentially dangerous.

Many children outgrow the epileptic tendency and treatment can be withdrawn after a few years without a recurrence of the convulsions.

EXOMPHALOS

A *congenital* abnormality in which there is a defect in the abdominal wall involving the umbilicus (navel) and surrounding tissue. It is apparent at birth, as part of the intestine can be seen covered with a thin membrane outside the abdominal cavity. Surgical repair is needed.

FALLOT'S TETRALOGY

This *congenital* heart disease is usually suspected if a child gradually becomes cyanosed (has blue lips and tongue) during the first year of life. The heart defect is complex, with a *ventricular septal defect*; *pulmonary valve stenosis*; an over-riding

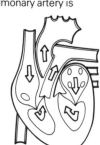

Fallot's tetralogy: **1**, narrowed pulmonary valve; **2**, ventricular septal defect (hole in partition between ventricles). Blood from both left and right ventricles enters the aorta. The blood flow to the pulmonary artery is reduced.

Structure of the normal heart (see page 143).

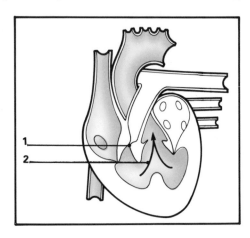

aorta, which receives blood simultaneously from both ventricles (lower chambers of the heart), and generalized thickening (hypertrophy) of the right ventricle. Children with Fallot's tetralogy require assessment and corrective cardiac surgery. Successful surgery gives very good results for health and long-term survival.

FAMILIAL HYPERCHOLESTEROLAEMIA

This disorder is relatively common and consists of a dominantly inherited tendency (see page 107) to a very high blood *cholesterol*. Affected individuals do not show symptoms in childhood but are prone to coronary heart disease in middle adult life. Detection of the condition in childhood, in individuals with a family history of early coronary disease, enables cholesterol-lowering treatment with diet or drugs to be started, and this can prevent the later onset of heart disease.

FEBRILE CONVULSIONS

Children between the ages of 9 months and 5 years are liable to have a convulsion if they develop a fever. About 5 per cent of children have at least one febrile convulsion between these ages. The convulsion is more likely to take place when the temperature is going up rather than when it has been raised for a while. The convulsion may happen without any prior warning that the child is ill. The child suddenly becomes unconscious, and the eyes may roll upwards. The whole body may be stiff for a short while, and then a series of jerks shakes the body and limbs. Febrile convulsions do not usually last more than about five or ten minutes. They end with the child becoming limp and starting to breathe normally, and very soon he regains consciousness.

If a child is having a convulsion he should be turned into the recovery position (see page 211). It is important that the clothing is removed to help him cool down, and he may also be cooled by a wet flannel or sponge. It is not necessary to put anything between the teeth.

Although the convulsion is usually short-lived and does not require any specific treatment the doctor should be consulted, and a cause for the fever found and treated. If a child has already had one febrile convulsion, prevention should be attempted if he seems unwell. This consists of taking his temperature, and if it is raised, making sure he is not wearing too much clothing and giving him paracetamol liquid to help to bring down his temperature. The temperature should be rechecked, and if it is still raised, sponging with cool water over the body is advised.

FISTULA

An abnormal connection between two hollow organs, or between a deep structure and the skin. Deep wounds that are infected or contain a foreign body often do not heal properly, but instead a fistula develops between the wound and the surface of the skin.

FIT see *Epilepsy*

FLAT FEET see page 175

FRACTURE see page 176

FROSTBITE (COLD INJURY)

When the outside temperature is very cold, as in arctic and sub-arctic areas, the limbs may become very cold in spite of protective clothing. The blood vessels going to the hands and feet constrict to prevent excess heat loss from the body; blood flow drops and inadequate oxygen and nutrients reach the peripheral tissues. Provided this does not last for too long no permanent harm is done, but the hands may be painful and red as they warm up again. Prolonged cold injury can lead to the death of tissue.

Chilblains, which usually occur on hands, feet or ears, are small areas of cold injury. The area is red and intensely itchy, particularly when it is warm, and persists for several days. Children should always be adequately clothed when the weather is cold, and should sleep in properly heated rooms. They should not be out of doors for long periods without coming into the warm to thaw out from time to time.

GALACTOSAEMIA

A rare metabolic error in which the sugar galactose, one of the constituents of milk sugar (lactose), cannot be metabolized properly. Affected children may vomit, lose weight and develop *jaundice* in the newborn period. If the child is changed to a feed free of lactose and galactose, the symptoms settle. The child always has to avoid milk sugar thereafter.

GAMMA GLOBULIN

Globulins are large-molecule proteins that occur naturally in the blood. The gamma group of globulins are antibodies that protect against infection. Gamma globulin can be obtained from blood donors or other volunteers to be given therapeutically to those at risk of serious infection.

GASTRO-ENTERITIS

Gastro-enteritis is common in childhood and consists of vomiting and/or diarrhoea due to disturbed bowel function. Direct infection of the alimentary tract is the usual cause in children, but infections elsewhere in the body may also present with the same symptoms. *Tonsillitis, otitis media* and urinary tract infections (see page 171) often present in this way in small children, and other infections may also have to be considered.

Vomiting of sudden onset, but usually without diarrhoea, can occur as a result of ingestion of irritant or unfamiliar foods, or foods which contain toxins from bacterial contamination. When irritant or contaminated food has been consumed the onset of symptoms is usually very rapid and occurs within an hour or two of ingestion.

In most cases of gastro-enteritis in children the gastro-intestinal tract itself is infected, due to the consumption of infected food or drink or close contact with another individual carrying pathogenic (disease-causing) micro-organisms. There are several different *bacteria, viruses* and protozoa that can give rise to gastro-enteritis. Some of those most frequently encountered are listed in the table on page 268. If the infection is affecting the stomach and small intestine vomiting is likely, while infection of the large intestine causes diarrhoea. Often both are affected together.

Acute gastro-enteritis is characterized by the sudden onset of vomiting and/or diarrhoea. Vomiting usually continues until the stomach is empty, but may recur if any drinks are given. Diarrhoea empties the bowel of its contents, but as the infection can cause excretion of fluid from the intestinal lining it may persist. In infants and small children dehydration is a serious risk and can occur within a few hours. If not prevented, it is a threat to life. The doctor should always be consulted about gastro-enteritis in children under the age of 2. Worldwide, diarrhoea is one of the major causes of infant mortality.

Even if an infant or small child with gastro-enteritis has been vomiting, a specially prepared glucose and electrolyte solution from a pharmacist given frequently by mouth in small amounts will often not provoke further vomiting, and will stop dehydration developing. If vomiting continues or if the child is dehydrated, admission to hospital and treatment with intravenous fluids may be required. Diarrhoea that is not accompanied by vomiting is less serious because dehydration can be prevented by administering clear fluids such as water, cola or electrolytic mixtures orally.

All cases of gastro-enteritis should be assumed to be infectious, and appropriate steps should be taken to prevent cross-infection; such steps include the sanitary disposal of vomit and stools in the toilet, and the thorough washing and dis-infecting of nappies.

Although gastro-enteritis is usually infective in origin *antibiotics* have little place in its treatment. Although they can temporarily improve the symptoms they do not eradicate the infection, and may prolong it. Drugs such as kaolin, codeine, loperamide and diphenoxylate reduce intestinal movement and are sometimes used for the symptomatic treatment of diarrhoea if it is prolonged.

The use of glucose and electrolyte solutions in the first twenty-four hours of infant diarrhoea is of great benefit, but there is no point in continuing it any longer, even if diarrhoea persists. Provided vomiting has stopped, the child can be restarted on solid food the next day, in gradually increasing amounts, and be given clear fluids to drink. Sometimes the diarrhoea becomes much worse on the reintro-duction of milk, because the infection has led to an inability to digest and absorb lactose, the sugar present in milk. The reintroduction of milk can be delayed if the child is obtaining other nutrients. A special lactose-free milk can be used until the ability to absorb lactose returns, which may take a few weeks.

COMMON CAUSES OF GASTRO-ENTERITIS

ORGANISM	FEATURES
Bacteria	
Escherichia coli	*E. coli* is a normal bowel inhabitant but disease-causing varieties causing acute (short-term) or chronic (long-term) diarrhoea exist.
Shigella species	Causes bacterial dysentery. Of sudden onset, with watery stools, and blood and mucus. Often causes abdominal cramps.
Salmonella species	Often causes a fever. Of gradual onset, with mucousy and foul-smelling stools.
Campylobacter	Causes a fever and water stools, often bloody.
Protozoon	
Giardia lamblia	Infests the duodenum and may cause chronic (long-term) diarrhoea, sometimes with malabsorption.
Virus	
Rotavirus	Affects mainly young children. Of sudden onset, with water diarrhoea lasting 5–7 days.

GERMAN MEASLES see *Rubella*

GLANDS

Glands are of two types: exocrine and endocrine. The exocrine glands are structures that produce secretions, and they are found widely in the mucous membranes, where they keep surfaces moist. Specialized exocrine glands such as the pancreas produce digestive secretions.

Endocrine glands produce hormones which are released into the bloodstream. The major endocrine glands are the pituitary, thyroid, parathyroid and *adrenal glands*; the gonads (ovaries and testes) and the pancreas also have an endocrine function. (When the *lymph nodes* become enlarged in the neck, armpits or groin they are sometimes erroneously called enlarged glands.)

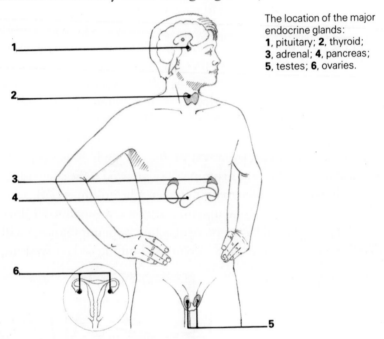

The location of the major endocrine glands:
1, pituitary; **2**, thyroid; **3**, adrenal; **4**, pancreas; **5**, testes; **6**, ovaries.

GLANDULAR FEVER

Glandular fever, also called infectious mononucleosis, is an infectious disease which usually affects children or young adults. It is due to infection with the EB (Epstein-Barr) virus, and symptoms are very variable. They are usually fever, malaise (a general feeling of being unwell), loss of appetite and sore throat. The *lymph nodes*, liver and spleen may be enlarged. Diagnosis can usually be confirmed by blood tests, as the blood film shows abnormal monocyte white blood cells, and in addition there is a special test that can be done – the Paul Bunnell test – which, if positive, makes the diagnosis certain.

The duration of glandular fever is very variable. Some people may recover within a week or two, but in many teenagers and young adults symptoms can linger for many weeks, and be accompanied by *depression* and emotional lability (instability).

There is no specific treatment, and quarantine is unnecessary.

GLUE EAR (SECRETORY OTITIS MEDIA)

Following an attack of *otitis media* the ear frequently returns to normal. Sometimes, however, the lining membrane of the middle ear goes on producing fluid which fills the middle ear. This is more likely to happen if the Eustachian tube, which connects the middle ear with the pharynx, is narrowed or blocked by congestion. The fluid in the middle ear is rather thick and sticky, and affects hearing as it impedes the movement of the eardrum and the ossicles or small bones which transmit sound. This is known as secretory otitis media, or more commonly as glue ear. Glue ear does not usually give rise to earache, although the ear may be uncomfortable and sometimes the child hears popping noises. As the hearing loss is partial it may pass unnoticed, but can lead to poor school progress.

On examination of the eardrum the doctor can see that it is grey and appears dull because of the fluid behind it. If left alone or treated with decongestants secretory otitis will gradually clear up. As this may take some time, and glue ear can be recurrent, a myringotomy operation is often recommended. This consists of making a small hole in the eardrum; then a minute plastic tube known as a grommet is inserted. The hole in the drum allows the thick secretions to drain out; with the grommet in place the secretions do not usually build up again and hearing improves. Adenoidectomy (removal of the adenoids – see page 189) is often performed at the same time as grommets are inserted if the adenoids are enlarged, to lessen the likelihood of recurrent infection. The grommets either fall out, or can be easily removed in the follow-up clinic after a few months. Children who have grommets in place should have a piece of cotton wool impregnated with petroleum jelly (Vaseline) inserted into the ear before swimming or hair washing.

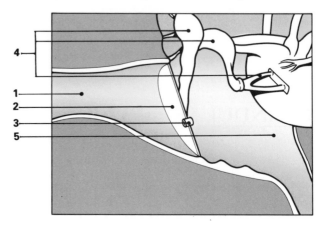

A grommet in position in the ear drum: **1**, outer ear; **2**, ear drum; **3**, grommet; **4**, ossicles; **5**, middle ear.

GLUE SNIFFING see *Solvent abuse*

GOITRE

The thyroid gland is situated at the front of the neck just below the larynx (voicebox). If it is enlarged it can be easily seen, and is known as a goitre. Small goitres are very common in young women in puberty and are usually of no significance. Larger goitres need investigation to see if the thyroid gland is working properly.

GROMMET see *Glue ear*

GUTHRIE TEST see page 23 and *Phenylketonuria*

HAEMOPHILIA

Haemophilia is a genetic disorder in which a person is unable to make adequate amounts of one of the factors necessary for blood clotting (see page 149). There are two main forms of haemophilia: classical haemophilia or haemophilia A, and Christmas disease or haemophilia B. Clinically the features are identical, but they differ in that in haemophilia A there is an inability to make blood clotting factor VIII, and in haemophilia B an inability to make factor IX.

Both haemophilia A and B are inherited as sex-linked recessive disorders (see page 108); only males suffer from the disease, females being the carriers. If a boy is found to have haemophilia it is imperative to determine whether his mother is a carrier, or whether the disorder arose from a new mutation. Sisters of haemophiliac boys may also be carriers. All the family should have blood tests to determine whether they are carriers and receive appropriate genetic counselling.

The clinical features of haemophilia depend on whether there is an almost complete absence of the clotting factor, or if it is present in significant but reduced quantities. Those boys with an almost complete absence of either factor VIII or IX will have spontaneous episodes of bleeding, frequently into a joint or the muscles. They may also bleed profusely from large cuts. Small cuts do not often cause problems as constriction of the blood vessels may be enough to stop the bleeding. More mildly affected boys will not bleed spontaneously into the tissues, but may bleed excessively following accidents or operations.

If haemophilia is suspected the doctor will want to do blood tests to determine whether there is a clotting factor deficiency.

Haemophilia can be treated by injection of the missing factor. For mildly affected boys factor replacement will only be needed before an operation or dental extraction, but in severe haemophilia most episodes of bleeding, whether into the tissues or outside, will require treatment. The factors used in treatment are extracted from donor blood, and a number of haemophiliacs contracted HIV infection before *AIDS* was known about. Now all blood donors are carefully screened and blood is treated to minimize the risk. Synthetic clotting factors are becoming available and these will remove all risk of infection.

HAEMORRHAGIC DISEASE OF THE NEWBORN

Occasionally bleeding from the bowel, umbilical cord or bladder occurs in babies a few days old due to defective clotting. This is almost always caused by a deficiency of some of the clotting factors in the blood which require vitamin K for their production. Vitamin K is normally synthesized by *bacteria* that live in the bowel, but production is not established until a week or so after birth. Most newborn babies are given an injection of vitamin K at birth to prevent haemorrhagic disease.

If an infant does have haemorrhagic disease this can be treated by an immediate injection of vitamin K, which will work within a few hours. However, if the disease causes heavy bleeding, an infusion of plasma (a blood extract) has an immediate effect on clotting.

HAIR LOSS see *Alopecia*

HARE LIP

Hare lip, or cleft lip, is a *congenital* failure of fusion of the upper lip, so that there is a split running from the edge of the lip up towards the nose, on one or both sides of the midline. It is often associated with *cleft palate*. The defect in the lip can be repaired by a plastic or paediatric surgeon when the baby is a few weeks old, and this causes a marked improvement in appearance.

HAY FEVER

An allergy to pollen, particularly grass pollen, which affects the nose and often also the conjunctivae, the membranes that cover the outside of the eyes and the inside of the eyelids. Symptoms consist of itchiness, watering and swelling of the eyes, and a continual watering and blockage of the nose. There may also be a cough.

The symptoms start in early summer when grasses are in flower. On dry days the pollen count is highest, and symptoms are likely to be more marked. Small children do not usually suffer from hay fever, but it is likely to come on between the ages of 5 and 10 years. Sufferers have often previously had *eczema* and/or asthma (see page 152), and may also have *allergic rhinitis* at other times of the year.

Attacks of hay fever can be treated with nose sprays and eye drops containing sodium cromoglycate, or locally acting steroids, or with *antihistamines*. Desensitizing injections can be given in courses during the preceding winter for those known to be prone to hay fever.

HEADACHE

Many children get headaches from time to time. Most are trivial and soon go away, either with or without simple treatment. They are usually due to such things as tiredness or upper respiratory infections. Some headaches are more severe. A severe headache associated with fever and other symptoms should be taken seriously and the doctor consulted. Although there are many infections that may give headaches, including *influenza* and *mumps*, headaches are also a prominent feature of *meningitis* and this needs to be taken into account.

Children who have recurrent headaches may be suffering from eye strain or sinus infection and these should be considered. If the headaches are frequent and interfering with normal life, the doctor should be consulted. Although parents often think of the possibility of a *brain tumour* if a child has recurrent headaches, the majority of headaches in childhood are not due to serious disease.

Some children have attacks of severe headaches, perhaps associated with dizziness or nausea, and these may recur frequently. In some these may be the beginnings of migraine, or they may be tension headaches. Severe and recurrent headaches in childhood are an indication of stress, either within the family, at school or within the child. Stress at home can come from problems in family relationships, worry over moving house, financial hardship, family illness or trouble with neighbours. At school bullying or an unsympathetic teacher may cause the child to worry, and this may show as headaches. Within the child causes may include trying to work very hard to be at the top of the class, or worrying about not having any friends or about personal appearance.

If headaches are not particularly severe, or only happen infrequently, treating the symptoms with paracetamol, making a fuss of the child, or sending him to bed early may be all that is required. *Aspirin* is not now recommended for children. If headaches are frequent or severe, the doctor should be consulted.

HEAD LICE see *Nits*

HEALTH CLINIC

Even when they are healthy, children need regular health surveillance to ensure that development is progressing satisfactorily, to check that they have no problems with vision, hearing or health, and to receive their immunizations when they become due. This follow-up may be performed by the family doctor, or can be carried out at a health clinic. The clinic is also likely to give useful information on many of the medical and social aspects of child care.

HEART MURMUR see page 145

HEMIPLEGIA

A weakness of one side of the body as a result of damage to the motor cortex, the part of the brain which is concerned with body movement. Hemiplegia is one of the patterns of weakness seen in some children with *cerebral palsy*.

HENOCH-SCHÖNLEIN PURPURA

A rare condition of childhood characterized by a rash due to bleeding points in the skin, affecting mainly the buttocks and the backs of the legs. Abdominal pain, bleeding from the rectum, joint pains and kidney inflammation may be associated. The cause is unknown. Most affected children make a full recovery in a few weeks without treatment.

HEPATITIS

Liver infection, or hepatitis, is due to a viral infection. There are two common forms, known as hepatitis A and hepatitis B. The most important in childhood is hepatitis A, or infectious hepatitis, which can spread from person to person, and occasionally causes small epidemics.

Hepatitis A is an infectious disease with an incubation period of about 4–6 weeks from exposure to the onset of *jaundice*. In the Western world it is relatively uncommon. However, in the countries of the developing world it is endemic and very common.

The first symptoms are malaise (a general feeling of being unwell) and loss of appetite, and these may be associated with nausea and vomiting, fever, abdominal pain and tenderness under the ribs on the right. The jaundice gradually appears over the next few days. The whites of the eyes become yellow, and the skin may also look yellow. In some people the infection is so mild that jaundice does not appear; in others it may be marked. At the same time as the jaundice, the urine becomes dark in colour, and the stools become pale.

The symptoms may only last for a few days, or may persist for two or three weeks depending on the severity of the infection. It is most infectious in the first few days, and the child should not mix more than is necessary with other people. There is no specific treatment, and recovery is usually straightforward. Rarely some liver damage persists.

If one person in a family has infectious hepatitis the others can be immunized with an injection of *gamma globulin* to protect them from the disease. This protection only lasts a few months.

Hepatitis B, also known as serum hepatitis, is spread from person to person by blood and blood products, so can be a complication of *blood transfusion*. It is common in intravenous drug users who share injecting equipment. It can also be transmitted by sexual contact, but otherwise does not usually spread from person to person. Individuals who have had hepatitis B may continue to carry the *virus* in the blood; carriers can be detected as they have a positive *Australia antigen* test. Pregnant mothers who are Australia antigen positive may transmit the disease to their baby after birth; the risk can be lessened by immunization of the baby against hepatitis in the newborn period.

HERNIA

A hernia, also known as a rupture, is where there is a weakness in the abdominal wall so that the abdominal contents can protrude. In children they are always the result of *congenital* weakness of the muscular abdominal wall. Umbilical hernias are very common in infants, particularly those of African and Afro-Caribbean origin. The umbilicus (navel) protrudes, and when the child cries, it becomes tense as the pressure rises in the abdomen. Such hernias are not painful, never become fixed or cause bowel obstruction, and almost always heal spontaneously by the age of 2 years, so no treatment is indicated.

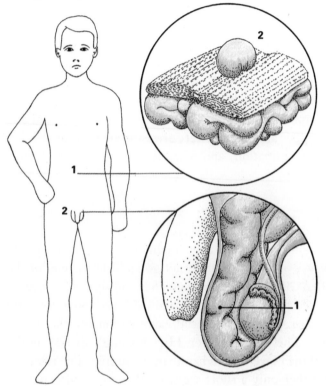

Common sites of hernias in childhood. An umbilical hernia (**top**) results from a weakness in the abdominal wall (**1**) at the umbilicus (navel) where a loop of intestine (**2**) pushes through to form a bulge under the skin. An inguinal hernia (**bottom**) is a congenital weakness in which a loop of bowel (**1**) forms a lump in either the groin or the scrotum (**2**).

In the groin, or inguinal region, the abdominal wall is sometimes deficient in boys, and an inguinal hernia results. The testicles arise from inside the abdominal cavity during fetal life, and then come through the abdominal wall into the scrotum. If the canal through the muscle does not close a hernia may result. Inguinal hernias may take the form of a lump in the groin, or part of the intestine may go down into the scrotum, which becomes swollen on that side. Inguinal hernias may get stuck in the inguinal canal and may become fixed and cause bowel obstruction, so they are usually repaired surgically soon after diagnosis. Inguinal hernias are very common in pre-term boys, and may close spontaneously in the first few months of life.

HERPES SIMPLEX

A *virus* which causes cold sores affecting the lips, which tend to recur whenever the sufferer is run down or has infection elsewhere. Herpes simplex can sometimes affect the mouth in small children; it is then called herpes stomatitis. There is ulceration, pain and swelling of the tongue, and difficulty in swallowing. Anti-viral ointment may be used to treat herpes simplex infections.

The genital herpes that sometimes affects adults is a different strain of the herpes simplex virus. *Chickenpox* is caused by a different virus, herpes zoster.

HIATUS HERNIA see page 165

HICCUPS

Spasmodic contraction of the diaphragm, the sheet of muscle separating the thorax from the abdomen, causes hiccups, which occur as a result of wind in the stomach or rapid swallowing of food, or sometimes with no obvious cause. There are many so-called remedies, none of which is reliable, but attacks are usually shortlived. Hiccups are occasionally a symptom of inflammation affecting the diaphragm due to an infection in the lung or upper abdomen. There are associated symptoms due to the condition causing the inflammation, and when this is treated the hiccups remit.

HIRSCHPRUNG'S DISEASE

In Hirschprung's disease there is a *congenital* abnormality of the nerve supply to the lower rectum, so that waves of contraction do not go right to the end of the bowel. As a result there is often constipation (see page 168) and signs of intestinal obstruction. Sometimes the child has diarrhoea (see page 168), and loose stools are likely to be passed if the doctor performs a rectal examination, or the baby's temperature is taken rectally. The treatment for Hirschprung's disease is the surgical removal of the part of the bowel which has no nerve supply. The extent of the operation depends on whether only a short segment of bowel is affected, or whether the problem is more extensive.

HIV see *AIDS*

HIVES see *Urticaria*

HOLE IN THE HEART see page 145

HUNTINGTON'S DISEASE

Huntington's disease, also known as Huntington's chorea, is an inherited condition in which people who have previously seemed normal develop a progressive neurological disease in mid-adult life. Both involuntary movements and dementia occur, and affected people die early. Huntington's disease is inherited in a dominant manner (see page 107), so that it can be passed by affected individuals to half of their offspring. There is no treatment.

Until recently individuals from a family where Huntington's disease affected some members did not know whether they would in due course develop the condition themselves, nor whether they could pass it on to their children. It is now possible in the majority of families to discover who is a carrier of the condition, so that meaningful genetic advice can be given, and there is a possibility of antenatal diagnosis.

HYALINE MEMBRANE DISEASE see page 40

HYDROCEPHALUS

In hydrocephalus there is an excess of fluid within the ventricles (cavities) of the brain. A blockage in the circulation of the cerebrospinal fluid, which bathes the brain and spinal cord, prevents its re-absorption, and consequently there is a build-up of both the volume and pressure of the fluid within the brain. The excess fluid causes the brain to expand, and when it is noted that the head is large and growing too fast, hydrocephalus is diagnosed.

Progressive hydrocephalus can be treated by inserting a plastic tube with a valve between the ventricles of the brain and the venous system so that the excess cerebrospinal fluid drains off, and normal brain growth and function return.

Hydrocephalus is frequently associated with *spina bifida*.

HYDROCOELE

Occasionally in small boys a layer of fluid around the outside of the testicle is present from early infancy; it is noticeable as it makes the scrotum larger than normal. This is known as a hydrocoele. No treatment is necessary, and the fluid gradually becomes absorbed as the boy grows bigger. Hydrocoeles are sometimes mistaken for *hernias*.

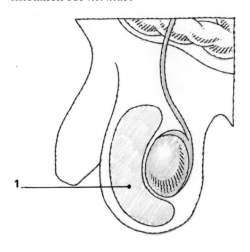

A hydrocoele (**1**) or swelling within the scrotum, caused by a layer of fluid around the outside of the testicle.

HYPERACTIVITY see page 78

HYPOGLYCAEMIA see page 43

HYPOSPADIAS

Normally in boys the urethra, the tube which carries urine away from the bladder, opens at the very tip of the penis. Occasionally there is a developmental abnormality and the opening is on the underside of the penis. This is known as hypospadias, and

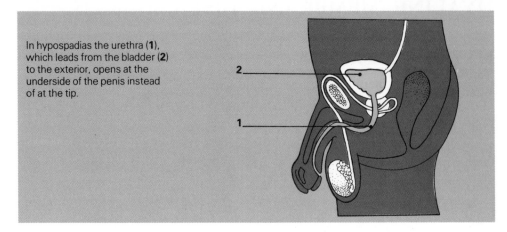

In hypospadias the urethra (**1**), which leads from the bladder (**2**) to the exterior, opens at the underside of the penis instead of at the tip.

there are varying degrees of severity, depending on how far down the penile shaft the opening is; it may even be on the perineum at the base of the penis. In hypospadias the prepuce (foreskin) is normally incomplete. Hypospadias can be corrected surgically; the more severe forms require more than one operation. Boys with hypospadias should not be circumcised, as the foreskin is used by the surgeon in the corrective operation.

HYPOTHYROIDISM

Under-activity of the thyroid gland; it may be present from birth, and if undetected can lead to mental handicap. Neonatal blood screening now tests for hypothyroidism as a matter of routine. In older children hypothyroidism can cause poor growth and perhaps a lack of energy, but there is no permanent effect on brain development. Once diagnosed, hypothyroidism is treated by hormone replacement.

HYPOXIA see *Anoxia*

ICTHYOSIS see page 191

IMPETIGO

A skin infection caused by the staphylococcus bacterium. Sore red patches that exude a yellowish, crusting secretion are characteristic of this type of infection. Impetigo responds promptly to treatment with an oral *antibiotic* or to antistaphylococcal ointment.

INFANTILE SPASMS

A rare form of *epilepsy* in which the child has episodes of flexing the trunk, about once a second and several times in succession, often with the arms held out. The child's development also regresses. Treatment with prednisolone may arrest the condition, but many children become mentally handicapped.

INFLUENZA

Infection with the influenza *virus* gives rise to a high fever, shivering attacks (rigors), a runny nose, cough and muscle aches. The condition is known as influenza, or 'flu. There are several strains of influenza virus, and new ones emerge from time to time, so that one attack does not confer immunity. Influenza vaccines boost immunity to a mixture of 'flu viruses for a few months. They are not recommended in children unless there is a particular reason to avoid influenza, such as chronic chest disease.

There is no specific treatment for influenza. Paracetamol will relieve the fever and some of the aches. The patient will probably prefer to be in bed most of the time during the attack, which lasts three or four days.

INSULIN

This natural hormone is produced by the pancreas and released into the blood-stream. It is important for regulating the amount of glucose in the blood, for transporting glucose to body cells, and for enabling glucose to be utilized for energy. Failure to produce insulin causes *diabetes mellitus*. Insulin with the same structure as human insulin but manufactured by molecular biological techniques is now available for the treatment of diabetes and in different types; the insulin is modified in various ways so that it is absorbed at different rates.
SEE ALSO illustration on page 258

INTOEING see page 175

INTUSSUSCEPTION

This uncommon condition is a form of intestinal obstruction caused by part of the bowel turning inside out within another part of the bowel. Infants are most commonly affected. Often they have had a slight cold for a day or two, and then

In intussusception part of the bowel turns inside out: **1**, normal bowel; **2**, intussuscepted bowel.

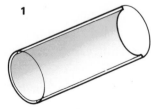
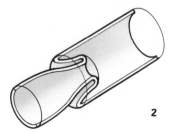

suddenly episodic colicky abdominal pain begins, recurring every few minutes. Sometimes bloody stools resembling redcurrant jelly are passed. The diagnosis can be made with a barium enema X-ray (see page 163), and this may also effect a cure. Sometimes an operation is needed.

IRON DEFICIENCY ANAEMIA

Iron deficiency anaemia may result either from inadequate amounts of iron in the diet or from blood loss. The full-term fetus has stores of iron in the body sufficient to last for several months, but in the latter part of the first year the amount of iron in the diet becomes important. Pre-term babies need to be given iron supplements throughout infancy as they grow rapidly and only have small iron stores. The richest sources of dietary iron are found in red meat, liver, egg yolk and green vegetables.

Iron deficiency anaemia is most common in childhood during the toddler period. At this age children who do not like eating red meat often have inadequate amounts of iron in their diet, and their initial iron stores have been used up in making more blood as they grow. Sometimes the anaemia passes unnoticed, but the child is likely to be pale, may be more prone to common infections, and if the anaemia is severe he may be lethargic. An unusual symptom of iron deficiency is pica, a tendency to eat strange things including earth, paper and plaster.

Blood loss may also give rise to iron deficiency anaemia. If the bleeding is apparent as, for example, after injury, the blood loss will be obvious and therefore recognized and treated. Slow bleeding, in which the amount lost is not readily seen, can give rise to anaemia. Repeated nosebleeds or bleeding from the bowel are another cause.

Iron deficiency anaemia can be treated by a suitable preparation of iron given by mouth, but the underlying cause should always be determined in case this also requires treatment.

IRRITABLE HIP

Some children, usually in mid-childhood, may suddenly develop either pain or a limp affecting one hip. The cause may be immediately apparent to a doctor, but often there may be no abnormalities apart from a slight limitation of movement of the hip. This is known as an irritable hip or observation hip, which is not a diagnosis but indicates that there is concern that something may be developing in the joint: this may be the beginning of either an infective *arthritis, Perthé's disease,* or chronic arthritis. In many cases it may simply represent strain caused by twisting or by a minor injury that has been forgotten. It is important to do blood tests and X-rays, and to observe the child closely over the next few days. Often the child is admitted to hospital until the diagnosis is clear and traction with weights is put on the leg to rest the joint by limiting movement. Many irritable hips settle without a diagnosis being made.

JAUNDICE

Jaundice is a yellow coloration of the skin and the whites of the eyes due to a build-up in the blood of the yellow pigment bilirubin. Bilirubin is formed in the body from the breakdown of the haemoglobin in red blood cells (see page 147). It is normally eliminated from the body by the liver, which extracts bilirubin from the blood and excretes it in the bile into the intestine. It is excreted bilirubin that gives stools their yellow-brown coloration.

Jaundice occurs in the newborn period (see page 28) and in some forms of *anaemia* where there is excess breakdown of red blood cells. Apart from these conditions, jaundice usually signifies liver disease; it may be due to the liver cells not working properly and failing to extract bilirubin from the blood, or to blockage of the bile ducts so that bile cannot be excreted.

The only common form of jaundice in childhood is infectious *hepatitis*.

KIDNEY DAMAGE/FAILURE see page 172

KNOCK KNEES see page 175

KOPLIK'S SPOTS

An early sign of *measles*, before the child has developed a rash, is the appearance inside the cheek of tiny white spots, surrounded by a red rim. These are known as Koplik's spots, and enable a confident diagnosis of measles to be made.

LARYNGITIS

Inflammation of the larynx or voice-box is known as laryngitis. It may be due to an infection spreading downwards from the nose or throat, or may occur alone. The larynx contains the vocal cords and mild infections are characterized by a hoarse and husky voice, perhaps associated with a sore throat. This lasts for a few days only. Severe inflammation of the larynx causes the airway to narrow and gives rise to symptoms of *croup*.

LAXATIVE

Laxatives should only be given to children on medical advice. They should be used regularly for children with constipation (see pages 62 and 168) rather than only when the child has not had his bowels open for several days. Laxatives are used as a means of establishing a regular bowel habit with the passage of soft stools and should be discontinued gradually once this is well established.

LAZY EYE see page 182

LEAD POISONING

Areas where children live and play should be painted with lead-free paint. Children can get lead poisoning from eating flakes of the paint on old buildings; often they chew away at a window sill or other area before they are noticed. Lead poisoning can cause abdominal pain and damage to the brain and nerves, and children must be prevented from eating lead-containing substances. The Asian cosmetic surma may contain lead and should not be used on children. Lead from car exhausts can pollute the atmosphere and the soil close to busy roads, but is not present in quantities large enough to cause definite symptoms.

LEUKAEMIA

There are several forms of leukaemia that occur in childhood. They are malignant diseases of the bone marrow cells that form white blood cells (see page 147). In early childhood the commonest form of leukaemia is acute lymphoblastic leukaemia, which primarily affects the bone marrow cells that form the lymphocytes. Acute lymphoblastic leukaemia responds well to treatment, and more than half of patients with the condition can now be cured. Acute myeloid leukaemia, which affects the marrow cells that form the granulocytes, tends to occur in later childhood, and also responds to treatment, but the results are not yet as good as with lymphoblastic leukaemia.

In leukaemia too many abnormal leukaemic cells are produced in the bone marrow, and this causes deficiencies of the normal cells. When red cell numbers are reduced there is *anaemia*; when white cells are reduced infections are common; and if the platelets are reduced the child develops bleeding into the skin and the alimentary tract. The liver, spleen and *lymph nodes* may also become enlarged because of infiltration with leukaemic cells.

Leukaemia in childhood may be noticed if the child is pale and lethargic, due to anaemia, because of infections caused by the shortage of functioning white blood cells, or because of a tendency to bleed. Sometimes all of these can occur in combination. The doctor will arrange a blood test and a bone marrow examination (see page 148) to establish or refute the diagnosis.

Once the diagnosis of leukaemia is made, treatment starts to try to eradicate all leukaemic cells from the body. The patient is given various drugs to kill off the abnormal cells, and supportive treatment with blood and platelet transfusions and *antibiotics*. Within a fortnight the patient is likely to be in remission, that is, the leukaemic cells will have disappeared from the blood. There then follows a period of consolidation in which an intensive regime of different chemotherapeutic drugs is continued to kill all or nearly all the residual leukaemic cells. Radiation is given to the head to prevent the leukaemia affecting the meninges, the protective membranes that surround the brain.

Maintenance treatment is needed for two or three years, but after this many children will remain healthy with no further treatment.

LISTERIA

An organism that can cause *meningitis* and *septicaemia* in newborn babies, but only rarely causes disease at other ages. If a mother contracts listeria during pregnancy she can pass it on to the fetus. Listeria is commonly found in soft cheese and may also be found in cooked meats that have been stored. One of the peculiarities of listeria is that it can grow at very low temperatures, so that it may spread even if food has been kept in an ordinary refrigerator. Pregnant women should avoid soft cheeses, and eating food that has been cooked and then stored for several days in a refrigerator.

LONG SIGHT see page 181

LYMPH NODES

Lymph nodes, also sometimes called lymph glands, are part of the body's defence system. They contain lymphocytes which fight infection and produce antibodies. Lymph nodes occur in clusters: in the neck, armpits and groin, as well as inside the chest and abdomen. With local infections the regional lymph nodes often become enlarged, and with generalized infections, such as some viral diseases, all the lymph nodes in the body may become swollen.

Enlarged lymph nodes are usually due to infection, but can also occasionally be caused by *leukaemia* or other malignancies. If lymph nodes enlarge without an obvious reason, the doctor should be consulted.

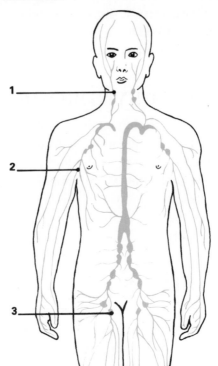

The lymphatic vessels carry fluid from the tissues towards the heart. Situated at intervals along the vessels are lymph nodes (sometimes called lymph glands). Lymph nodes are present in the neck (**1**), armpits (**2**) and groin (**3**) as well as internally. With infection bacteria may enter the lymphatic system, and the nodes then enlarge and produce cells and antibodies to help overcome the infection.

MALABSORPTION

Malabsorption of nutrients can arise in many different disorders. They tend to be characterized by poor growth and weight gain, together with diarrhoea. If the appetite is also affected, the intake of nutrients may be low and diarrhoea is not then a prominent symptom.

In some conditions the digestion and absorption of sugars may be deficient — lactose or milk sugar in *gastro-enteritis*, for instance. The non-absorbed sugar acts rather like a laxative so that large watery stools are passed. The stool can be tested for sugars to make the diagnosis. There is also often an increase in wind as some of the sugar is broken down by *bacteria* in the large intestine to acids and carbon dioxide. Elimination of the sugar from the diet relieves the symptoms.

In *coeliac disease* the protein *gluten*, which occurs in wheat and rye, damages the lining of the small intestine, so that it does not absorb food properly. Symptoms vary from marked weight loss and failure to thrive with associated diarrhoea and abdominal distension, to slow growth alone. The diagnosis is made by studying a sample (obtained by passing a tube down to the intestine) of the lining of the small intestine under a microscope, and the disease can be treated by the imposition of a gluten-free diet.

Intolerance of the protein in cow's milk can also damage the intestinal lining, and may look similar to coeliac disease. Fortunately most children who are initially allergic to cow's milk protein grow out of their sensitivity and can later take a full diet.

One of the characteristics of *cystic fibrosis* is a malabsorption syndrome due to the absence of the pancreatic digestive enzymes (see page 163); this can be treated with pancreatic supplements.

Other malabsorption syndromes do occur in childhood, but are rare.

MARFAN'S SYNDROME

This uncommon condition is an inherited disorder of collagen, part of the connective tissue. Patients with Marfan's syndrome are often tall, have long spindly fingers and may have a high, arched palate. The important features are possible eye problems, as the supporting tissue for the lens is weak, and also possible cardiovascular disease (disease of the heart and blood vessels), because of weakness in the wall of the aorta, the main artery taking blood from the heart around the body.

MASTOIDITIS

The mastoid bone (part of the skull, just behind the ear) contains air-filled cavities which connect with the middle ear. Infection of these cavities is known as mastoiditis, formerly a serious, common complication of *otitis media* but now very rare thanks to the availability of antibiotics.

MEASLES

A highly infectious viral illness. At the onset the child develops a runny nose and fever, and becomes gradually more ill over the next two days, with increasing fever, *conjunctivitis*, cough and a purulent nasal discharge which may be blood-stained. The typical measles rash appears on the third or fourth day, but the diagnosis can be made before this if *Koplik's spots* are found inside the mouth. The rash consists of large red blotches that start behind the ears and on the forehead, but spread rapidly to cover the whole body. The rash fades after two or three days, and following this, the skin may flake over the next week.

There is no specific treatment for measles. The temperature can be reduced by taking paracetamol at regular intervals, and a good fluid intake is useful. Secondary infection of the ears or chest is common after measles, and may need *antibiotic* treatment. An attack of measles confers lifelong immunity.

Measles is an unpleasant infection which can be prevented by immunization. The vaccine is usually administered at around 1 year of age. If a child is known to have been exposed to measles before this age the attack can, if necessary, be prevented or eased by an injection of *gamma globulin*, which confers temporary immunity.

MECONIUM see page 25

MENINGITIS

The brain is surrounded by protective membranes called meninges. Infection of the meninges is called meningitis and may be due to either a viral or bacterial infection.

At the onset the symptoms of meningitis are indefinite, with malaise (a general feeling of being unwell) and fever. The child may vomit, and very soon a *headache* develops, which may be severe. The child may complain that the light hurts his eyes, and may become drowsy. Occasionally fits occur. On examination the doctor will be particularly interested in whether head movements are restricted; if the

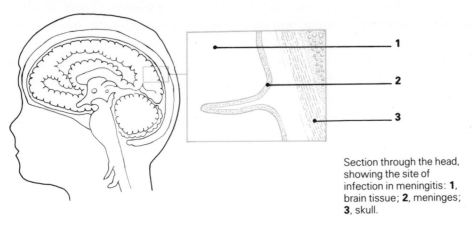

Section through the head, showing the site of infection in meningitis: **1**, brain tissue; **2**, meninges; **3**, skull.

meninges are inflamed, it is generally impossible to lower the chin on to the chest.

If meningitis is suspected the child will be hospitalized and a lumbar puncture performed (see page 157). This will ascertain whether or not inflammation is present and will give an indication of the organism causing the problem. Viral meningitis does not require treatment, but bacterial meningitis should be treated promptly with appropriate *antibiotics*. Usually these are given intravenously.

Provided treatment is started promptly, most children with meningitis make a full recovery, although convalescence may be prolonged.

MENINGOCOCCAL SEPTICAEMIA

Only a few people who come in contact with the meningococcus bacterium develop an infection. Many are symptomless carriers for a few days and then the bacteria disappear again. Sometimes, however, an overwhelming infection develops. The child rapidly becomes ill, with a high fever, malaise (a general feeling of being unwell) and lethargy. A rash appears, which rapidly spreads to form large blotches like bruises over the skin. This is due to the rapid spread of the micro-organism throughout the body, carried in the blood. Urgent *antibiotic* treatment is required, but is not always successful in controlling the infection.

MENTAL HANDICAP see page 160

MICROCEPHALY

The term used to describe a head that is much smaller than normal. Poor head growth is secondary to poor growth of the brain, and microcephalic patients always have some degree of mental handicap (see page 160).

MIGRAINE

Migraine is a form of severe *headache*, characterized by pain mainly on one side of the head during an attack, although both sides may be affected in different attacks. In childhood the headache may not be definitely one-sided. There is often associated nausea and vomiting, and sometimes visual symptoms such as flashing lights or zigzags.

Young children do not often get migraine, but it may occur over the age of around 8 years. There is often a family history. The headache may be relieved by paracetamol or other analgesics (pain killers) if given early in the attack. Often the accompanying nausea or vomiting stops the drug being absorbed, so treatment with analgesic and an anti-emetic is needed. Lying down is likely to give the best relief and many children sleep off an attack. If a child has frequent headaches, the doctor should be consulted in case stress is precipitating the attacks.

MILIA see page 29

MUMPS

A viral infection with an incubation period of around 2 – 3 weeks. Typically the onset is noted because of painful swelling of the parotid salivary gland, which is located just in front of and below the ear. One side usually swells first, but the other is likely to swell within a few days. The child will have a mild fever. The infection persists for up to two weeks, symptoms gradually lessening. There is no specific treatment. One attack confers life-long immunity.

The mumps virus can also affect other parts of the body. The principal sites are the other salivary glands, which are located under the lower jaw, the pancreas (giving rise to abdominal pain and perhaps vomiting), the testicles and the meninges, the protective membranes which surround the brain.

The testicles may be affected with mumps. This condition is known as mumps orchitis and mainly occurs after the onset of puberty. It is characterized by painful swelling of the testicles, fever and malaise (a general feeling of being unwell) and usually affects one testicle only. The swelling can persist for up to a week and then gradually subsides. Fertility is usually normal following mumps orchitis.

Mumps is one of the viruses that can cause viral *meningitis*. The meninges are usually affected before the other features of mumps appear. The child will have a severe *headache* and a stiff neck, and will vomit; tests to establish the cause of the meningitis will need to be undertaken.

MURMUR see page 145

MUSCULAR DYSTROPHY

An inherited progressive weakness of some or all of the muscles of the body. The severe form that occurs in childhood, known as Duchenne muscular dystrophy, is inherited as a sex-linked disorder (see page 108) and only affects boys. The first problems are likely to be noted in mid-childhood, the child gradually finding difficulty in running and climbing stairs. As the weakness progresses, his abilities become more limited, and most affected boys need to use a wheelchair by the beginning of their teens. There is no cure at present, but a lot of research is in progress.

MUSIC THERAPY

Management of mental handicap (see page 160) and some other disorders concentrates on trying to teach a child to communicate with others. Speech is one form of communication, but there are many others. Making and listening to music with people who are handicapped can improve their ability to communicate and enhance their social skills. Music therapy is becoming established in the management of many handicapped patients.

MYCOPLASMA INFECTION

Mycoplasma is a micro-organism that can cause epidemics of respiratory infection. It is not highly infectious and has a very long incubation period, so that within a family there may be several weeks between one member and another contracting the disease. A cough is the principal symptom, and it persists for a long time if correct treatment is not given. Mycoplasma organisms are neither *bacteria* nor *viruses*, but are somewhere in between. They are sensitive to the *antibiotics* erythromycin and tetracycline and a course of erythromycin may cut short the attack.

NAPPY RASH see pages 29 and 63

NECROTIZING ENTEROCOLITIS see page 44

NEPHRITIS

An inflammation of the kidney which may follow certain infections, particularly those caused by streptococci *bacteria*, but can also occur in other diseases. It is characterized by albumin (a protein) and sometimes blood in the urine, reduced urine output and high blood pressure. Many forms of nephritis are transient, but occasionally chronic (persistent) nephritis develops.

NEPHROBLASTOMA

A rare malignant tumour of the kidney which occurs in infancy. Parents may notice an abdominal swelling when changing or bathing the child, or there may be malaise (a general feeling of being unwell) and loss of weight. Nephroblastoma needs surgical and drug treatment in a special centre, and is often completely curable.

NEPHROTIC SYNDROME

Fluid retention secondary to the abnormal loss of large amounts of protein through the kidney. It gives rise to puffiness of the face, especially around the eyelids, to abdominal swelling and swollen legs. In childhood the nephrotic syndrome is treated with the drug prednisolone, and it usually remits entirely after a variable length of time.

NITS

Head lice are tiny insects that live in the scalp. They lay eggs which are attached to the base of the hair, and as the hair grows these eggs gradually mature and come nearer to the ends of the hair. They can be seen as little white oval particles, and are known as nits. It is much less common to see the insects themselves, but they may make their presence known by causing itchiness of the scalp.

Regular hair washing is not adequate to remove or prevent nits, and if a child is found to be infested all the family should have their hair treated with an insecticide lotion; malathion and carbaryl are both suitable. There are also insecticide shampoos, but these are less effective as the insecticide does not stay in contact with the hair for long enough to leave a residue.

NYSTAGMUS

Rapid involuntary eye movements sometimes seen in people with visual or neurological co-ordination problems.

OBESITY see page 98

OCCUPATIONAL THERAPIST

Occupational therapists are concerned with helping children with handicaps to participate to the full in normal activities. Mobility, feeding, toileting and bathing are all major areas where the therapist has special skills both in teaching the child and in knowing about special modifications that may be useful.

OEDEMA

Excess fluid in the space between the cells in tissues. It may be the result of local inflammation, or generalized fluid retention due to kidney, heart or liver disease.

OESOPHAGEAL ATRESIA

A *congenital* blockage of the oesophagus, or gullet, so that the child is unable to swallow. It is often associated with an abnormal connection between the gullet and the trachea (windpipe), a tracheo-oesophageal fistula. Babies with oesophageal atresia are likely to cough and splutter when given their first feed. Both oesophageal atresia and tracheo-oesophageal fistula are surgically correctable.

OPHTHALMOLOGIST see page 124

ORTHOPAEDICS see page 124

ORTHOPTIST

Orthoptists are concerned with the treatment of squints (see page 182), lazy eyes (page 182) and other eye problems of children. They work closely with ophthalmic surgeons.

OSTEOMYELITIS

A bacterial infection of the bone; the commonest organism causing the infection is the staphylococcus which reaches the bone via the blood stream. Sometimes there is a history of boils or other skin infection some weeks before. The *bacteria* set up an area of local inflammation which, if not treated promptly, can proceed to an abscess and result in destruction of an area of the bone. Infection may spread into an adjacent joint. Pain and fever are the usual initial symptoms. There may be localized tenderness over the affected area of bone which helps in making the diagnosis. Prompt treatment with antibiotics usually settles the infection, but sometimes surgery is needed to drain the pus from the bone. Antibiotic treatment needs to be prolonged to enable the infection to be eradicated.

OTITIS EXTERNA

Infection occasionally affects the external ear canal. The ear will be painful, there may be purulent (pussy) discharge, and often there is slight bleeding. Hearing may be impaired. Otitis externa is more common in children prone to *eczema* and other allergic skin conditions.

Otitis externa is usually treated with *antibiotic* ear drops, sometimes also containing hydrocortisone to help settle the inflammation; it usually clears up rapidly.

OTITIS MEDIA

Inflammation of the middle ear is called otitis media; it may be due to infection caused by *bacteria* or by *viruses*. Infection can spread to the ear from the throat by travelling up the Eustachian tube which connects the middle ear with the pharynx. Infection is especially likely when the adenoids are enlarged. The symptoms vary with the virulence of the infecting organism. Infection with streptococcal or pneumococcal bacteria can produce severe symptoms. The patient develops a temperature and pain in the ear. The throat is also likely to be sore. Hearing in the infected ear will be impaired, and it is likely that some of the *lymph nodes* in the neck will be enlarged. With less virulent organisms, symptoms are less pronounced, but earache, fever and temporary hearing loss are common. Otitis media does not always cause symptoms involving the ear, especially in young children. This is why the doctor often routinely examines children's ears in case there is hidden infection.

Under examination the eardrum will appear red in colour, and the throat may show infection. Sometimes the eardrum perforates because of a build-up of pus behind it. Fortunately when otitis media is due to bacterial infection response to *antibiotics* is usually rapid, and the child is restored to health in two or three days. Viral infection clears without treatment. A perforated eardrum usually heals spontaneously, but will need to be followed up to ensure that healing does take place. Hearing soon returns to normal, unless fluid persists in the middle ear, a condition known as *glue ear*.

If a child has repeated episodes of middle ear infection and has enlarged adenoids it may be worth considering removal of the latter to try to prevent further attacks (see Adenoidectomy, page 189).

SEE ALSO illustration on page 184

PAEDIATRICIAN see page 123

PAINKILLER see *Analgesic*

PARAPLEGIA

A weakness or total paralysis of both legs. It occurs in *cerebral palsy* and in *spina bifida*.

PATENT DUCTUS ARTERIOSUS see page 44

PERIODS, ABSENCE OF see *Amenorrhoea*

PERTHÉ'S DISEASE

Perthé's disease, or osteochondritis of the hip, is an uncommon condition affecting children aged between 5 and 9 in which the head of the femur, or thigh-bone, becomes softened and deformed as a result of interruption of the blood supply. Treatment is directed at maintaining the shape of the femoral head as near normal as possible while waiting for recovery to take place, which can take up to two years. Treatment may involve resting the joint, and sometimes an operation.

PHENYLKETONURIA

A rare inherited metabolic disorder which involves an inability to handle normal amounts of protein in the diet. Phenylalanine, an amino acid (amino acids are the building blocks of proteins), builds up in the blood and can cause mental handicap. All newborns should have a blood test (the Guthrie test, see page 23) in the first week of life for phenylketonuria. If the disorder is detected early, dietary treatment prevents the onset of the mental handicap.

PHOTOTHERAPY see page 37

PHYSIOTHERAPIST

With children physiotherapists are concerned with encouraging development, strengthening muscles, preventing deformities, and improving co-ordination, as well as using other physical methods of treatment in a wide variety of acute and persistent conditions.

PNEUMONIA

Infection of the lung; it is sometimes also called pneumonitis. The infection may be the result of a primary infection, due to organisms like the pneumococcus bacterium or *mycoplasma*, or may be secondary to blockage of the minor airways or the retention of secretions. Pneumonia is treated with *antibiotics*, with or without chest physiotherapy.

SEE ALSO *Bronchopneumonia*

PNEUMOTHORAX see page 42

POLIOMYELITIS

This infectious disease has been almost eradicated from developed countries by immunization programmes, but is still present in the Third World. Most children who become infected with the *virus* do not suffer permanent consequences, but in some the nerve cells that work the muscles are destroyed and permanent paralysis results.

POLYCYSTIC KIDNEYS

An inherited condition in which the kidneys gradually become damaged due to the growth of multiple fluid-filled *cysts* within the kidney. Some forms of polycystic disease give rise to symptoms in childhood, while others do not cause problems until mid-adult life. If there is a family history of polycystic disease an opinion from a specialist geneticist can be obtained.

POLYP

An outgrowth of tissue from a mucous surface; polyps may be tumours or sometimes a reaction to chronic (persistent) inflammation. Multiple bowel polyps may indicate a tendency to develop *cancer* in adult life, and regular surveillance of affected patients is needed so any complications can be treated if and when they develop.

PTOSIS

Sagging of the upper eyelid, which results from failure of development or damage to the nerve supply of the muscles around the eye. If needed, a small operation can improve the appearance.

PULMONARY VALVE STENOSIS

A *congenital* lesion of the heart, in which there is narrowing (stenosis) of the pulmonary valve at the exit of the right ventricle which may obstruct the flow of blood. The narrowing of the valve gives rise to a heart murmur (see page 145), which enables the diagnosis to be made. If there is an obstruction which may impose strain on the heart, an operation to relieve the narrowing may be recommended.

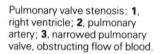

Pulmonary valve stenosis: **1**, right ventricle; **2**, pulmonary artery; **3**, narrowed pulmonary valve, obstructing flow of blood.

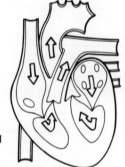

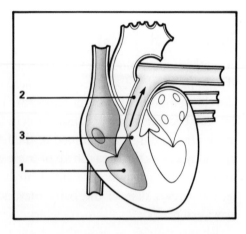

Structure of the normal heart (see page 143).

PURPURA

A rash due to multiple small areas of bleeding within the skin. It may be due to blood vessel weakness or to a deficiency of the blood platelets (see Chapter 13). There may also be bleeding from the nose, bladder or bowel.

PYLORIC STENOSIS see page 164

QUADRIPLEGIA see *Diplegia*

RABIES

A serious disease, transmitted by the bite of an infected animal, in which the nervous system is progressively attacked. There is a long incubation period between the bite and the onset of symptoms, and vaccine treatment during this time prevents the onset of the disease.

RECESSIVE INHERITANCE see page 108

RENAL DAMAGE/FAILURE see page 172

RESPIRATORY DISTRESS SYNDROME see page 40

RETROLENTAL FIBROPLASIA

Damage to the eye due to overgrowth of the blood vessels behind the lens and in the retina, the light-sensitive membrane lining the back of the eye; it can be caused by excess oxygen given to pre-term babies (see page 41). The oxygen level in the blood needs to be carefully monitored to prevent serious degrees of retrolental fibroplasia.

REYE'S SYNDROME see *Analgesic; Aspirin*

RHESUS DISEASE

A mother whose blood group is rhesus negative may have rhesus positive children if her partner's blood group is rhesus positive; this may cause the mother to develop antibodies to the rhesus factor. This is not a problem in the first pregnancy, but can become an increasing problem in subsequent pregnancies as the maternal antibody can damage the blood of the fetus. This is known as rhesus disease. The antibody causes the breakdown of some of the baby's red blood cells, giving rise to *anaemia* which may be present at birth, and *jaundice* that develops soon after. In severe rhesus disease the baby may need to be given *blood transfusions* in the newborn period.

Rhesus disease is now almost entirely prevented by giving rhesus negative mothers an injection following delivery or abortion to prevent them becoming sensitized to the rhesus factor.

RICKETS

A deficiency of vitamin D gives rise to rickets, a weakness of the bones. Rickets usually occurs between the ages of 6 and 18 months, and can be signalled by thickened wrists, bowing of the legs, or knock knees. The child is miserable and gains weight poorly. This is an age when growth is rapid and so the body requirement for vitamin D is high. Rickets can be diagnosed by an X-ray or blood test and is treated by giving vitamin D. The bones strengthen again, and any deformities will lessen as the child grows.

The prevention of rickets is important. Manufactured baby milks all have added vitamins, including vitamin D, and a child will not get rickets while being fed such milk. Drops containing vitamins A, B, C and D are recommended for babies up to the age of 2 years. Vitamin D can also be synthesized in the skin if it is exposed to sunlight. Breast milk contains vitamin D if the mother has an adequate vitamin D intake, or has manufactured enough in the sun.

RIGORS

Episodes of shivering due to infection. They occur when the temperature is rising, and are particularly common with urinary tract infections (see page 171) and with malaria (page 118).

RINGWORM

An infection of the scalp due to the fungus *Tinea capitis*. A temporary patch of baldness results. Ringworm can be cured with an antifungal treatment called griseofulvin.

ROSEOLA INFANTUM

An uncommon minor viral infection of infants and young children. The child has a fever, and a rash develops as the child is getting better. No treatment is needed.

ROUNDWORM

Intestinal infestation with roundworms is seldom seen in developed countries, but does occur in the tropics. The worms are apparent in the stools, and resemble small earthworms. They can be eradicated with medication.

RUBELLA

Rubella, or German measles, is a trivial infection except in early pregnancy when it can cause disastrous damage to the fetus with the possibility of mental handicap, deafness, visual handicap and heart disease. Rubella will be gradually eradicated if all children are immunized in infancy.

The incubation period is 2–3 weeks.

The illness consists of a mild fever and malaise (a general feeling of being unwell), and the development of a rash of small separate spots over the face and trunk. The *lymph nodes* at the back of the neck may be enlarged. Rubella can be mimicked by other viral infections and a definite diagnosis can only be made by isolating the *virus* or testing the blood for evidence of recent rubella infection. An attack of rubella and immunization give prolonged immunity.

RUPTURE see *Hernia*

SALMONELLA

There are various different *bacteria* in the Salmonella family, most of which give rise to diseases of the alimentary tract. The most severe is typhoid, which is rarely seen in countries with good sanitation and water supply. Infection with other Salmonellae, which give rise to *gastro-enteritis*, is more common. Infection may be passed from someone who is suffering from or carrying the bacteria. The Salmonella is excreted in the stools, and personal hygiene, including adequate hand washing, is very important in cutting down the spread of infection. Infection may also come from eating infected food, and poultry and shellfish are often contaminated. They must be properly cooked, and the cook must wash his or her hands thoroughly after preparing the meat for cooking.

Gastro-enteritis due to Salmonella is usually only associated with slight vomiting, but diarrhoea can be severe and sometimes prolonged, and there may be fever and crampy abdominal pains. Although Salmonella is a bacterium, treatment with *antibiotics* does not eradicate the infection and may prolong the carrier state, so they are not routinely used.

SCABIES

An intensely itchy rash provoked by a tiny insect burrowing in the skin to lay eggs. In adults the affected parts tend to be the webs between the fingers, but they can be all over the body in infants. Scabies should be considered if children develop any unexplained itchy rash. It can be eradicated by skin treatment with an insecticide.

SCARLET FEVER

Scarlet fever, or scarlatina, is a red rash covering the whole body, although often sparing the areas around the mouth. It is due to infection of the throat with certain strains of streptococci *bacteria* which produce a toxin that gives the rash. Since the advent of *antibiotics* scarlet fever has ceased to be a serious infection.

SCHOOL PHOBIA

School phobia is different from truancy. Truancy tends to be a problem with teenage children; it arises because of a lack of interest in school work, and from a sense of excitement at taking time off. In school phobia the child develops anxiety symptoms when thinking about going to school. These symptoms may include dizzy feelings, nausea and vomiting. They tend to become more marked as the time for school approaches, or may happen at school, making the child's return home necessary.

Anxiety may be provoked by something at school or at home, or can come from within the child. Things at school that can precipitate anxiety include worries over an inability to understand school work, poor relationships with the peer group, bullying, or a teacher who is perceived as stern or frightening. The child may be anxious about going to school because he cannot be sure that things will be all right at home if he is not there. This can be caused by concern over a sick relative, or because of unsettled relationships within the family. Children may also worry about themselves and whether they will be able to do the school work, or may feel concerned about their appearance or their inability to make friends.

When it is realized that a child's symptoms are related to school phobia the cause may be apparent and it may be possible for the family to overcome the difficulties.

If the child continues to be phobic towards school, professional help from a child guidance team or a psychologist may be helpful.

SCOLIOSIS

A spinal deformity with sideways curving and a twisting of the spine. There is a secondary deformity of the rib cage, which appears asymmetric. Scoliosis may arise because one or more of the bones of the spine has not formed properly. This is known as a structural scoliosis, and is likely to be noted in early childhood. It needs to be monitored as the child grows in case the deformity becomes more marked, but very often no treatment is required.

Children with abnormalities of the muscles may develop scoliosis as the spine gets pulled out of position. This can occur with muscular weakness, as in *muscular dystrophy*; or with abnormal muscular action, as may occur in *cerebral palsy*.

Teenage girls occasionally develop a scoliosis during the puberty growth spurt (see page 82). It is not known why this occurs, or why boys are hardly ever affected. If any spinal deformity is noted at this age a medical opinion should be obtained. Sometimes the spinal twisting is merely due to bad posture, but if it is a true scoliosis it will need frequent monitoring to ascertain whether it is likely to give rise to progressive deformity. If this is the case a spinal brace may be needed during the period of growth to prevent the scoliosis worsening.

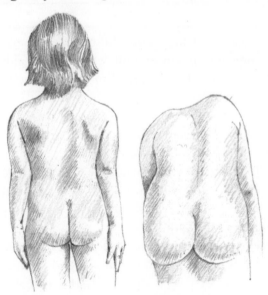

When a child is standing upright the spine may appear curved (**left**). This may be due to the child's posture, or to scoliosis, a curvature of the spine. With scoliosis the defect becomes more obvious when the child bends forwards (**right**) as an assymetry of the rib cage is apparent.

SEBORRHOEIC ECZEMA AND CRADLE CAP

Seborrhoeic eczema differs from *atopic eczema* in its age of onset and remission, its distribution, and in that it is not itchy. Seborrhoeic eczema usually begins during the first few weeks of life. It may persist throughout the first year, but usually remits completely after this.

The first sign is often the development of a brown greasy crusting of the scalp at the top of the head, the so-called cradle cap. This can be the only feature, but in many children a red, scaly rash may develop which involves the face, behind the ears and around the neck. The rash may be present on the upper trunk and is often florid in the nappy area. Seborrhoeic eczema is not itchy, and although the skin may look very sore, the infant is usually not upset by the rash.

Cradle cap can be treated with olive or arachis (peanut) oil applied to the scalp to loosen the crusts before shampooing with a baby shampoo. With this treatment every three or four days the cradle cap will gradually improve. The patches of eczema respond to treatment with hydrocortisone cream.
SEE ALSO *Atopic eczema*

SEIZURE see *Epilepsy*

SEPTICAEMIA

A generalized bacterial infection carried in the blood. Usually it starts as a localized infection, such as an *abscess*, but the infection may become generalized because the body's immune system is overwhelmed.

SEX-LINKED INHERITANCE see page 108

SEXUAL ABUSE

It has become apparent in recent years that the sexual abuse of children is not uncommon. This is not a new phenomenon, and many adult women, some elderly, are only now able to recount sexual abuse that happened to them in their own childhood.

The main victims are girls, although boys may also be abused; almost all the abusers are male. In the vast majority of cases the male is either part of, or well known to, the family. The form the abuse takes is very variable, but is often accompanied by threats not to tell, so that the child may have to suffer repeated abuse over a prolonged period. Other adults within the family are unlikely to know what is going on, but if one child is being abused it may be happening, or may have happened, to other children in the family.

Parents, nursery staff and teachers should all be aware that sexual abuse is prevalent, and if a child wants to talk about something of a sexual nature they should be prepared to listen in case she is trying to disclose it. If sexual abuse is suspected, further consideration is needed, and if the suspicion is confirmed the child needs to be protected. The family doctor or social services should be alerted, and the inquiry should be conducted by skilled, tactful and specially trained staff.

SHINGLES

Shingles (herpes zoster) is rare in childhood. It is a localized rash which appears around the trunk or on the face, and is due to infection of one of the nerves in the skin by the herpes zoster virus, which also causes *chickenpox*. The raised red spots turn into vesicles (blisters), and then scab over. The rash is intensely painful. The symptoms may be ameliorated by treatment with anti-viral ointment. Shingles is more common in adults, and a non-immune child can catch chickenpox from an adult with shingles.

SHORT SIGHT see page 181

SICKLE CELL ANAEMIA

Sickle cell anaemia, also called sickle cell disease, is a genetic condition found in people of West African or Afro-Caribbean origin. People who inherit the sickle cell gene (see Chapter 8) produce a variant type of haemoglobin, the pigment in blood which transports oxygen round the body; this variant is known as sickle haemoglobin or haemoglobin S. Ordinary adult haemoglobin is known as haemoglobin A. In the fetus and newborn infant there is also haemoglobin F. Haemoglobin genes, like other genes, occur in pairs. An individual carrying dissimilar genes, one for haemoglobin A and one for S, will produce both types of haemoglobin. Individuals where both genes are for haemoglobin S will only produce sickle haemoglobin.

Molecules of haemoglobin S can transport oxygen in the same way as haemoglobins A and F but as the haemoglobin S molecule gives up its oxygen it assumes an abnormal shape. Red blood cells containing only haemoglobin S assume a crescent or sickle shape in areas of low oxygen concentration because of the molecular deformation of the haemoglobin. These sickle cells are broken down rapidly in the spleen and other tissues, so that the patient is always anaemic. Furthermore the abnormally shaped red cells sometimes cause blockage of blood vessels, with a small area of tissue becoming damaged or dying as a result of the blood supply being cut off.

Children who have both haemoglobin genes of the S type have sickle cell disease. They are always moderately anaemic, although this does not usually cause many symptoms. From time to time they are also likely to develop painful episodes due to the blockage of small blood vessels by a mass of distorted red cells. These painful crises may affect hands and feet, arms or legs, and sometimes the abdomen and other parts. The pain usually persists for a few days and may be severe; painkillers need to be given. Sometimes the blockage of small vessels may cause lasting problems if the brain or the bones are affected. Patients with the disease are prone to infections, particularly with the pneumococcus bacterium.

There is no curative treatment for sickle cell disease. Treatment with folic acid, a vitamin, makes sure that the body can keep up a high production of red cells to replace those being rapidly destroyed. Continuous treatment with penicillin prevents infection with the pneumococcus. Iron medicines have no effect on this type of anaemia and should not be taken.

In winter it is important to prevent the child from becoming cold, as the resulting sluggish circulation in arms or legs can precipitate painful crises. If any operation is needed it is important to tell the surgeon and anaesthetist about the sickle cell disease. Children with the disease should be regularly supervised by the doctor to make sure they remain as healthy as possible.

People who have one sickle gene and one normal haemoglobin gene are often described as having sickle trait. They do not normally have symptoms. They are mildly anaemic, and may develop occlusions (blockages) of blood vessels if they become very short of oxygen. This is only likely to happen with severe illness or during operations. They are, however, carriers of the sickle gene, and if their partner is also a carrier they may have children with sickle cell disease.

All people with sickle cell trait or disease need to be given genetic advice so that they are aware of any implications the condition may have for them.

SINUSITIS

The maxillary sinuses are air-filled spaces in the bones of the cheek, and they connect with the nasal airway. They do not develop until mid-childhood. They occasionally become infected and this can cause *headache* and persistent nasal discharge. If *antibiotics* do not clear sinusitis a decongestant drug may be used in addition.

SMALLPOX

This previously dreaded disease with a high mortality has been totally eradicated by a world-wide immunization programme. It is no longer necessary for children or travellers to receive smallpox vaccination.

SNAKE BITE

Bites from venomous snakes are serious and require prompt expert medical treatment. Specific anti-venoms for most venomous snakes are now available. Children should be taught not to pick up snakes if they come across them. Many snake bites are caused by neglect of this rule.
SEE ALSO page 225

SOLVENT ABUSE

Solvent abuse or glue sniffing is a dangerous craze which has been taken up by young teenagers and some even younger children. Solvents from glue, cleaning fluid or lighter fuel are inhaled to induce intoxication. Many of these substances are very toxic, and can cause cardiac arrest. Vomiting while intoxicated can lead to vomit being sucked into the lungs and to the person choking.

All adults should be watchful, and if parents know that solvent abuse is prevalent in their area they should be active in trying to stop it. Children who abuse solvents may develop a rash around the mouth from a reaction to the solvent, may at times smell aromatic, and may have glue spilt on their clothes. They may have lighter fuel, typewriter correction fluid solvent or adhesives in their possession without a legitimate reason, and this should alert suspicion.

Parents need advice and help from a doctor or social worker if they find their child is abusing solvents, and should also try to make sure that the appropriate authorities are alerted so that the craze can be curtailed.

SORE THROAT

Infection of the tonsils and the pharynx is common, and may result from *viruses* or *bacteria*, particularly the streptococcus bacterium. If a sore throat is accompanied by a fever and enlarged *lymph nodes* in the neck it is probably bacterial, and an *antibiotic* may be needed. There is no specific treatment for viral infections.

SPEECH THERAPIST

Speech therapists have special training and experience in the development of language, in the workings of the muscles and other structures of the tongue, mouth and lips, and in the production of speech. They can help with feeding and vocalizing problems of children with *cleft palates* from a very early age. Children whose language development is delayed, or who have problems of speech or pronunciation also benefit from speech therapy.

SPINA BIFIDA

A *congenital* defect in which the lower part of the spine, and often the spinal cord, does not develop fully, so that at birth a defect is present in the lower back. The defect involves the skin and underlying bone, and may also involve the membranes around the spinal cord which may protrude as a fluid-filled sac known as a

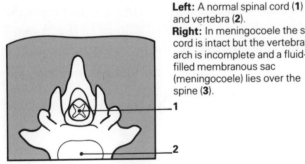
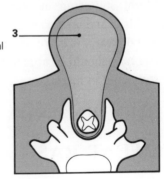

Left: A normal spinal cord (**1**) and vertebra (**2**).
Right: In meningocoele the spinal cord is intact but the vertebral arch is incomplete and a fluid-filled membranous sac (meningocoele) lies over the spine (**3**).

meningocoele. Often the spinal cord is also involved, and the sac is then known as a myelomeningocoele. If the legs or anal sphincter are weak, there is certainly some damage to the spinal cord. The damage may be partial, with variable loss of power and sensation below the spinal defect, in severe cases the legs, bladder and bowel may be totally paralysed and sensation absent over the legs.

In spina bifida the skin defect over the spinal defect can be closed surgically to prevent infection, but this does not restore function. Furthermore, closure of the defect often leads to progressive *hydrocephalus* which will also require surgical treatment. Even with treatment most children are left with some residual disability.

SQUINT see page 182

STERNOMASTOID TUMOUR

The sternomastoid muscles are large muscles in the neck that run from behind the ear to the breastbone (sternum). In the newborn a lump is sometimes found within the sternomastoid muscle on one side, and the baby is likely to have difficulty in turning the head to the opposite side. This lump, or sternomastoid tumour, is the result of injury to the muscle during delivery. There is some bleeding into the muscle, and a reaction around the area of bleeding. The lump will gradually disappear over the space of a few months. If neck movement is limited, regular gentle manipulation may help to restore it, and a *physiotherapist* should demonstrate the required technique.

STICKY EYES see page 29

STICKY UMBILICUS see page 29

STILLBIRTH see page 136

STUTTERING

Slight stuttering or stammering on occasion is very common in pre-school children and is of no great importance. More severe stuttering, particularly in the school years, is more of a problem and may be associated with facial *tics*. A *speech therapist* should be able to help the child and prevent the nervousness that leads to stuttering in many cases.

SUDDEN INFANT DEATH SYNDROME see page 137

SWEAT RASH see page 29

TAY-SACHS DISEASE

This recessively inherited disease (see page 108) is mainly seen in Ashkenazi Jews.

Due to a metabolic defect there is the gradual build-up of an abnormal substance in the nervous system and progressive brain damage results. Affected children become blind in infancy, and develop muscle weakness and progressive mental handicap. Eventually they die. There is no treatment. The carrier state can be tested for before conception in those thought to be at risk.

TEETHING see page 194

TETANUS see page 114

THALASSAEMIA

A genetic anaemia due to defective haemoglobin production (haemoglobin is the pigment in blood which transports oxygen round the body). Thalassaemia occurs in people of Mediterranean or Asian stock, and is especially common in those from Cyprus and the eastern Mediterranean.

Possession of the thalassaemia gene interferes with the production of haemoglobin A, ordinary adult haemoglobin. The heterozygous individual, with one normal and one thalassaemia gene, has mild or moderate anaemia, as only about half the normal quantity of haemoglobin can be made. This state is sometimes referred to as thalassaemia minor. The homozygous individual, who has a pair of thalassaemia genes, is unable to form any haemoglobin, apart from fetal haemoglobin during life in the womb and early infancy. This condition is known as thalassaemia major, and without treatment is fatal in infancy.

Infants with thalassaemia major become severely anaemic during their first year of life. They feed poorly, become breathless and fail to thrive. The liver and spleen enlarge so the babies have distended abdomens. Treatment is by *blood transfusions* to correct the anaemia, and these need to be continued for life. Transfusions mean that the children can be kept well, but also entail injections of a drug to prevent the build-up of excess iron in the body.

It is now possible to make a diagnosis of thalassaemia major during early pregnancy, so that the pregnancy can be terminated if the fetus is affected, and if the couple so wish. Couples who were not previously prepared to risk pregnancy in case their child had thalassaemia major are now able to plan a family. All those who are or might be carriers of the thalassaemia gene should receive advice.

THREADWORM

Threadworms live in the lower bowel and come out of the anus at night to lay eggs on the skin. They cause itchiness around the anus, but do not cause abdominal pain or loss of appetite. The worms can often be seen moving in a freshly passed stool; they are thread-like and 1-2cm (⅓-¾in) long. They can be eradicated by treatment with the drug piperazine for ten days, or by a single dose of merbendazole. All the family should be treated, even if only one member is known to be infested.

THRUSH see page 29

TIC

Tics are sudden, short, jerky movements of the face, head or arm. They are involuntary and become worse at times of anxiety or stress. They are not due to disease of the nervous system, but are emotional in origin. If they only happen occasionally treatment may not be necessary, but a doctor should be consulted if they are frequent or troublesome.

TONGUE TIE

Under the tip of the tongue is a fold of mucous membrane, the frenum, which connects the tongue with the floor of the mouth. If the tongue is not very mobile it may be because the frenum is not as lax as usual; this is known as tongue tie. Provided the tip of the tongue can pass through the teeth the frenum will not prevent the development of speech or interfere with swallowing, and no treatment is required.

TONSILLECTOMY see page 189

TONSILLITIS

A sore throat and sometimes a fever characterize infection of the tonsils, known as tonsillitis. The tonsils will look large and reddened. Sometimes they are coated in a purulent (pussy) discharge. The *lymph nodes* in the neck may also be enlarged. Most episodes of tonsillitis are due to bacterial infection, often from the streptococcus bacterium, and settle rapidly and completely with *antibiotic* treatment. Provided the tonsils go back to normal after an attack, no further treatment is indicated. However, in cases where a child suffers frequent attacks of tonsillitis, or the tonsils remain chronically infected, removal of the tonsils may be necessary (see Tonsillectomy, page 189).

TOOTH DECAY see page 194

TORSION OF THE TESTICLE

Sometimes the testicle may rotate and obstruct the veins and arteries. This is known as torsion and gives rise to severe pain as the testicle becomes congested with blood and swells up. The arterial supply is gradually cut off and unless the condition is relieved within a few hours the testicle may be damaged. If the diagnosis is confirmed by the doctor, an urgent operation is required to untwist the testicle and to fix it so that torsion cannot happen again. In individuals who have had torsion there is significant risk of a recurrence but on the other side. It is usual, therefore, at the time of operation to fix the other testicle in position also.

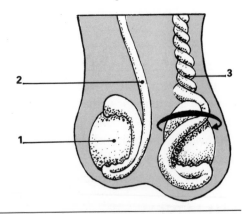

Torsion of the testicle. The testicle on the left in the diagram (**1**) is in normal alignment with the blood vessels and spermatic duct (**2**) leading to it. In torsion the testicle twists on its pedicle of blood vessels (**3**) which cuts off the blood supply.

TRACHEOSTOMY

An operation which involves cutting a hole in the front of the trachea (windpipe) and inserting a tube to establish an airway with the outside. It is an operation that is occasionally needed in children for upper airway obstruction.

TRANSPLANTATION

Techniques of transplantation have been worked out for many organs including the kidneys, liver, heart, lungs and bone marrow. The suppression of the body's immune system so that the transplanted organ is not rejected is also well tried now, and rejection can be prevented in most cases. These advances have opened up a new era of medical treatment, and transplantation offers hope to many individuals with different diseases, most grafts being successful and functioning for many years.

TRANSPOSITION OF THE GREAT VESSELS

Transposition is a severe heart abnormality in which the aorta, the main artery, rises from the right ventricle (one of the lower chambers of the heart), and the pulmonary artery from the left ventricle, instead of the other way round. The baby

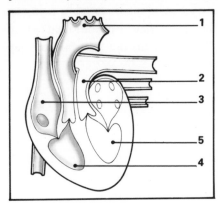

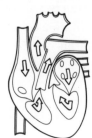

Structure of the normal heart (see page 143).

Transposition of the great vessels: **1**, aorta; **2**, pulmonary artery; **3**, right atrium; **4**, right ventricle; **5**, left ventricle.

is blue because there is very little oxygen in the blood circulating around the body. Babies affected by this condition need urgent investigation and surgical treatment to correct the flow of blood.

TRAVEL SICKNESS

Many young children become motion sick in cars, trains, boats or planes. Arranging where possible for frequent breaks in the journey, preventing the atmosphere from becoming stuffy, and making sure the child can see out of a window all help. Some children will still develop motion sickness in spite of these precautions and should be given travel sickness medication before any long journey. Preparations containing the drug hyoscine or *antihistamines* are suitable.

TRUANCY see *School phobia*

TUBERCULOSIS

Tuberculosis (TB) is now a rare disease in developed countries with good public health systems, as effective *antibiotic* treatment is readily available; it remains a major health problem in underdeveloped countries. In children infected with TB there is a risk that the infection can spread around the body – so-called miliary TB – or give rise to *meningitis*. Children may be found to have acquired the infection before they develop any symptoms because they are known to have been in contact with a confirmed case of tuberculosis. Provided TB is diagnosed early, treatment with antibiotics is effective in eradicating the infection, although tuberculous meningitis remains a serious disease.

TURNER'S SYNDROME see page 67

ULCER

An inflamed area characterized by a loss of the overlying skin or mucous membrane. Mouth ulcers, also called aphthous ulcers, are common in childhood and can be painful. Their cause is unknown. The soreness can be eased by using an application containing a local anaesthetic, and the ulcers may be encouraged to heal with an ointment containing carbenoxalone. Children do not get varicose leg ulcers, and stomach ulcers are rare.

ULCERATIVE COLITIS

Ulcerative colitis is rare in childhood. The disease is an inflammation of the mucous membrane which lines the large intestine, with patches of ulceration which bleed. The symptoms consist of the passage of frequent loose stools containing blood and mucus. The patient feels weak and unwell, and loses weight.

Diagnosis is established by barium enema X-rays (see page 163) and by endoscopy (see page 163), and removal of some tissue for study under a microscope. Treatment utilizing various drugs will usually control symptoms, but surgery is occasionally required.

UNDESCENDED TESTICLE

The testicles form inside the abdominal cavity during fetal life and migrate into the scrotum via the inguinal canal in the groin at around thirty-two weeks of pregnancy. The testicle may fail to descend at all, be held up in the inguinal canal, or go off course so that it remains in the groin. Establishing that the testicles are in the scrotum should be part of the medical checks in infancy. If one or both testicles are undescended after the age of 1 year an operation will be needed to position it/ them in the scrotum. This is preferably done some time before the age of 5. By the time the first changes of puberty start (see Chapter 6), the testicles need to be in the correct position.

The position of the testicles: **1**, normal; **2**, undescended.

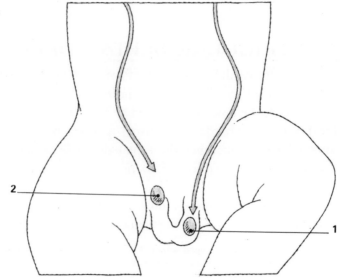

UPPER RESPIRATORY TRACT INFECTION
see page 152

URINARY TRACT INFECTION see page 171

URTICARIA

A skin rash (also known as hives) which resembles that caused by a stinging nettle. Urticarial rashes usually indicate an *allergy*. The skin shows red blotches and weals (pale, fluid-filled raised areas). The skin is itchy. Calamine lotion or *antihistamines* are soothing. It is important to try to ascertain the cause of the rash and avoid contact with the allergen in future.

VAGINAL BLEEDING

A small amount of vaginal bleeding is not uncommon in baby girls in the newborn period. Maternal hormones, oestrogens, may have crossed the placenta and caused overgrowth of the mucous membrane in the fetal uterus (womb); this membrane is shed after birth. Bleeding at other times may be due to injury, or to hormonal upset. The doctor should be consulted.

VAGINAL DISCHARGE

Slight vaginal or vulval discharge is very common in young girls and is usually associated with redness and soreness of the vulva. It may be due to localized infection. If the discharge has an offensive odour the infection is likely to be an organism which has come from the bowel. Soreness and discharge may also be due to chemical irritation caused by soap or bubble bath.

An *antibiotic* cream may settle the vulval discharge, but if it is persistent a specialist opinion should be obtained.

VENTRICULAR SEPTAL DEFECT (VSD)

Ventricular septal defect is a form of *congenital* heart disease in which there is a hole in the septum or partition between the left and right ventricles, the lower chambers of the heart; the hole allows blood to flow from left to right. As a consequence the heart works harder than usual as extra blood gets pumped to the lungs unnecessarily. Sometimes the septal defect is so large that the baby becomes breathless and is unable to feed properly, in which case surgical treatment is required. Many children with a murmur (see page 145) due to a VSD have no symptoms, and in some the hole closes spontaneously during childhood. If the defect is large and does not close an operation may be needed.

Ventricular septal defect: **1**, aorta; **2**, pulmonary artery; **3**, right atrium; **4**, left atrium; **5**, right ventricle; **6**, left ventricle; **7**, defect or hole in partition between ventricles, allowing blood to flow from left to right.

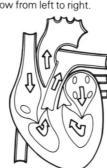

Structure of the normal heart (see page 143).

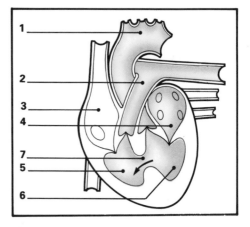

VERNIX see page 26

VERRUCA see *Warts and verrucas*

VIRUS

Many common diseases of childhood, including colds (see page 152), *influenza*, *rubella* (German measles), *measles*, *chickenpox* and *mumps*, are due to viral infections. Viruses are very small micro-organisms that only grow inside living cells. They are not killed by *antibiotics*, and there are few antiviral treatments, although some are available for herpes virus infections. Vaccines can be produced for some virus diseases such as measles, mumps and rubella (see Chapter 9).

VITAMIN DEFICIENCY see page 93

VOMITING see page 164

WARTS AND VERRUCAS

Warts are localized overgrowths of skin tissue caused by infection with the wart virus. Warts on the hands are often multiple. Warts on the sole of the foot grow inwards rather than outwards, and may be painful to pressure; they are known as verrucas or plantar warts and are caused by the same virus as ordinary warts.

Left alone, most warts would gradually disappear over the space of a few months. The process can be speeded up by treatment. Preparations containing salicylic acid applied directly to the wart gradually kill the outer layers, which then flake off. Repeated applications can eventually kill the wart completely. The doctor may freeze multiple or resistant warts with liquid nitrogen. This kills off some of the wart tissue and induces a blister to form under the wart. The skin over the blister and the wart are shed after a few days. As the skin rewarms after freezing it can be very painful, but this does not last long.

The genital warts that adults contract are caused by a different type of virus from skin warts.

WHOOPING COUGH

Whooping cough, or pertussis, is a serious infection caused by a bacterium. The incubation period is between 1 and 2 weeks. It starts with the signs of upper respiratory infection: a runny nose and slight cough and perhaps a slight fever. Instead of clearing in a couple of days, the cough gets worse and becomes paroxysmal: coughing occurs in bouts which may last more than a minute, the child becoming increasingly distressed and going red in the face. At the end of the paroxysm there may be a drawing in of breath that makes the characteristic 'hoop' sound. This is often followed by the vomiting of thick, stringy mucus.

These coughing paroxysms can occur many times during the day and night at the height of the attack, and this can go on for several weeks. Even after the symptoms seem to be lessening they may return and be just as bad as before if the child develops a cold or other respiratory infection. Coughing can continue for several months after the onset of pertussis.

Although whooping cough is caused by a bacterial infection, *antibiotics* do not help the symptoms nor is anything known that reliably gives relief from the paroxysms. All children should be immunized against whooping cough, unless there are very strong contra-indications (see page 115).

WORMS see *Roundworms; Threadworms*

INDEX

For Jenny, with love

This edition published in 1991 by
The Hamlyn Publishing Group Limited,
part of Reed International Books,
Michelin House, 81 Fulham Road,
London SW3 6RB

Reprinted 1992

ISBN 0 600 57137 8

Conceived and produced by Breslich & Foss,
Golden House, 28-31 Great Pulteney Street,
London W1R 3DD

Designed by Edward Kinsey
Design Assistant Sarah Crouch

Illustrators: Stan Johnson, Sally Launder,
Simon Roulstone and John Woodcock

Project editor: Tessa Rose
Copy editor: Wendy Lee
Proofreader: Diana Vowles
Indexer: Peter Barber

Typeset by Angel Graphics, London
Produced by Mandarin Offset in Hong Kong

ACKNOWLEDGEMENTS

The author wishes to thank Chris Bungay MSCP and Mary
John MSc for their contribution to this book and also Roger
Bradford, Wendy Lee and St George's Hospital and
Medical School, London.

The publishers wish to thank the following organizations
and individuals for supplying photographs to this book:

Chris Bungay: page 134
Everaids: page 132
Chris Fairclough Colour Library: pages 13 (top), 17, 25,
26, 29, 30, 32, 35, 36, 51, 52, 57, 75, 79, 97, 106, 114,
121, 125, 129, 144, 173, 177, 180, 185, 187, 192, 197

Edward Kinsey: page 21
Science Photo Library: pages 28, 49 (Chris Priest/Mark
Clarke); 104 and 115 (Jim Selby); 158 (Alexander Tsiaras);
160 (Larry Mulvehill)
Spastics' Society Uphill/Downhill Ski Club: page 135
Dr Richard West: pages 13 (bottom), 19, 20, 37, 60, 101,
123, 134, 146, 157, 174 and 182
Jennie Woodcock: pages 24, 45, 59, 67, 68, 87, 122
Tim Woodcock: pages 64, 70, 78, 85, 90, 194 and 206
ZEFA Picture Library (UK) Limited: pages 88
(O. Bench); 92 (R. Wagoner); 98 (Boiselle); 199 and 202
(C. Voigt); 203 (J. Flowerdew).